Series Editors:
Steven F. Warren, Ph.D.
Marc E. Fey, Ph.D.

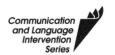

Communication
and Language
Intervention
Series

SPEECH & LANGUAGE
DEVELOPMENT &
INTERVENTION
in Down Syndrome
& Fragile X Syndrome

D0921943

Also in the *Communication
and Language Intervention Series*

*Dual Language Development and Disorders:
A Handbook on Bilingualism and Second Language Learning*
by Fred Genesee, Ph.D.,
Johanne Paradis, Ph.D.,
and Martha B. Crago, Ph.D.

*Phonological Disorders in Children:
Clinical Decision Making in Assessment and Intervention*
edited by Alan G. Kamhi, Ph.D.,
and Karen E. Pollock, Ph.D.

Treatment of Language Disorders in Children
edited by Rebecca J. McCauley, Ph.D.,
and Marc E. Fey, Ph.D.

Clinical Decision Making in Developmental Language Disorders
edited by Alan G. Kamhi, Ph.D.,
Julie J. Masterson, Ph.D.,
and Kenn Apel, Ph.D.

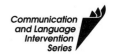

Communication
and Language
Intervention
Series

Speech & Language Development & Intervention

in Down Syndrome & Fragile X Syndrome

edited by

Joanne E. Roberts, Ph.D.
FPG Child Development Institute
The University of North Carolina at Chapel Hill

Robin S. Chapman, Ph.D.
Waisman Center
University of Wisconsin–Madison

and

Steven F. Warren, Ph.D.
Schiefelbusch Institute for Life Span Studies
The University of Kansas, Lawrence

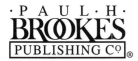

·P A U L·H·
BROOKES
PUBLISHING CO®

Baltimore • London • Sydney

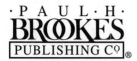

Paul H. Brookes Publishing Co.
Post Office Box 10624
Baltimore, Maryland 21285-0624

www.brookespublishing.com

Typeset by Spearhead Global, Inc., Bear, Delaware.
Manufactured in the United States of America by
Sheridan Books, Inc., Chelsea, Michigan.

The information provided in this book is in no way meant to substitute for a medical or
mental health practitioner's advice or expert opinion. Readers should consult a health or
mental health professional if they are interested in more information. This book is sold
without warranties of any kind, express or implied, and the publisher and authors dis-
claim any liability, loss, or damage caused by the contents of this book.

All photographs in this book and on the cover are used by permission of the individuals
pictured or their parents/guardians.

Library of Congress Cataloging-in-Publication Data

Speech and language development and intervention in Down syndrome and fragile
X syndrome / edited by Joanne E. Roberts, Robin S. Chapman, and Steven F. Warren.
    p.   cm.   (Communication and language intervention series)
  Includes bibliographical references and index.
  ISBN-13: 978-1-55766-874-5 (pbk.)
  ISBN-10: 1-55766-874-4 (pbk.)
    1. Speech therapy for children. 2. Language disorders in children—Treatment.
3. Down syndrome—Patients—Language. 4. Fragile X syndrome—Patients—Lan-
guage. I. Roberts, Joanne Erwick, 1950– II. Chapman, Robin S. III. Warren, Steven F.
IV. Title. V. Series: Communication and language intervention series (Unnumbered)
[DNLM: 1. Language Disorders—etiology. 2. Language Disorders—rehabilitation. 3.
Down Syndrome—complications. 4. Fragile X Syndrome—complications. WL 340.2
S741 2008]

  RJ496.S7S625 2008
  618.92'85506—dc22   2007012612

British Library Cataloguing in Publication data are available from the British Library.

Contents

Series Preface

The purpose of the *Communication and Language Intervention Series* is to provide meaningful foundations for the application of sound intervention designs to enhance the development of communication skills across the life span. We are endeavoring to achieve this purpose by providing readers with presentations of state-of-the-art theory, research, and practice.

In selecting topics, editors, and authors, we are not attempting to limit the contents of this series to viewpoints with which we agree or that we find most promising. We are assisted in our efforts to develop the series by an editorial advisory board consisting of prominent scholars representative of the range of issues and perspectives to be incorporated in the series.

Well-conceived theory and research on development and intervention are vitally important for researchers, educators, and clinicians committed to the development of optimal approaches to communication and language intervention. The content of each volume reflects our view of the symbiotic relationship between intervention and research: Demonstrations of what may work in intervention should lead to analysis of promising discoveries and insights from developmental work that may in turn fuel further refinement by intervention researchers. We trust that the careful reader will find much that is of great value in this volume.

An inherent goal of this series is to enhance the long-term development of the field by systematically furthering the dissemination of theoretically and empirically based scholarship and research. We promise the reader an opportunity to participate in the development of this field through debates and discussions that occur throughout the pages of the *Communication and Language Intervention Series*.

Editorial Advisory Board

About the Editors

Joanne E. Roberts, Ph. D., Senior Scientist, FPG Child Development Institute, and Professor of Speech and Hearing Sciences and Research Professor of Pediatrics, The University of North Carolina at Chapel Hill, 105 Smith Level Road, Chapel Hill, NC 27599-8180

Joanne E. Roberts's research focuses on the language development of children with disabilities and children at risk for language and learning difficulties. She studies the speech and language development of children with fragile X syndrome and children with Down syndrome and the potential mechanisms underlying speech and language development. Dr. Roberts also studies the role of language in the literacy skills and school success of African American children as well as the role of otitis media in children's language and school achievement. She has published more than 125 articles and chapters in speech and hearing, pediatric, child development, education, and early childhood journals and books. Dr. Roberts is particularly interested in translating research findings into assessment and intervention practices. She has served on journal editorial boards as well as several national multidisciplinary research panels.

Robin S. Chapman, Ph.D., Professor Emerita, Department of Communication Disorders, and Principal Investigator, Waisman Center, University of Wisconsin–Madison, 1500 Highland Avenue, Madison, Wisconsin 53705

Robin S. Chapman received the 2006 Career Research Scientist Award from the Academy on Mental Retardation in May 2007. The award was made for her outstanding contributions to research in mental retardation and developmental disabilities. She has carried out research on language learning in children and adolescents with Down syndrome, demonstrating strengths in vocabulary learning, ongoing acquisition of complex syntax in expressive language in adolescence, and longitudinal losses in syntax comprehension in young adults. Dr. Chapman is a faculty member of the Post-Doctoral Training Program in Developmental Disabilities Research at the Waisman Center. She was a codeveloper of SALT, a computer program for systematic analysis of language transcripts; a teacher of undergraduate, graduate, and doctoral students at the University of Wisconsin–Madison; and a researcher on topics in language acquisition in typically developing children, children with specific language impairment, and children and adolescents with Down syndrome. She is also a poet, with nine published collections of poetry, and a watercolor painter.

Steven F. Warren, Ph.D., Director, Schiefelbusch Institute for Life Span Studies, and Director, Kansas Intellectual and Developmental Disabilities Research Center, The University of Kansas, 1000 Sunnyside Avenue, 1052 Dole, Lawrence, Kansas 66045

From 1982 through 1999 Steven F. Warren served as a faculty member in the Department of Special Education and Psychology at Peabody College, Vanderbilt University. While at Vanderbilt he served as the Director of the Mental Retardation Research Training Program from 1988 to 1999 and as Deputy Director of the John F. Kennedy Center for Research on Human Development from 1991 through 1999. In January 2000, Dr. Warren returned to The University of Kansas, where he is presently Director of the Schiefelbusch Institute for Life Span Studies, Director of the Kansas Intellectual and Developmental Disabilities Research Center, and Professor of Applied Behavioral Science. Dr. Warren has conducted extensive research on early communication and language development and intervention. He has published more than 100 papers and a dozen books on these and related topics. He has been particularly instrumental in the development of the milieu teaching approach. In 1999, the National Down Syndrome Congress awarded Dr. Warren the Theodore D. Tjossem National Research Award in recognition of his research on early language intervention. Dr. Warren is the former editor of the *Journal of Early Intervention* and served as President of the American Association on Mental Retardation from 2001 to 2002. His present research remains focused on communication and language development and intervention with young children.

Contributors

Leonard Abbeduto, Ph.D.
Professor of Educational Psychology
Associate Director for Behavioral
    Sciences
Director, University Center for
    Excellence in Developmental
    Disabilities
Waisman Center
University of Wisconsin–Madison
1500 Highland Avenue
Madison, Wisconsin 53705

Elizabeth F. Barnes, Ph.D.
Assistant Professor
North Carolina State University
Department of Communication
201 Winston Hall
Raleigh, North Carolina 27695

Nancy C. Brady, Ph.D.
Associate Research Professor
Schiefelbusch Institute for
    Life Span Studies
The University of Kansas
1000 Sunnyside Avenue
Lawrence, Kansas 66045

**Shelley L. Bredin-Oja, M.A.,
    CCC-SLP**
Speech-Language Pathologist
The University of Kansas
1000 Sunnyside Avenue
Lawrence, Kansas 66045

**Sue Buckley, B.A., CPsychol,
    AFBPsS**
Professor and Director for Research
The Down Syndrome Educational
    Trust
Belmont Street
Portsmouth PO5 1NA
Hampshire, United Kingdom

Anna J. Esbensen, Ph.D.
Assistant Scientist
Waisman Center
University of Wisconsin–Madison
1500 Highland Avenue
Madison, Wisconsin 53705

Randi J. Hagerman, M.D.
Professor
Department of Pediatrics
Director
MIND Institute
University of California Medical
    Center
2825 50th Street
Sacramento, California 95817

Mina C. Johnson-Glenberg, Ph.D.
President
Neuronfarm, LLC
Honorary Fellow
Waisman Center
University of Wisconsin–Madison
4284 Jordan Drive
McFarland, Wisconsin 53558

Ray D. Kent, Ph.D.
Professor Emeritus
University of Wisconsin–Madison
Waisman Center
Room 435
1500 Highland Avenue
Madison, Wisconsin 53705

Libby Kumin, Ph.D., CCC-SLP
Professor of Speech Language
    Pathology
Loyola College in Maryland
4501 North Charles Street
Baltimore, Maryland 21210

Ira Lott, M.D.
Professor of Pediatrics and
  Neurology
Associate Dean of Clinical
  Neurosciences
Chief, Pediatric Neurology
  Division
University of California, Irvine
  School of Medicine
UCI Medical Center
101 The City Drive South
ZZ 4482
Orange, California 92868

Gary E. Martin, M.A.,
  CCC-SLP
Speech-Language Pathologist
FPG Child Development Institute
The University of North Carolina at
  Chapel Hill
Division of Speech and Hearing
  Sciences
Campus Box 8180
Chapel Hill, North Carolina 27599

Andrea McDuffie, Ph.D.,
  CCC-SLP
Assistant Professor
School of Education
Indiana University
201 North Rose Avenue
Bloomington, Indiana 47405

Lauren Moskowitz, B.S.
Clinical Psychology Doctoral
  Student
Stony Brook University
Stony Brook, New York 11794

David Patterson, Ph.D.
Senior Scientist
Eleanor Roosevelt Institute
Professor
Department of Biological Sciences
University of Denver
1899 Gaylord Street
Denver, Colorado 80206

Marsha Mailick Seltzer, Ph.D.
Professor
School of Social Work
Director
Waisman Center
University of Wisconsin–Madison
1500 Highland Avenue
Madison, Wisconsin 53705

Johanna R. Price, Ph.D.
Assistant Professor
Mississippi University for Women
1100 College Street, MUW-1340
Columbus, Mississippi 39701

Audra Sterling, M.A.
Doctoral Student
Schiefelbusch Institute for
  Life Span Studies
The University of Kansas
1000 Sunnyside Avenue
Room 1052
Lawrence, Kansas 66045

Carol Stoel-Gammon, Ph.D.
Professor
Department of Speech and Hearing
  Sciences
University of Washington
1417 Northeast 42nd Street
Seattle, Washington 98105

Foreword

I am very pleased to write a foreword for this innovative book that provides a detailed account of the language and communication characteristics of individuals with Down syndrome (DS) and fragile X syndrome (FXS). The format of this book provides an excellent mechanism for comparing and contrasting these two genetic syndromes. The genetics of each syndrome has received increased attention since the early 1990s, and it is clear that each is caused by very different mechanisms. The genotypes involve a single gene mutation (FMR1) in FXS, versus the overexpression of multiple genes on chromosome 21, the interaction of differing alleles with one another, and the genetic makeup of other chromosome pairs in DS that affect almost every organ system in the body. This volume brings together the most current research on the behavioral phenotype of the language and communication for each syndrome as well as suggestions for behavioral interventions to optimize developmental outcomes. This is truly a remarkable work, reflecting the advances in identifying the causes of intellectual disability.

Early research on language and communication in children with intellectual disability focused on cognitive impairments as a general construct, ignoring, out of necessity, specific etiologies. Outcomes of this research were intended to address language learning for individuals with intellectual disability as a group even though it was well understood that intellectual disability was a classification resulting from a variety of causes: genetic, metabolic, prenatal injury, substance abuse, and environmental deprivation. We should remember that while this was not that long ago, it reflected genetic and metabolic research of the time. In the 1960s, fewer than 30% of individuals with intellectual disability had a specific diagnosis such as DS. Indeed, FXS was identified in the late 1960s, but the specific gene, FMR1, was not identified until 1991. DS has been recognized as a specific syndrome associated with intellectual disability for many years, but the specific genetics are still being investigated. In a relatively short period of time, we have moved language and communication research on children with intellectual disability from investigating the outcomes of cognitive deficits in general to documenting the behavioral phenotype for the language and communication of a specific genotype, that is, documenting the language learning outcomes of specific brain syndromes.

The work presented in this volume describes the language and communication outcomes for each syndrome, in particular their uniqueness and similarities. Children with FXS have difficulty with social reciprocity resulting in significant difficulty with conversational exchange and response to communication partners. Children with DS have difficulty mastering the grammar of language but do much better with comprehending language than with production. These statements are overgeneralizations that must be understood relative to children's developmental progression. That is, they most reflect the performance of children 4–12 years of age, may not be evident in the early developmental period, and may diminish with the onset of adolescence. You can imagine that research studies in the early 1980s that included children with FXS and DS as well as other syndromes in single experimental groups yielded mixed results. A major question of the day was whether the language and communication of children with intellectual disability would follow the same developmental course as typically developing children but at a slower pace or if their language was unique, disordered, or different. The picture emerging from this work was of language developing in the same sequence as typical children but at a slower pace. Those studies arguing for disordered language faced the difficult task of defining exactly what "disorder" meant, usually citing slower development as "disorder" or asynchronies in development across language domains. Either of these definitions can be reinterpreted as evidence for supporting a general development view. While grammar may lag behind other language domains in the production in children with DS, it still follows the same developmental course as typical children. It is evident that focusing research on specific etiologies has revealed different language and communication outcomes for different causal constructs.

The past major research question, is language development in children with intellectual disability delayed or disordered, has been redefined to focus on how language development in people with cognitive impairments fits current developmental theory. The current overarching question then becomes which theory of language acquisition is supported by the language development data accumulated on each syndrome. A recent paper by Leonard Abbeduto and Robin Chapman (2005) addressed this question directly. They contrasted modularity theory with the social-interactionist account of language learning. The modularity account presumes strong innate constraints on development, a minimal and circumscribed role for experience, and a relative independence of language development from other facets of development. In contrast, the social-interactionist account proposes intimate bidirectional influences between language development and nonlinguistic developments like social cognition and a critical role for experiences, particularly experiences in social interaction with supportive competent language users. Abbeduto and Chapman argued that language development data on both syndromes support the social-interactionist account of language learning in these children. The asynchronies observed in the language development of each syndrome could not be accounted for by a modular view of development that would predict synchrony in development. Nor could modularity account for the preponderance of evidence that nonverbal cognition is tightly linked to advancing language skills. The social-interactionist account suggests that language and communication can be shaped by environmental interventions to optimize language and communication development.

The current view of language development in both FXS and DS can be characterized as following the same course of development as typical children at a pace dictated by advancing nonverbal cognitive skills. There are notable asynchronies that are distinct for each syndrome: the social use of language and syntax. Of crucial importance is the wide variability in both language and cognitive abilities within each syndrome. Why some children with DS and FXS are functioning within age group norms and others have profound impairments remains to be illuminated. In FXS, boys are more significantly affected than girls and some individuals with the FMR1 mutation are not affected at all. In DS, children face perceptual, motor, and cognitive challenges that affect language learning. It seems clear that research on genetic and environmental predictors of developmental progress will need to evaluate multiple factors at the same time. This will require collaboration among molecular and behavioral scientists to provide detailed phenotypic data to map advancing genetic description. This argues for longitudinal research to map the course of language development, which spans 12–18 years in typical children and two to three times that in children with cognitive deficits. Semilongitudinal or cross-sectional research designs limit our ability to identify predictors of language and communication development. We know that language and communication development is a sensitive indicator of a variety of sensory, motor, cognitive, and environmental impairments.

Another area of overlap in the two syndromes is deficits in speech intelligibility. Speech intelligibility presents a clear challenge for researchers studying language and communication production. It is time to consider how speech intelligibility affects subject selection as well as how it may affect performance on language production tasks. Research documents that typically developing children with speech intelligibility problems may alter word choice and sentence length to produce utterances that are more intelligible. It is also time to investigate the origins of the speech problems in these two syndromes to improve our understanding of the nature of the deficits that may lead to improved speech. Speech intelligibility improvements have been noted for individuals with DS through adolescence and young adulthood (Miller, Leddy, & Leavitt, 1999).

The specific detail of the language and communication development of each syndrome presented in this volume is energizing, providing motivation for further research and new ways to conceptualize intervention programs. This volume provides an in-depth review of the research on these developmental disabilities, documenting a critical shift in our conceptualization of causal constructs affecting language and communication development.

Jon F. Miller, Ph.D.
Professor Emeritus
Department of Communicative Disorders
Investigator, Waisman Center
University of Wisconsin–Madison

REFERENCES

Abbeduto, L., & Chapman, R. (2005). Language development in Down syndrome and fragile X syndrome: Current research and implications for theory and practice. In P. Fletcher & J. Miller (Eds.), *Developmental theory and language disorders*. Philadelphia: John Benjamins Publishing.

Miller, J.F., Leddy, M., & Leavitt, L.A. (Eds.). (1999). *Improving the communication of people with Down syndrome*. Baltimore: Paul H. Brookes Publishing Co.

Foreword

Since the late 1950s a large body of research has been devoted to understanding the nature and course of language development in children. Competing theories have been offered and tested, hundreds of observational studies have been conducted, and a wide variety of interventions have been evaluated. Researchers now have a good understanding of developmental processes and the efficacy of a variety of intervention models.

Much remains to be learned, however, about the genetic and biological components of speech and language development. One of the most fruitful ways of understanding genetic and biological factors is to study individuals with known genetic or chromosomal abnormalities, and it is from this context that Roberts, Chapman, and Warren offer this informative text. Down syndrome (a chromosomal abnormality, usually a spontaneous mutation resulting in an extra copy of chromosome 21) and fragile X syndrome (an inherited mutation in the FMR1 gene on the X chromosome) are two of the most commonly occurring known genetic causes of intellectual disability. They result in very different developmental and behavioral profiles. In both conditions, speech and language development is affected, but in different ways. These differences have important implications not only for treatment but also ultimately for understanding the genetic bases of speech and language development.

Some might suggest that etiology is irrelevant in planning interventions for children with disabilities, arguing that individualized assessment of abilities and learning styles should provide sufficient information from which an experienced clinician can determine appropriate intervention strategies. This book makes it clear that etiology does indeed matter, playing an important role in shaping the nature and course of speech-language development, the manifestation of delays or abnormality in speech-language development, and the differential implications for intervention. The book contains a useful and thorough overview of what is known about Down syndrome and fragile X syndrome, how speech and language development vary (and are similar) across the two, and the implications for treatment.

Throughout the chapters is reinforced the notion that language development is a complex interplay between biology and experience. The authors draw on an extensive literature specific to these two conditions but then step back and look at how the broader fields of language development, cognitive processes, social milieu, therapeutic and educational interventions, and family processes and adaptation all contribute to communicative competence. Professionals from a number of disciplines will find this book both informative and thoughtful, not only as it applies to children with these two conditions but as a model for examining other disorders as well.

Donald B. Bailey, Jr., Ph.D.
Distinguished Fellow, RTI International
Research Triangle Park, North Carolina

Preface

Down syndrome (DS) is the most common genetic cause of intellectual disability, and fragile X syndrome (FXS) is the most common inherited genetic cause of intellectual disability. Individuals with DS or FXS generally have speech and language difficulties, but the specific profile of skills and the potential mechanisms underlying the speech and language difficulties usually differ in these two populations. Understanding the similarities and differences in the speech and language phenotype of individuals with DS and FXS and the potential mechanisms underlying these individual differences has important implications for language assessment and intervention.

This book focuses on speech and language development in individuals with DS and FXS. Communicating a message is the ultimate goal of language. Language is composed of a code of symbols and the rules for combining those symbols. Language requires a means for expression. Speech, the production of vocal sound patterns, is the most common means of human communication. The ability to produce and use language is critical for successful functioning in all aspects of life. An individual's language skills affect interactions with family members, peers, and others at home, in school and in the neighborhood, and beyond. Language skills predict academic achievement as well as many other aspects of development.

This book presents a comprehensive review of the latest research on speech and language development in individuals with DS and individuals with FXS; discusses the implications of this research for assessment, intervention, and family involvement for each disorder; and suggests future directions for research. We draw on new research as well as current findings on DS and FXS. We believe this book is timely for several reasons. These include recent findings in molecular genetics; the recognition of the importance of studying the role of and interactions of genes, brain, behavior, and the environment; recent and ongoing longitudinal research defining the language phenotype in DS and FXS; and the increasing recognition of the importance of optimizing the success in educational, home, vocational, and community settings of individual with disabilities.

Section I is intended to describe the status, recent research, and future directions for research on the etiology, diagnosis, and clinical phenotype in DS and FXS. David Patterson and Ira Lott (Chapter 1) discuss for DS the genetics, diagnosis, effects on development and neurodegeneration (e.g. Alzheimer's disease), and the phenotype of DS as related to health care issues. Randi J. Hagerman (Chapter 2) reviews for FXS the genetics, diagnosis, neurobiology, development, neuroimaging findings, associated medical conditions, and interventions focused on medical and behavioral problems.

Section II reviews research findings on speech and language profiles in FXS and DS from infancy through adulthood, implications for speech and language assessment and intervention, and future directions for research. Audra Sterling and Steven F. Warren (Chapter 3) review communication and language development in infants and toddlers with DS and FXS from birth to age 3 years, focusing on prelinguistic communication development through use of single words. They discuss oral-motor development, phonological development, sign language and gestures, joint attention, and imitation in infants and toddlers with FXS or DS; the impact of these characteristics on interactions with parents and other caregivers; and implications for assessment and intervention. Joanne E. Roberts, Robin S. Chapman, Gary E. Martin, and Lauren Moskowitz (Chapter 4) review receptive and expressive development of language during the preschool and school age years for typically developing children, children with DS, and children with FXS. These authors describe findings in vocabulary, syntax, and pragmatics for children with DS and FXS, underlying mechanisms such as hearing loss, cognitive profile, autistic characteristics, speech motor function that may explain language difficulties in each population, and strategies for language assessment and intervention and parent involvement. In Chapter 5, Andrea McDuffie, Robin S. Chapman, and Leonard Abbeduto describe language profiles in adolescents and young adults with DS and FXS. The authors review receptive and expressive language development in vocabulary, syntax, and pragmatics in DS and FXS and how language development in FXS is affected by gender and autism. They also suggest strategies for assessment, intervention, and parent involvement to support language development. In the final chapter of this section (Chapter 6), Joanne E. Roberts, Carol Stoel-Gammon, and Elizabeth F. Barnes review speech development of typically developing children, children with DS, and children with FXS. They summarize the literature on prelinguistic vocal development, single-word productions, connected speech, and speech intelligibility of individuals with DS and FXS; describe factors that may cause or contribute to speech difficulties; and present guidelines for speech assessment and intervention and parent involvement.

Section III presents interventions, research findings, and directions for research to increase language skills in individuals with DS and FXS. Nancy C. Brady, Shelley L. Bredin-Oja, and Steven F. Warren (Chapter 7) describe prelinguistic and early language interventions for children with DS and FXS. This chapter describes prelinguistic and early linguistic development in typically developing children and in children with DS and FXS and prelinguistic and early linguistic interventions that have been used with children with DS, FXS, and other developmental disabilities. Libby Kumin (Chapter 8) presents a clinical perspective on intervention methods to develop complex language for individuals with DS and FXS who use an average length of utterance of three or more words. She describes intervention strategies for different language ages and stages and specifically for vocabulary, syntax, and pragmatics for individuals with DS and FXS from a clinical perspective. In Chapter 9 Johanna R. Price and Ray D. Kent focus on interventions to increase speech intelligibility in individuals with DS and FXS. The authors discuss speech intelligibility, methods to measure intelligibility, study findings on speech intelligibility in children with DS and children with FXS, and interventions to increase speech intelligibility in both populations.

Sue Buckley and Mina C. Johnson-Glenberg (Chapter 10) describe interventions to increase literacy learning in individuals with DS and FXS. This chapter discusses literacy development for individuals with DS and FXS, the effects of literacy instruction on speech-language and memory skills in DS, and methods to increase literacy learning for both populations. Nancy C. Brady (Chapter 11) describes augmentative and alternative communication systems for children with

DS or FXS. The chapter presents different augmentative and alternative communication approaches such as manual sign systems, the Picture Exchange Communication System, and voice output communication aids that have been used with children with disabilities and describes specific applications for children with DS or FXS. In the last chapter of this section (Chapter 12), Anne J. Esbensen, Marsha Mailick Seltzer, and Leonard Abbeduto discuss the impact on families of raising a child with DS or FXS. Topics covered include the effects of genetic syndromes on families; family well-being at diagnosis and during childhood, adolescence, and adulthood when a family member has DS or FXS; the well-being of siblings of individuals with DS; and the well-being of carriers in FXS. An appendix at the end of the book lists key DS, FXS, and related organizations.

Our hope is that this book will deepen the knowledge of practitioners, families and other caregivers, and researchers about speech and language development and intervention for both individuals with DS and FXS. These genetic disorders have different causes and some unique characteristics. However, like human beings in general, they share far more similarities than differences. Most important among these is the ability to grow and develop into citizens with meaningful and productive lives. To help individuals with DS and FXS achieve this potential, it is essential that we do everything possible to enhance their communication and speech and language development.

Acknowledgments

This book is the result of the efforts of many individuals and agencies. First, we greatly appreciate each of the chapter authors for contributing their research reviews and thoughtful perspectives. Second, we acknowledge with great gratitude Anne Taylor and Sarah Henderson for their assistance and great attention to detail in the preparation of the book. We also appreciate the assistance of colleagues of the FPG Child Development Institute, especially Don Bailey, Anne Harris, Anne Edwards, Cheryl Malkin, and Kristin Cooley. We give very special thanks to the funding agencies who have supported our research, particularly the National Institute of Child Health and Human Development (Grants R01 HD044935, RO1 HD038819, R01 HD23353, P30 HD02528, and P30 HD003110-38S1), the National Fragile X Foundation, National Down Syndrome Society, March of Dimes, and The Ireland Family Foundation. These funding agencies are not responsible for the content or opinions expressed in the book. We also want to thank the many editors and staff of Paul H. Brookes Publishing Co. who worked with us during this project. We are especially grateful to the children with Down syndrome and children with fragile X syndrome and their families who continually teach us and motivate us to learn more. In addition, Joanne Roberts would like to express her sincerest thanks to her children, Justin and Matthew, and husband, Barry, for their patience and support throughout this project. Robin Chapman thanks her husband, Will Zarwell, for his support during the preparation of this book, and her sons, John and Josh Chapman, who taught her about language learning 3 decades ago. Steve Warren would like to express his thanks to his daughters Marie and Lena and wife Eva for their continuing support and encouragement in ways both large and small and to his mother Ruth—his first language teacher.

*To my mother, Trudy Erwich, because of her love of family,
passion for life, and never-ending support and encouragement*

—*JER*

Identification and Development in Down Syndrome and Fragile X Syndrome

CHAPTER 1

Etiology, Diagnosis, and Development in Down Syndrome

DAVID PATTERSON AND IRA LOTT

Down syndrome (DS) is the most common genetic cause of significant intellectual disability, occurring in approximately 1 in 700 to 1 in 800 live births (Centers for Disease Control and Prevention, 2006; Roizen & Patterson, 2003), and it was the first chromosomal disorder of humans to be defined. In this chapter we discuss 1) the nature and origin of the chromosomal anomaly (most often an extra copy of an intact human chromosome 21); 2) the origins of the extra chromosome; 3) the genes on chromosome 21 and their possible role in DS; 4) the diagnosis of DS; 5) how human development is affected in individuals with DS, including the essentially novel relationship of DS to Alzheimer's disease; and 6) the phenotype of DS as related to health care issues. We describe some of the more recent experiments attempting to elucidate how the extra chromosome 21 leads to DS. These include new insights into chromosome structure and function and the use of mouse models to study DS. We also consider issues related to prenatal diagnosis and screening for DS and the status of clinical trials meant to ameliorate the effects of the extra chromosome 21. We conclude with some considerations concerning future directions in research about DS and its potential significance for the issues confronting individuals with DS and their families.

THE GENETICS OF DOWN SYNDROME

The fundamental cause of DS is trisomy of a set of genes located on chromosome 21. The phenotype of DS, however, may not involve contributions from all trisomic genes, as discussed in this section.

The Chromosomal Abnormality Causing Down Syndrome

DS is caused by trisomy (the presence of three copies instead of the typical two) of all or part of chromosome 21, the smallest human chromosome. Trisomy of the entire chromosome is present in about 95% of DS cases. In a small fraction of

This work was supported by grants to Dr. Ira Lott (AG21912, AG16573, and the My Brother Joey Clinical Neuroscience Fund) and to Dr. David Patterson (the Jerome Lejeune Foundation, the Bonfils-Stanton Foundation, and the Alvin Itkin Foundation).

cases (5% or less), trisomy of part of chromosome 21—often a translocation involving chromosomes 13, 14, 15, 21, or 22—leads to DS, and rarely other translocations involving chromosome 21 lead to DS. In addition, 1% to 3% of individuals with DS are mosaic; that is, some cells in the individual are trisomic for chromosome 21 and some are not (Devlin & Morrison, 2004). Individuals with mosaicism of chromosomes 21 may have a milder form of DS depending upon the extent of mosaicism.

The extra chromosome 21 in DS arises when, during development of the sperm or egg, the two copies of chromosome 21 do not separate properly (nondisjunction), resulting in sperm or eggs with either zero or two copies of chromosome 21. Almost invariably, cells with zero copies of chromosome 21 cannot lead to a viable individual. During fertilization, however, an egg or sperm with two copies of chromosome 21 can fuse with the egg or sperm with one copy of the chromosome, resulting in a fertilized egg with three copies of the chromosome. The origin of the nondisjunction event in DS is maternal in 95% of cases, and the incidence of DS births shows a striking increase with increasing maternal age, the cause of which is unknown (Lamb & Hassold, 2004). Interestingly, there is an increased risk of birth of a second child with DS to mothers who have had a child with DS, but this seems limited to women younger than 40 years old. The increased risk of having a second child with DS for a woman 30 years old is approximately sixfold (Morris, Mutton, & Alberman, 2005). Recent evidence suggests that the increased risk of chromosomal nondisjunction can involve other chromosomes and that some women may have a higher risk for nondisjunction than others (Warburton et al., 2004).

The Genes on Chromosome 21 and the Phenotype of Down Syndrome

Although it is clear that trisomy of at least a part of chromosome 21 is responsible for DS, how trisomy of the genes on the chromosome leads to the phenotype of DS remains unclear. A crucial step in understanding how the genes on chromosome 21 lead to DS was the publication of the essentially complete DNA sequence of the long arm of chromosome 21 (21q) and the annotation of this sequence (Hattori et al., 2000). At that time, annotation of the sequence revealed 127 known genes, 98 predicted genes, and 59 pseudogenes (DNA regions that have some of the characteristics of genes but are unlikely to be functional). Annotation of the sequence of chromosome 21 is, however, an ongoing process, and as of this writing, about 430 genes and gene models have been identified (see http://chr21db.cudenver.edu for more information).

Two primary hypotheses exist regarding the relationship of the genes on chromosome 21 to the phenotype. The first, known as the *gene dosage hypothesis*, posits that elevated expression of specific genes on chromosome 21 leads to the phenotype (Korenberg et al., 1990). In the most straightforward version of this hypothesis, each gene on chromosome 21 would be expressed at 150% of that found in individuals with two copies of chromosome 21. This hypothesis does not make any predictions regarding how many genes on chromosome 21 may be involved in causation of the phenotype. The second hypothesis is the *genetic homeostasis hypothesis.* This hypothesis states that the expression of extra genes, regardless of their identity or function, lead to perturbations in the timing and sequence of development. The larger the number of trisomic genes, the more severe the phenotypic outcome would be (Shapiro, 1983). Clearly, numerous combinations of these hypotheses are possible. For example, it could be that overexpression of a relatively small set of genes on chromosome 21 has a direct connection to some aspects of the phenotype of DS, whereas the overexpression of a large number of extra genes could also disturb normal development.

If there is a correspondence between particular genes and particular aspects of the phenotype, it should be possible to correlate trisomy of these particular genes with particular aspects of the phenotype. Rarely, DS is caused by a translocation or rearrangement (e.g., ring 21) in which only part of chromosome 21 is trisomic. Indeed, attempts have been made to correlate the trisomic region of chromosome 21 with particular phenotypes associated with DS (Delabar et al., 1993; Korenberg et al., 1994). In general, this has been a very difficult approach because some features of DS can be correlated with specific regions of chromosome 21, but others, for example intellectual disability, cannot. Recent work on mouse models of DS also indicates that the issue of genotype to phenotype correlations is quite complex and not yet understood (Olson, Richtsmeier, Leszl, & Reeves, 2004).

THE DIAGNOSIS OF DOWN SYNDROME

Even though a physician may suspect a diagnosis of DS at birth based on physical features of the newborn, the definitive diagnosis of DS is made by detection of trisomy of all or a part of chromosome 21 by cytogenetic analysis. Cytogenetic analysis is a procedure by which the number and structure of chromosomes is analyzed microscopically. Because each chromosome can be identified unambiguously using this technique, it is considered the gold standard for diagnosis of chromosome abnormalities. In a 2004 retrospective study of 197 cases of trisomy DS, 90% were correctly diagnosed by physical features; however, only 37.5% of mosaic cases were correctly diagnosed on this basis (Devlin & Morrison, 2004). Thus, a definitive diagnosis requires cytogenetic analysis.

The phenotypic features of DS have shown considerable variability in case comparison studies (Fryns, 1990; Jones, 1997; Kava, Tullu, Muranjan, & Girisha, 2004; Kumar & Delatycki, 2001). Certain aspects of the phenotype in DS appear to occur in every person, whereas other traits are more highly variable (Antonarakis, Lyle, Dermitzakis, Reymond, & Deutsch, 2004). For example, cognitive impairment is ubiquitous, albeit with variable severity, among individuals with DS. Congenital heart defects, by contrast, occur in only 40% of those with DS. Certain other conditions—such as duodenal atresia, Hirschsprung disease, and acute megakaryocytic leukemia—are increased in individuals with DS compared with the general population. Explanations for this phenotypic variability have included transcriptional changes in gene expression on chromosome 21 (Mao, Zielke, Zielke, & Pevsner, 2003), developmental instability caused by a global chromosome 21 dosage imbalance (Shapiro, 1983, 1997), or an imbalance related to a small number of chromosome 21 genes in the critical DS region (Korenberg et al., 1990).

The cognitive phenotype in DS is characterized by a disproportionate deficiency in language development as opposed to social intelligence (Chapman, Seung, Schwartz, & Kay-Raining Bird, 1998). There is some evidence of a plateau in cognitive functioning seen within the first 2 decades of life (Brown, Greer, Aylward, & Hunt, 1990). Expressive and receptive language measures, as well as expressions of theory of mind (the ability to understand that others have beliefs, desires, and intentions that are different from one's own), have been reported to be more involved in DS as opposed to individuals with fragile X syndrome (Abbeduto et al., 2001). Motoric aspects of speech production in DS, as measured by canonical babbling (repetitive sequences of vowels and consonants prior to speech development), appear to contribute to the subsequent expressive language disorder (Lynch et al., 1995). The evaluation of cognitive functioning in DS can be complicated by the presence of hearing impairments or sleep disorders (Roizen & Patterson, 2003).

Variability of Gene Expression as a Factor in the Down Syndrome Phenotype

The availability of the complete DNA sequence of the human genome presents enormous opportunities to understand chromosome 21 and how an extra copy of this chromosome leads to the phenotype of DS and to the variability of the phenotype. This is one of the essential tasks of the functional genomics of chromosome 21 (determination of how the genome functions to affect phenotype). Antonarakis and colleagues (2004) have taken a novel and interesting approach to the question of phenotypic variability raised in Deutsch and colleagues (2005). Deutsch and colleagues hypothesized that in any human population there will be variation in the expression levels of many genes. Furthermore, they argued that if the variation in expression in the general population of a gene on chromosome 21 exceeds the 1.5-fold expression elevation expected by the gene dosage hypothesis, then this gene may not be related to the phenotype or may only be related to the phenotypes of DS that are not universally present. If, however, the expression level of a particular chromosome 21 gene is tightly regulated in individuals with two copies of chromosome 21, then a change in expression of 1.5-fold might be directly related to the more consistently present phenotypes of DS, such as intellectual disability. Antonarakis and colleagues presented evidence that variation of expression levels of a significant fraction of genes on chromosome 21 is indeed greater than twofold in the typical population, raising the possibility that these genes may not be causal for the more universally present features of DS.

DEVELOPMENT AND DOWN SYNDROME

The development of virtually every organ system is affected by DS over the lifespan. Developmental consequences of particular significance are discussed in this section.

Brain Structure and Function in Down Syndrome

Structural brain anomalies in DS, as revealed by autopsy studies, have included low brain weight, brachycephaly (an abnormally widened brain structure), underdevelopment of the cerebellum and frontal and temporal lobes, simplification of the sulci, and a narrow superior temporal gyrus (Becker, Mito, Takashima, &

Onodera, 1991; Coyle, Oster-Granite, & Gearhart, 1986; Wisniewski, 1990). Dendritic abnormalities in cortical pyramidal neurons are considered to be the most common microscopic finding in the disorder (Benavides-Piccione et al., 2004), with attenuated branching suggesting a "tree in winter" appearance (Mrak & Griffin, 2004). High-resolution MRI studies have allowed quantitative explorations of brain structure in living individuals with DS. Several of the originally reported postmortem findings have been confirmed by neuroimaging, including small hippocampal neocortical structures and a disproportionately small cerebellum (Pinter, Eliez, Schmitt, Capone, & Reiss, 2001; White, Alkire, & Haier, 2003). Unexpectedly, the parahippocampal gyrus appears to be larger than age-matched controls in DS (Kesslak, Nagata, Lott, & Nalcioglu, 1994), a finding of uncertain significance as of this writing.

Down Syndrome and Alzheimer's Disease

Brain changes of Alzheimer's disease (AD) accumulate across the lifespan in DS, and by age 40 years, virtually all individuals with DS have neuropathological findings of the disorder (Mann & Esiri, 1989). These pathological changes include extracellular aggregates consisting primarily of a fragment of the amyloid precursor protein (APP), the gene for which is located on chromosome 21 (beta-amyloid plaques), and abnormal fibrils found within neuritis that are largely composed of the microtubule-associated protein tau (neurofibrillary tangles). Abeta pathology begins to accumulate in childhood (as young as 8 years) and rises progressively with increasing age (Leverenz & Raskind, 1998). Acceleration in AD pathology between 35 and 45 years also occurs (Wisniewski, Wisniewski, & Wen, 1985). Interestingly, the changes of AD in DS do not appear to be associated with atherosclerosis (Lott & Head, 2005), despite the fact that adults with DS are often sedentary and obese, with abnormal lipid profiles. Although the clinical signs of dementia increase with age in DS, not all adults undergo obvious cognitive decline. Tyrrell and colleagues (2001) reported a prevalence of dementia in 13.3% of individuals with DS at age 54.7 years. This percentage increases with age. Early events of beta-amyloid accumulation in the brains of individuals with DS have been an interest in current research. Both soluble and intracellular beta-amyloid accumulation may occur before extracelluar beta-amyloid (senile plaques) are present in DS (Head & Lott, 2004). Increased levels of beta-amyloid in DS may reflect the increased expression in protein levels of a beta-site amyloid precursor protein cleavage enzyme 2 (BACE2) on chromosome 21, although recent studies also suggest that BACE2 may actually decrease the production of Abeta (Sun et al., 2005). The impact of the accumulation of beta-amyloid may have differential effects on development and aging in DS. Intracellular accumulation of Abeta is associated with caspase activation in DS, suggesting that an apoptotic program leading to cell death is activated within seemingly benign senile plaques containing morphologically normal appearing neurons (Head, Lott, Cribbs, Cotman, & Rohn, 2002). Inflammatory factors and the presence of the apolipoprotein E E4 allele have been identified as risk factors for dementia in DS (Lott & Head, 2005). Health morbidities also increase with age for individuals with DS at risk for dementia (McCarron, Gill, McCallion, & Begley, 2005) and need to be considered in both diagnosis and treatment of individuals presenting with cognitive decline (Roizen & Patterson, 2003).

Neuropsychological Findings Associated with Down Syndrome

DS and autistic disorder are commonly encountered disorders in clinical practice. Autistic disorder has been reported to occur in approximately 1 in 1,000 children, and the more broadly defined autistic spectrum disorder (ASD) occurs in 3–6 per 1,000 children (Rutter, 2005). In individuals with DS, the comorbidity rate of ASD has ranged from 0% to 16.7% (Fombonne, 2003). Capone and colleagues (2005) used the *Diagnostic and Statistical Manual of Mental Disorders, Fourth Edition* (*DSM-IV;* American Psychiatric Association, 1994), criteria as a measure of autism and the Aberrant Behavior Checklist (ABC; Aman, Singh, Stewart, & Field, 1985) in 61 children with DS and ASD. Compared with children with typical DS, children with DS who met *DSM-IV* criteria for ASD had significantly greater cognitive impairment (87% with IQ score < 40 versus 0% in typical DS) and more maladaptive behaviors as measured by the ABC. More than 80% of the DS and ASD participants were male. Clinical descriptions included increased impairment in body and object use as well as decreased social relatedness (Capone, 1999, 2002). In a study using multiple diagnostic measures of autistic disorder, Doran and colleagues (2004) found that children with DS and autistic disorder met the standard research criteria for autistic disorder. The children differed from the autistic disorder group in having relatively preserved abilities in social interactions and nonverbal communication. Lower levels of intellectual functioning and more impairment in play behavior were observed in the dual diagnosis group. These findings suggest that children with comorbid DS and autistic disorder have a distinctive behavioral phenotype incorporating features of both conditions.

Although exhibiting less comorbid psychiatric disease than individuals with other forms of developmental disabilities, children and adults with DS do show an increased incidence of hyperactive and aggressive behaviors (Myers & Pueschel, 1991). Evidence exists that depression is a risk for people with DS as they age. Older adolescents with DS may show decreased externalizing symptoms and subtle increases in withdrawal, possibly as an early sign of depression (Dykens, Shah, Sagun, Beck, & King, 2002). Often the presenting signs of dementia in DS involve a primary emotional change characterized by a decline in social discourse, conversational style, literal understanding, and verbal expression in social contexts (Nelson, Orme, Osann, & Lott, 2001). Some evidence suggests that functional decline in adults with DS may be helped, at least temporarily, by selective serotonin reuptake inhibitor medication (Geldmacher et al., 1997).

Summary of Health Care Issues for Individuals with Down Syndrome

Health care for individuals with DS begins with the establishment of a diagnosis by karyotype analysis. The physical expression of the syndrome is widely variable, and the diagnosis may be missed if too much reliance is made on the typical Down syndrome facies. In addition to confirming the diagnosis, karyotping can provide a degree of closure for the parents and provides some information concerning the genetic risk of having another child with DS (Holzgreve, Nippert, Ganshirt-Ahlert, Schloo, & Miny, 1993). Congenital heart defects are present in approximately 40% of infants with DS (Antonarakis et al., 2004). The long-term prognosis is best when an infant with a cardiac defect is referred to a pediatric cardiologist or cardiac surgeon (Clark, 1996).

A variety of gastrointestinal defects have been associated with DS, including conditions causing intestinal blockage such as duodenal atresia (obliteration of the lumen of the duodenum during fetal development) or Hirschprung disease (in which there is a dilated section of the colon due to absence of fetal nerve development in this tissue). These conditions may manifest as difficulties with feeding or stooling. Infants with DS may have reflux from the gastrointestinal tract and chronic constipation. Because of the midfacial malformations, drainage from the eustachian tubes and sinuses may be impaired. As a result, young children with DS are particularly prone to middle-ear infections and inflammation of the sinuses. It has been recommended that children with DS have auditory brainstem response testing for hearing loss by the age of 6 months. Obstructive sleep apnea also is common in DS, with 30%–60% of children having chronic obstructive hypoventilation (Shott et al., 2006). In a 5-year longitudinal study, up to 80% of children with DS were found to have abnormalities on a polysomnogram (a type of sleep recording). The abnormalities on the sleep tracings did not correlate well with the parents' impression of sleep problems in their children. For this reason, it has been suggested that children with DS have a baseline polysomnogram between ages 3 and 4 years.

Because of the pervasive low muscle tone in DS, individuals with DS are prone to instability of the atlantoaxial junction (a region of the cervical spine). Specific X-ray studies with flexion and extension views of the cervical spine have been recommended (Cohen, 2006) between 3 and 5 years of age. More controversial is whether instability of the cervical spine in asymptomatic children should preclude participation in sports (Pueschel et al., 1995). Most observers agree that children who present with symptoms of neck instability should be examined immediately for cervical spinal cord compression resulting from atlantoaxial dislocation. These symptoms include head tilt, neck pain, deterioration of gait, unexplained urinary incontinence, or complaints of sensory symptoms in the arms or legs.

Endocrine disorders, particularly thyroid disease, are more common in infants with DS. Symptoms of low-functioning thyroid mimic the developmental disability associated with DS. For this reason a sensitive thyroid-stimulating hormone test has been recommended on an annual basis (Pueschel et al., 1995). Gonadal dysfunction and growth hormone deficiency also can occur in DS (McCoy, 1992). Growth hormone treatment increases growth velocity in DS but does not increase brain size (head circumference) or neurodevelopmental parameters (Anneren et al., 1999).

Because children with developmental disabilities may be heavily affected by sensory loss, it is important to check visual functioning as well as hearing. Congenital cataracts occur more frequently in DS, which requires a funduscopic examination at birth. A variety of other congenital ocular problems occur in DS, including nystagmus, strabismus, and keratoconus. These problems may require a referral to a pediatric ophthalmologist (Cooley & Graham, 1991). Transient increase in white blood cell count (leukemoid reaction) occurs in approximately 10% of newborns with DS and is extremely rare in other infants (Cooley & Graham, 1991). A substantially increased risk of acute lymphoblastic and nonlymphoblastic leukemias exists in the disorder (1%). Mutations in the GATA-1 gene have been found, rendering the leukemias extremely sensitive to chemotherapy but also raising the risk of drug toxicity (Webb, 2005).

Seizures occur in up to 10% of children with DS and tend to have a bimodal occurrence. In early infancy, seizures are often associated with West syndrome (infantile spasms and hypsarhythmia), whereas the onset of seizures in mid–adult life often heralds the onset of dementia (Menendez, 2005). Common dental problems in DS include delayed eruption of molars, unusually shaped teeth, enamel defects, and periodontal disease (Sterling, 1992).

The transition to adult life for individuals with DS brings some additional potential problems. Mental illness occurs in approximately 30% of adults with DS, with the most common symptoms related to depression, obsessive-compulsive disorder, and conduct disorder (Prasher, 1995). Self-talk, or soliloquy, is fairly common in adults with DS who are undergoing a stressful situation and is usually mental-age appropriate (McGuire & Chicoine, 1996). As an isolated symptom, self-talk should not be considered to be pathological hallucinatory behavior.

Dementia of the AD type increases with age in individuals with DS, with up to 75% prevalence after age 60 years (Van Dyke, Harper, & Dyken, 1998). It is necessary to rule out conditions in DS that may mimic the onset of dementia, including hypothyroidism and mental illness. Signs of dementia include changes in behavior, loss of ability to carry out daily living functions, gait dyspraxia, new onset seizures, urinary incontinence, and pathological reflexes on examination (Lott, 2002).

MECHANISMS OF VARIABILITY IN GENE EXPRESSION IN DOWN SYNDROME

The mechanisms behind variability in gene expression are undoubtedly complex. Some unexpected possibilities are being revealed through analysis of genome structure and function. Some of these are as follows.

Copy Number Polymorphisms

Copy number polymorphisms (CNPs) result when a small, cytogenetically undetectable region of DNA is either duplicated or deleted in some individuals. Thus, individuals may vary in the number of copies of this region of DNA they possess, and these DNA regions are said to be polymorphic. Polymorphisms can also result if, for example, a particular gene or DNA region varies in its nucleotide sequence from individual to individual. One possible mechanism that might result in variability in gene expression as measured by messenger RNA (mRNA) levels is CNPs. That is, it is possible that small, perhaps even single-gene, regions of the genome have been duplicated or lost in some individuals and that these duplications or deletions represent polymorphic (variable) loci in the genome. Indeed, this appears to be the case for genes on chromosome 21. A 2006 study presents evidence that duplication of a small region of chromosome 21, including the amyloid precursor protein (APP) gene, can lead to familial AD (Rouvelet-Lecrux et al., 2006). This evidence is consistent with the idea that trisomy of APP may explain, at least in part, the observation that individuals with DS virtually always develop the neuropathology associated with AD. It appears likely that several hundred

CNPs exist throughout the human genome, as assessed by comparative genomic hybridization using DNA microarrays of various types.

Transcription Factors and Variability of Expression

For a gene to produce an active protein and, therefore, have an effect in a cell, the information in the gene must be copied into an mRNA molecule—a process called transcription. The number of copies of an mRNA molecule from a particular gene present in a cell (transcript levels) is one way of assessing how active a gene is. Transcription factors are proteins that control or regulate the transcription of genes. It is beyond the scope of this chapter to discuss the role of transcription factors in the regulation of gene expression. Suffice it to say, however, that at least 10 transcription factor genes are present on chromosome 21. It is highly likely that these are important in the regulation of many genes, both on chromosome 21 and on other chromosomes. Analysis of regulation of chromosome 21 encoded genes by transcription factors is an ongoing area of intense research (Arron et al., 2006; Gardiner, 2006).

Posttranscriptional Regulation

Assessments of transcript levels are crucial for understanding DS and other conditions. Transcript levels do not, however, always accurately reflect the levels of proteins made from a particular transcript. Therefore, regulatory processes that occur after the gene is transcribed (posttranscriptional regulatory mechanisms) clearly play important roles. Some unexpected mechanisms of posttranscriptional regulation have been revealed by functional genomics studies.

MicroRNAs

MicroRNAs are endogenous, small RNA molecules approximately 22 nucleotides long and derived from larger transcripts (Bartel, 2004; Kosik & Krichevsky, 2005). Hundreds of microRNAs have been identified by genomic approaches (Nam et al., 2005). Some microRNAs appear to target mRNAs for destruction or for repression of the process of producing functional proteins from these mRNAs (a process known as translation; Bartel, 2004; Bartel & Chen, 2004; Fahr et al., 2005). An intriguing hypothesis is that microRNAs serve to dampen translation of mRNAs. In this capacity, they may be able to exert more rapid and subtle modifications of protein levels than transcriptional control mechanisms (Bartel & Chen, 2004; Kosik & Krichevsky, 2005). A number of putative microRNAs are encoded by genes on chromosome 21. Their role in DS is unknown at the time of this writing.

Conserved Noncoding Regions

As the essentially complete genomic sequences of mammals, including humans, have become available, genomic sequence comparisons have revealed some unexpected characteristics of mammalian genomes. One of these is the existence of a large number of conserved noncoding regions (CNCs; Dermitzakis, Reymond, & Antonarakis, 2005). CNCs are regions of DNA that are not genes but that have DNA sequences that are highly conserved from organism to organism. CNCs are not repetitive sequences, and the vast majority are not transcribed (copied into RNA; Dermitzakis et al., 2005). Chromosome 21 was the first chromosome completely analyzed for CNCs, and 2,262 were identified. Possible functions for CNCs include controlling the function of genes or elements required for chromatin or chromosome structure (Dermitzakis et al., 2004). It is interesting to consider the possible interplay among CNCs, microRNAs, and CNPs in conditions such as DS.

MOUSE MODELS TO STUDY THE ETIOLOGY OF DOWN SYNDROME

Rationale for Mouse Models

The rationale for the use of mouse models to study the etiology of DS has been discussed at length in the past 5 years, and the reader is referred to these works for in-depth discussions of this point (Gardiner, Fortna, Bechtel, & Davisson, 2003; Patterson & Costa, 2005). It is worth stressing some points here. The intrinsic value of mouse models is that mice genetically and biochemically are quite similar to humans. This is important when one is attempting to determine the genetics and biochemistry of any human disease. This similarity extends to the level of chromosomes. That is, many large chromosome regions in the mouse are very similar to specific human chromosomes (such regions are said to be *syntenic*). Of particular relevance for the study of DS, a large region of mouse chromosome 16 is very similar to a large region of human chromosome 21. This region of similarity corresponds to about half of the genes on human chromosome 21. Even the order of the genes on the chromosomes is the same. Extensively validated tests of learning and memory in mice exist. Moreover, many experiments cannot be done in humans or in simpler systems such as tissue culture.

DS presents particular problems because the phenotype is likely to involve many genes and biological pathways. In general, three types of mouse models have proven useful for study of DS. These are 1) mice in which one or more human chromosome 21 genes have been introduced into the mouse genome (transgenic mice), 2) mice carrying mouse chromosomal segments or indeed whole chromosomes homologous to part of chromosome 21 (or human chromosome 21 itself) in an extra copy, and 3) mice in which the mouse equivalents of chromosome 21 genes have been inactivated by targeted mutagenesis (knockout mice).

Validity of Mouse Models

Even though mice and humans are similar biochemically and genetically, they are not identical. For example, species-specific genes that appear on human chromosome 21 are not present in the mouse, and there appear to be mouse genes on mouse chromosome 16 that are not present in humans (Gardiner et al., 2003). Although the number of these genes is small, their effect is not clear. Indeed, with the complexity of nonprotein coding genes and regions that are being revealed, it seems likely that additional differences between the genomes of mice and humans will be uncovered.

Even if the genes involved are similar in mice and humans, the functions of those genes may not be quite the same, or their regulation may be different in the two species. For example, a pathway of great interest is that of folate and one-carbon metabolism—metabolic systems that are known to be important for learning and memory. It appears that the tissue specificity of critical genes in these biological systems is different in mice and in humans (Butler, Bowersox, Forbes, & Patterson, 2006; Liu et al., 2005; Whetstine, Flatley, & Matherly, 2002), implying that these pathways serve slightly different functions in humans and in mice. Information of this nature will be critical for proper interpretation of results from studies of transgenic mice and should be taken into account in the design of these mice. For example, in some situations, it may be more appropriate to make mice triplicated for mouse genes rather than mice containing a copy of the cognate human gene.

Partially Trisomic Mice

Human chromosome 21 has syntenic regions on three mouse chromosomes: 16, 17, and 10. So far, the most thoroughly studied mouse models carry an extra copy of all or part of mouse chromosome 16. Mice trisomic for the entire mouse chromosome 16 die during fetal development or shortly after birth, so they are not useful for studies of learning and memory.

The most studied mouse model of DS is the Ts65Dn mouse, which is trisomic for about half of the genes located on human chromosome 21 (Gardiner et al., 2003). These mice have learning and memory impairments such as those seen in individuals with DS. For example, Ts65Dn mice have impairments in performance in the Morris Water Maze and impairments in learning and remembering features of their environment (Hyde, Frisone, & Crnic, 2001; Stasko & Costa, 2004). A very simplified description of this test is as follows: A tub is filled with water made opaque with a nontoxic substance (e.g., nontoxic latex paint). A platform is placed in the tub. The platform can be either hidden or visible. The mouse is then placed in the tub and asked, over repeated trials, to learn where the platform is. If the platform is hidden below the surface of the water, the mouse is forced to use distal visual cues placed in the testing room. This is thought to be a test of visual-spatial learning, which requires hippocampal function. There are many additional complexities and complications of this test, and these are elegantly discussed in *What's Wrong with My Mouse?* by J. Crawley (2007). These are tasks thought to reflect hippocampal function, and similar difficulties appear to be present in individuals with DS (Pennington, Moon, Edgin, Stedron, & Nadel, 2003). It is possible to ameliorate these difficulties, for example, by treatment with estrogen or minocycline (Granholm et al., 2002; Hunter, Bachman, & Granholm, 2004). Deficient hippocampal neurogenesis has been observed in Ts65Dn mice, and this appears to be alleviated by fluoxetine (Clark, Schwalbe, Stasko, Yarowsky, & Costa, 2006).

Ts65Dn mice show abnormalities in craniofacial and cerebellar development, which resembles what is observed in individuals with DS (Baxter, Moran, Richtsmeier, Tronosco, & Reeves, 2000; Richtsmeier, Zumwalt, Carlson, Epstein, & Reeves, 2002). Indeed, one abnormality in cerebellar development was first found in the Ts65Dn mice and then later found in individuals with DS (Baxter et al., 2000). As might be expected given the abnormalities seen in the cerebellum of Ts65Dn mice, these mice have motor difficulties such as those occasionally seen in individuals with DS (Hampton, Stasko, Kale, Amende, & Costa, 2004). Again, it appears to be possible to ameliorate the defective cerebellar development seen in Ts65Dn mice with drugs (Roper et al., 2006).

Because studies with the Ts65Dn mice indicate that the impairments in hippocampal and cerebellar development and function can be corrected with drug treatment, these studies provide optimism that such goals may be achievable in humans with DS as well. These studies also amply justify continued study of these mice and attempts to create additional mouse models mimicking aspects of DS.

Several other mouse models with triplication of smaller regions of mouse chromosome 16 have been made, and their analysis has begun (Olson et al., 2004). Mice have also been produced in which a large part of human chromosome 21 has been introduced (Kazuki et al., 2003; O'Doherty et al., 2005). These mice again have many features reminiscent of DS. So far, however, all the viable mice of this type are mosaic; that is, varying fractions of cells in different tissues have the human chromosome. The usefulness of these mice remains to be determined.

Single-Gene Transgenic Mice

Single-gene transgenic mice are extremely useful for analysis of the role of trisomy of individual genes. Transgenic mice have been created for several chromosome 21 genes, and more are being reported rapidly. A number of these mice have learning and memory impairments and other abnormalities reminiscent of DS. Moreover, transgenic mice can often demonstrate unexpected complexity in relating specific genes to phenotypes. A few examples out of many possibilities are described briefly here to illustrate these points.

A particularly elegant study demonstrated the role of the DYRK1A gene in learning and memory impairments and in synaptic plasticity (Ahn et al., 2006). These researchers were very careful to ensure that only a single extra copy of the DYRK1A gene was introduced into the transgenic mice. In many other cases, multiple copies of the transgene have been introduced into the mice. This can be useful in terms of understanding gene function, but it is not a precise model of DS, in which only one extra copy of each gene is present. These mice have significant impairments in hippocampal function, for example, in the Morris Water Maze task, which is known to be abnormal in people with DS, and in the Ts65Dn mouse model of DS. Interestingly, single-gene transgenic mice also have abnormalities in functioning of synapses, the regions at which neurons connect to each other, which is observed in Ts65Dn mice as well. These mice provide a simpler model than the Ts65Dn mice in which to study synapse function. This simplicity is not, however, what is seen in DS or in the Ts65Dn mice.

An example that illustrates this point is a report of attempts to produce transgenic mice with the human DSCR1 (Down Syndrome Critical Region 1) gene, a gene also thought to be involved in synapse function (Keating, Chen, & Pritchard, 2006; Kluetzman, Perez, & Crawford, 2005). Even though the DSCR1 gene is present in an extra copy in the Ts65Dn mice, so far it has been essentially impossible to produce transgenic mice containing the normal form of the human DSCR1 gene as the only extra gene (Kluetzman et al., 2005). This suggests the possibility that another gene (or genes) on human chromosome 21 or mouse chromosome 16 can counteract the lethal effects of an extra copy of DSCR1.

Knockout Mice

In recent years it has become possible to inactivate specific mouse genes by a procedure called targeted mutagenesis. In this procedure, DNA similar to the gene of interest but without the function of the gene can be introduced into mouse embryonic stem cells. Occasionally this DNA replaces all or part of the active mouse gene, rendering it inactive. This is called "knocking out" the mouse gene, and such mice are called *knockout mice*. Knockout mice have the potential to reveal a great deal about the function of the gene that has been knocked out because they no longer have that function. Because many genes on chromosome 21 (and elsewhere in the genome) are of unknown function, this approach can provide valuable information.

This approach can also be used in combination with Ts65Dn mice. For example, as implied previously in the discussion of the DSCR1 gene, it is becoming clear that synaptic function, and especially a process called *endosome function*, is an early target in AD and in DS (Cataldo et al., 2004; Keating et al., 2006; Nixon, 2005). It turns out that dosage of the APP gene modulates these abnormalities (Cataldo et al., 2003). Thus, Ts65Dn mice, which have an extra copy of the APP gene, have endosomal abnormalities. Mice transgenic for a mutant form of the APP gene known to cause AD in humans do not possess these abnormalities. Mice in which the APP gene has been knocked out are viable and fertile (Zheng et al., 1995). By breeding the APP knockout mice with Ts65Dn mice, it is possible to produce mice that have only two copies of the APP gene but that have three copies of all the other genes present in three copies in the Ts65Dn mice. These mice do not possess the endosomal abnormalities seen in the Ts65Dn mice (Cataldo et al., 2003). Thus, trisomy of the APP gene is necessary but not sufficient to produce the endosomal dysfunction that appears to be an early feature of AD and perhaps is related to the intellectual disabilities of individuals with DS.

PRENATAL DIAGNOSIS AND SCREENING FOR DOWN SYNDROME

Amniocentesis and Chorionic Villus Sampling

Because DS is a chromosomal disorder, prenatal diagnosis by analysis of fetal cells is feasible. The incidence of DS shows a dramatic increase with the age of the mother, so many physicians recommend amniocentesis (analysis of fetal cells taken from the amniotic fluid) or chorionic villus sampling (CVS; analysis of fetal cells taken from the membrane surrounding the fetus) to pregnant women older than 35 years of age. Generally, but not always, these procedures are performed so that the parents have the option of pregnancy termination of an affected fetus.

Amniocentesis for diagnosing DS has been available since 1966 (Steele & Breg, 1966), and CVS has been available since 1983 (Simoni et al., 1983). As of this writing, the risk of fetal loss with either procedure is estimated to be 0.5%–1% (Brambati & Tului, 2005). CVS is advantageous because it can be carried out in the first trimester, when the risk of maternal mortality from pregnancy termination is about 1.1/100,000 as opposed to second trimester, when the risk is about 7–10/100,000 (Lawson et al., 1994; Simpson, 2005). Amniocentesis is not performed until the second trimester (Pinette et al., 2004).

Biochemical and Ultrasonographic Screening

Because of the risk of fetal loss and maternal mortality associated with amniocentesis and CVS, and because neither of these diagnostic tests is practical as a screening test, development of a less invasive test suitable for screening all pregnancies for DS and other chromosomal anomalies is an ongoing area of clinical and basic research. To date, second trimester screening commonly uses three or perhaps four markers. The triple screen measures alpha-fetoprotein, human chorionic gonadotrophin, and unconjugated estriol. The quadruple screen adds measurement of inhibin A to this battery (Malone et al., 2005).

Clearly, a first trimester screening protocol would have significant advantages in terms of the safety, ease, and privacy of pregnancy termination. Moreover, in the large majority of cases, the results will be negative, thus offering reassurance to the family that the fetus is not affected. In 1992, measurement of enlarged fetal nuchal translucency (NT) by ultrasonography was introduced as a screening test for chromosomal anomalies (Nicolaides, Azar, Byrne, Mansur, & Marks, 1992). More recently, NT measurements have been combined with measurement of the serum markers pregnancy-associated plasma protein A (PAPP-A) and the free beta subunit of human chorionic gonadotrophin (f-beta-hCG; Malone, 2005).

All screening methods described so far have significant false positive rates, and none detect all cases of DS. Two large studies comparing various screening protocols have been reported: the Serum, Urine, and Ultrasound Screening Study (SURUSS) of 47,053 singleton pregnancies (Wald, Rodeck, Hackshaw, & Rudnicka, 2005) and the First and Second Trimester Evaluation of Risk (FASTER) study of 38,167 pregnancies (Malone et al., 2005). Both studies found that first trimester screening including NT was superior to second trimester screening. Both studies determined that the protocol with the highest detection rate and the lowest false positive rate was the integrated protocol. In this protocol, a first trimester screen including NT, PAPP-A, and f-beta-hCG was performed, followed by a quadruple screen in the second trimester. Results were calculated on the basis of all tests, and none were released after the first trimester screening. Both studies found that integrated screening without the NT test in the first trimester could be a reasonable alternative given the potential obstacles to adding NT screening (Malone, 2005).

Integrated screening requires that test results from the first trimester screening not be revealed. This has the obvious difficulty that diagnosis with amniocentesis will, out of necessity, be delayed until after the second trimester test. The FASTER study found that stepwise sequential screening can be quite effective. In this protocol, first trimester screening is carried out and the results provided, allowing high-risk individuals to proceed with CVS if they desire. Second trimester screening (the quadruple test) is then carried out and a single combined risk is calculated. The detection rate is similar to fully integrated screening, but the false positive rate is estimated to increase to 4.9%.

Detection of Fetal Cells in the Mother's Blood

In the 1960s, evidence was presented suggesting the presence of fetal cells in maternal blood samples (Tepper & Verso, 1964; Wagner, Schunck, & Isebarth, 1964). By 1975, the possibility that these cells could be used for prenatal diagnosis, thus avoiding invasive procedures, had been raised (Raafat, Brayton, Apgar, & Borgaonkar, 1975), and by 1979, fetal cells had been separated from maternal blood using fluorescence-activated cell sorting (FACS; Herzenberg, Bianchi, Schroder, Cann, & Iverson, 1979). In 1993, magnetic cell sorting was introduced as an alternative way to isolate fetal cells from maternal blood, and the method was used to detect trisomies of chromosomes 21 and 18 (Ganshirt-Ahlert et al., 1993). This method is considerably less expensive and demanding than FACS-based methods and appears to produce superior results (Bianchi et al., 2002). This approach, however, is not yet adequate for clinical use. In a large multicenter study, the National Institute of Child Health and Human Development Fetal Cell Isolation Study (NIFTY-1), the detection rate of finding at least one aneuploid cell (a cell with an abnormal number of chromosomes) in samples from known aneuploid pregnancies was only 74.4% (Bianchi et al., 2002).

Some fetal cells persist for years in the maternal blood, making analysis of multiple pregnancies problematic. Partly for this reason, there is considerable interest in isolating and analyzing fetal nucleated red blood cells (NRBC). These cells do not persist long in the maternal circulation. Moreover, they are nucleated, so, in principle, they could be analyzed for chromosome number and structure either by standard approaches or by molecular approaches such as fluorescent *in situ* hybridization (FISH), a procedure in which fluorescently labeled DNA probes specific for individual chromosomes or chromosome regions are used. Again, proof of principle experiments demonstrate that this can be achieved. Very significant technical problems, however, remain to be overcome before this method can be considered for clinical use.

Molecular Methods Other than Fluorescent *in situ* Hybridization

A promising new technology for molecular detection of chromosomal aneuploidies is quantitative fluorescent PCR. PCR, or polymerase chain reaction, is a procedure by which thousands or even millions of copies of a small, specific region of DNA can be produced in the laboratory. This procedure provides enough DNA of the target region to analyze using a number of different approaches. In this procedure, DNA samples from amniotic fluid, CVS samples, or other sources are subjected to PCR analysis using primers that amplify highly polymorphic small tandem repeat (STR) markers (El Mouatassim et al., 2004; Ogilvie, Donaghue, Fox, Docherty, & Mann, 2005). These tests appear to be rapid, easily amenable to high throughput, and extremely accurate. In addition, it appears that DNA from fetal NRBCs is more amenable to PCR analysis than to FISH (Babochkina et al., 2005).

It seems likely that both diagnosis and screening methods will continue to evolve and to employ new technologies.

CLINICAL TRIALS

The ultimate goal of understanding the etiology and development of DS is to improve the lives of individuals with DS and their families. This will, of course, have very significant societal benefits as well. This will require rigorous clinical trials of possible therapies for DS. Clinical trials have been late in coming to individuals with DS. In the area of brain functioning, the most active trials have been directed toward enhancing cholinergic dysfunction, a problem most marked in the dementia process. Treatment with acetylcholinesterase inhibitors have been shown to improve cognitive functioning in individuals with DS and dementia (Lott, Osann, Doran, & Nelson, 2002; Prasher, Huxley, & Haque, 2002). Some preliminary evidence suggests that cholinergic treatment may improve language functioning in individuals with DS prior to the onset of dementia (Heller et al., 2003; Johnson, Fahey, Chicoine, Chong, & Gitelman, 2003), but double-blind studies have not been carried out to date. At least since the 1960s, nutritional interventions, including vitamin supplementation, have been popular but controversial in DS (Roizen & Patterson, 2003). Clinical trials of nutritional supplements have had methodological problems and have shown no efficacy (Ani, Grantham-McGregor, & Muller, 2000; Salman, 2002). Piracetam, a psychoactive drug therapy hypothesized to improve cognitive function in children with DS (Holmes, 1999), has been shown to be ineffective and associated with adverse side effects (Lobaugh et al., 2001).

CONCLUDING CONSIDERATIONS

An important consideration in understanding the etiology of DS is to relate molecular findings to the clinical phenotype of the disorder. Specifically with regard to speech and language, evidence suggests that specific genes, for example FOXP2 (a gene that is not on chromosome 21 and not thought to be related to the speech problems seen in DS but nonetheless illustrates the point), may play a critical role in speech and language and that alterations in copy number of functional genes may be sufficient to alter speech and learning ability (Enard et al., 2002; Fisher, 2005). It is not known whether there are genes on chromosome 21 that directly influence speech and language when their copy number is altered. Clearly, a better understanding of variations in gene expression, the role of conserved nongenic sequences, copy number polymorphisms, and microRNAs in the etiology of DS (and other genetic conditions) must be understood. Answers to these questions will likely require new technologies (e.g., proteomics), increased use of computational modeling and bioinformatics systems biology approaches, and improved mouse models.

It will be important to develop a more complete understanding of the development of DS throughout the lifespan. DS provides one of the few models in medicine in which processes of development and aging are linked. This is of critical importance, as the life expectancy of individuals with DS continues to increase. It seems likely that the natural history of DS will alter as continued improvements in clinical care occur. For example, improved understanding of the role of sleep apnea may well allow for improved development of speech and language even without detailed understanding of the etiology of the sleep apnea at the molecular level. Again, improved mouse models and continued characterization of existing mouse models may be enlightening in terms of how various aspects of the phenotype of DS develop.

It seems certain that eventually a reliable and inexpensive screening method for DS will be developed. The application of such a screening method will be a societal issue, especially as the life prospects for individuals with DS continue to improve.

REFERENCES

Abbeduto, L., Pavetto, M., Kesin, E., Weissman, M.D., Karadottir, S., O'Brien, A., et al. (2001). The linguistic and cognitive profile of Down syndrome: Evidence from a comparison with fragile X syndrome. *Down Syndrome Research and Practice, 7,* 9–15.

Ahn, K.-J., Jeong, H.K., Choi, H.-S., Ryoo, S.-R., Kim, Y.J., Goo, J.-S., et al. (2006). DYRK1A BAC transgenic mice show altered synaptic plasticity with learning and memory deficits. *Neurobiology of Disease, 22*(3), 463–472.

Aman, M.G., Singh, N.N., Stewart, A.W., & Field, C. (1985). The Aberrant Behavior Checklist: A behavior rating scale for the assessment of treating effects. *American Journal of Mental Deficiency, 89,* 485–491.

American Psychiatric Association. (1994). *Diagnostic and statistical manual of mental disorders* (4th ed.). Washington, DC: Author.

Ani, C., Grantham-McGregor, S., & Muller, D. (2000). Nutritional supplementation in Down syndrome: Theoretical considerations and current status. *Developmental Medicine and Child Neurology, 42,* 207–213.

Anneren, G., Tuvemo, T., Carlsson-Skwirut, C., Lonnerholm T., Bang, P., Sara, V.R., et al. (1999). Growth hormone treatment in young children with Down's syndrome: Effects on growth and psychomotor development. *Archives of Disease in Childhood, 80,* 334–338.

Antonarakis, S.E., Lyle, R., Dermitzakis, E.T., Reymond, A., & Deutsch, S. (2004). Chromosome 21 and Down syndrome: From genomics to pathophysiology. *Nature Reviews Genetics, 5,* 725–738.

Arron, J.R., Winslow, M.M., Polleri, A., Chang, C.P., Wu, H., Gao, X., et al. (2006) NFAT dysregulation by increased dosage of DSCRI and DYRKIA on chromosome 21. *Nature, 441,* 595–600.

Babochkina, T., Mergenthaler, S., De Napoli, G., Hristoskova, S., Tercanli, S., Holzgreve, W., et al. (2005). Numerous erythroblasts in maternal blood are impervious to fluorescent in situ hybridization analysis, a feature related to a dense compact nucleus with apoptotic character. *Haematologica, 90,* 740–745.

Bartel, D.P. (2004). MicroRNAs: Genomics, biogenesis, mechanism, and function. *Cell, 116,* 281–297.

Bartel, D.P., & Chen, C.-Z. (2004). Micromanagers of gene expression: The potentially widespread influence of metazoan microRNAs. *Nature Reviews Genetics, 5,* 396–400.

Baxter, L.L., Moran, T.H., Richtsmeier, J.T., Tronosco, J., & Reeves, R.H. (2000). Discovery and genetic localization of Down syndrome cerebellar phenotypes using the Ts65Dn mouse. *Human Molecular Genetics, 9,* 195–202.

Becker, L., Mito, T., Takashima, S., & Onodera, K. (1991). Growth and development of the brain in Down syndrome. *Progress in Clinical Biology Research, 373,* 133–152.

Benavides-Piccione, R., Ballesteros-Yanez, I., de Lagran, M.M., Elston, G., Estivill, X., Fillat, C., et al. (2004). On dendrites in Down syndrome and DS murine models: A spiny way to learn. *Progress in Neurobiology, 74,* 111–126.

Bianchi, D.W., Simpson, J.L., Jackson, L.G., Elias, S., Holzgreve, W., Evans, M.I., et al. (2002). Fetal gender and aneuploidy detection using fetal cells in maternal blood: Analysis of NIFTY I data. *Prenatal Diagnosis, 22,* 609–615.

Brambati, B., & Tului, L. (2005). Chorionic villus sampling and amniocentesis. *Current Opinions in Obstetrics and Gynecology, 17,* 197–201.

Brown, F.R., III, Greer, M.K., Aylward, E.H., & Hunt, H.H. (1990). Intellectual and adaptive functioning in individuals with Down syndrome in relation to age and environmental placement. *Pediatrics, 85,* 450–452.

Butler, C., Bowersox, J., Forbes, S., & Patterson, D. (2006). The production of transgenic mice expressing human cystathionine beta-synthase to study Down syndrome. *Behavior Genetics, 36*(3), 429–438.

Capone, G.T. (1999). Down syndrome and autistic spectrum disorder: A look at what we know. *Disability Solutions, 3,* 8–15.

Capone, G.T. (2002). Down syndrome and autistic spectrum disorders. In W.I. Cohen, L. Nadel, & M.E. Madnick (Eds.), *Visions for the 21st century: Down syndrome* (pp. 327–336). New York: Wiley-Liss.

Capone, G.T., Grados, M.A., Kaufmann, W.E., Bernad-Ripoll, S., & Jewell, A. (2005). Down syndrome and comorbid autism-spectrum disorder: Characterization using the Aberrant Behavior Checklist. *American Journal of Medical Genetics A, 134,* 373–380.

Cataldo, A.M., Petanceska, S., Peterhoff, C.M., Terio, N.B., Epstein, C.J., Villar, A., et al. (2003). App gene dosage modulates endosomal abnormalities of Alzheimer's disease in a segmental trisomy 16 mouse model of Down syndrome. *The Journal of Neuroscience, 23,* 6788–6792.

Cataldo, A.M., Petanceskca, S., Terio, N.B., Peterhoff, C.M., Durham, R., Mercken, M., et al. (2004). Abeta localization in abnormal endosomes: Association with earliest Abeta elevations in AD and Down syndrome. *Neurobiology of Aging, 25,* 1263–1272.

Centers for Disease Control and Prevention. (2006). Improved national prevalence estimates for 18 selected major birth defects—United States, 1999–2001. *Morbidity and Mortality Weekly Report, 54,* 1301–1305.

Chapman, R.S., Seung, H.K., Schwartz, S.E., & Kay-Raining Bird, E. (1998). Language skills of children and adolescents with Down syndrome: II. Production deficits. *Journal of Speech Language and Hearing Research, 41,* 861–873.

Clark, E.B. (1996). Access to cardiac care for children with Down syndrome. In B. Marino & S.M. Pueschel (Eds.), *Heart disease in persons with Down syndrome* (pp. 145–150). Baltimore: Paul H. Brookes Publishing Co.

Clark, S., Schwalbe, J., Stasko, M.R., Yarowsky, P.J., & Costa, A.C.S. (2006). Fluoxetine rescues deficient neurogenesis in hippocampus of the Ts65Dn mouse model for Down syndrome. *Experimental Neurology, 200*(1), 256–261.

Cohen, W.I. (2006). Current dilemmas in Down syndrome clinical care: Celiac disease, thyroid disorders, and atlanto-axial instability. *American Journal of Medical Genetics, Part C, 142C,* 141–148.

Cooley, W.C., & Graham, J.M. (1991). Down syndrome: An update and review for the primary pediatrician. *Clinical Pediatrics, 30,* 233–253.

Coyle, J.T., Oster-Granite, M.L., & Gearhart, J.D. (1986). The neurobiologic consequences of Down syndrome. *Brain Research Bulletin, 16,* 773–787.

Crawley, J.N. (2007). *What's wrong with my mouse?* Hoboken, NJ: John Wiley and Sons.

Delabar, J.-M., Theophile, D., Rahmani, Z., Chettouh, Z., Blouin, J.L., Prieur M., et al. (1993). Molecular mapping of twenty-four features of Down syndrome on chromosome 21. *European Journal of Human Genetics, 1,* 114–124.

Dermitzakis, E.T., Kirkness, E., Schwarz, S., Birney, E., Reymond, A., & Antonarakis, S.E. (2004). Comparison of human chromosome 21 conserved nongenic sequences (CNGs) with the mouse and dog genomes shows that their selective constraint is independent of their genic environment. *Genome Research, 14,* 852–859.

Dermitzakis, E.T, Reymond, A., & Antonarakis, S.E. (2005). Conserved non-genic sequences: An unexpected feature of mammalian genomes. *Nature Reviews Genetics, 6,* 151–157.

Deutsch, S., Lyle, R., Dermitzakis, E.T., Attar, H., Subrahmanyan, L., Gehrig, C., et al. (2005). Gene expression variation and expression quantitative trait mapping of human chromosome 21 genes. *Human Molecular Genetics, 14,* 3741–3749.

Devlin, L., & Morrison, P.J. (2004). Mosaic Down's syndrome prevalence in a complete population study. *Archives of Diseases of Childhood, 89,* 1177–1181.

Doran, E., Osann, K., Spence, M.A., Modahl, C., & Lott, I.T. (2004). Double phenotype of Down syndrome with Autistic Disorder: Specific neuropsychological findings. *Annals of Neurology 62(Supplement 5),* A66.

Dykens, E.M., Shah, B., Sagun, J., Beck, T., & King, B.H. (2002). Maladaptive behaviour in children and adolescents with Down's syndrome. *Journal of Intellectual Disabilities Research, 46,* 484–492.

El Mouatassim, S., Becker, M., Kuzio, S., Ronsin, C., Gil, S., Nouchy, M., et al. (2004). Prenatal diagnosis of common aneuploidies using multiplex quantitative fluorescent polymerase chain reaction. *Fetal Diagnosis and Therapy, 19,* 496–503.

Enard, W., Przeworski, M., Fisher, S.E., Lai, C.S.L., Wiebe, V., Kitano, T., et al. (2002). Molecular evolution of FOXP2, a gene involved in speech and language. *Nature, 418,* 869–872.

Fahr K.K.-L., Grimson, A., Jan, C., Lewis, B.P., Johnston, W.K., Lim, L.P., et al. (2005). The widespread impact of mammalian microRNAs on mRNA repression and evolution. *Science, 310,* 1817–1821.

Fisher S.E. (2005). On genes, speech, and language. *New England Journal of Medicine, 353,* 1655–1657.

Fombonne, E. (2003). Epidemiological surveys of autism and other pervasive developmental disorders: An update. *Journal of Autism and Developmental Disorders, 33,* 365–382.

Fryns, J. (1990). Chromosome 21, trisomy 21. In M. Buyse (Ed.), *Birth defects encyclopedia* (pp. 391–393). Cambridge, MA: Center for Birth Defects Information Services, Inc. and Blackwell Scientific Publications.

Ganshirt-Ahlert, D., Borjesson-Stoll, R., Burschyk, M., Dohr, A., Garritsen, H.S.P., Helmer, E., et al. (1993). Detection of fetal trisomies 21 and 18 from maternal blood using triple gradient and magnetic cell sorting. *American Journal of Reproductive Immunology, 30,* 194–201.

Gardiner, K. (2006). Transcriptional dysregulation in Down syndrome: Predictions for altered protein complex stoichiometries and post-translational modifications and consequences for learning/behavior genes ELK, CREB, and the estrogen and glucocorticoid receptors. *Behavioral Genetics, 36,* 439–453.

Gardiner, K., Fortna, A., Bechtel, L., & Davisson, M.T. (2003). Mouse models of Down syndrome: How useful can they be? Comparison of the gene content of human chromosome 21 with orthologous mouse genomic regions. *Gene, 318,* 137–147.

Geldmacher, D.S., Lerner, A.J., Voci, J.M., Noelker, E.A., Somple, L.C., & Whitehouse, P.J. (1997). Treatment of functional decline in adults with Down syndrome using selective serotonin-reuptake inhibitor drugs. *Journal of Geriatric Psychiatry and Neurology, 10,* 99–104.

Granholm, A.C., Ford, K.A., Hyde, L.A., Bimonte, H.A., Hunter, C.L., Nelson, M., et al. (2002). Estrogen restores cognition and cholinergic phenotype in an animal model of Down syndrome. *Physiology and Behavior, 77,* 371–385.

Hampton, T.G., Stasko, M. R., Kale, A., Amende, I., & Costa, A.C. (2004). Gait dynamics in trisomic mice: Quantitative neurological traits of Down syndrome. *Physiology and Behavior, 82,* 381–389.

Hattori, M., Fujiyama, A., Taylor, T.D., Watanabe, H., Yada, T., Park, H.S., et al. (2000). Chromosome 21 mapping and sequencing consortium: The DNA sequence of human chromosome 21. *Nature, 405,* 311–319.

Head, E., & Lott, I.T. (2004). Down syndrome and beta-amyloid deposition. *Current Opinions in Neurology, 17,* 95–100.

Head, E., Lott, I.T., Cribbs, D.H., Cotman, C.W., & Rohn, T.T. (2002). Beta-amyloid deposition and neurofibrillary tangle association with caspase activation in Down syndrome. *Neuroscience Letters, 330,* 99–103.

Heller, J.H., Spiridigliozzi, G.A., Sullivan, J.A., Doraiswamy, P.M., Krishnan, R.R., & Kishnani, P.S. (2003). Donepezil for the treatment of language deficits in adults with Down syndrome: A preliminary 24-week open trial. *American Journal of Medical Genetics A, 116,* 111–116.

Herzenberg, L.A., Bianchi, D.W., Schroder, J., Cann, H.M., & Iverson, G.M. (1979). Fetal cells in the blood of pregnant women: Detection and enrichment by fluorescence-activated cell sorting. *Proceedings of the National Academy of Sciences of the United States of America, 76,* 1453–1455.

Holmes, L.B. (1999). Concern about piracetam treatment for children with Down syndrome [letters to the editor]. *Pediatrics, 103,* 1078.

Holzgreve, W., Nippert, I., Ganshirt-Ahlert, D., Schloo, R., & Miny, P. (1993). Immediate and long-term applications of technology. *Clinical Obstetrics and Gynecology, 36,* 476–484.

Hunter, C.L., Bachman, D., & Granholm, A.C. (2004). Minocycline prevents cholinergic loss in a mouse model of Down syndrome. *Annals of Neurology, 56,* 675–688.

Hyde, L.A, Frisone, D.F., & Crnic, L.S. (2001). Ts65Dn mice, a model for Down syndrome, have deficits in context discrimination learning suggesting impaired hippocampal function. *Brain and Behavior Research, 118,* 53–60.

Johnson, N., Fahey, C., Chicoine, B., Chong, G., & Gitelman, D. (2003). Effects of donepezil on cognitive functioning in Down syndrome. *American Journal of Mental Retardation, 108,* 367–372.

Jones, K. (1997). Down syndrome (Trisomy 21 syndrome). In K. Jones (Ed.), *Smith's recognizable patterns of human malformation* (pp. 8–13). Philadelphia: W.B. Saunders.

Kava, M.P., Tullu, M.S., Muranjan, M.N., & Girisha, K.M. (2004). Down syndrome: Clinical profile from India. *Archives of Medical Research, 35,* 31–35.

Kazuki, Y., Schulz, T.C., Shinohara, T., Kadota, M., Nishigaki, R., Inoue, T., et al. (2003). A new mouse model for Down syndrome. *Journal of Neural Transmission Supplement, 67,* 1–20.

Keating, D.J., Chen, C., & Pritchard, M.A. (2006). Alzheimer's disease and endocytic dysfunction: Clues from the Down syndrome-related proteins, DSCR1 and ITSN1. *Ageing Research Reviews, 5,* 388–401.

Kesslak, J.P., Nagata, S.F., Lott, I.T., & Nalcioglu, O. (1994). Magnetic resonance imaging analysis of age related changes in the brains of individuals with Down's syndrome. *Neurology, 44,* 1039–1045.

Kluetzman, K.S., Perez, A.V., & Crawford, D.R. (2005). DSCR1 (ADAPT78) lethality: Evidence for a protective effect of trisomy 21 genes? *Biochemical and Biophysical Research Communications, 337,* 595–601.

Korenberg, J.R., Chen, X.-N., Schipper, R., Sun, Z., Gonsky, R., Gerwehr, S., et al. (1994). Down syndrome phenotypes: The consequences of chromosomal imbalance. *Proceedings of the National Academy of Sciences of the United States of America, 91,* 4997–5001.

Korenberg, J.R., Kawashima, H., Pulst, S.M., Ikeuchi, T., Ogasawara, N., Yamamoto, K., et al. (1990). Molecular definition of a region of chromosome 21 that causes features of the Down syndrome phenotype. *American Journal of Human Genetics, 47,* 236–246.

Kosik, K.S., & Krichevsky, A.M. (2005). The elegance of the microRNAs: A neuronal perspective. *Neuron, 47,* 779–782.

Kumar, R.K., & Delatycki, D.M. (2001). Down syndrome. In S. Gupte (Ed.), *Recent advances in paediatric neurology* (pp. 1–13). New Delhi, India: Jaypee Brothers.

Lamb, N.E., & Hassold, T.J. (2004). Nondisjunction: A view from ringside. *New England Journal of Medicine, 351,* 1931–1934.

Lawson, H.W., Frye, A., Atrash, H.K., Smith, J.C., Shulman, H.B., & Ramick, M. (1994). Abortion mortality, United States, 1972 through 1987. *American Journal of Obstetrics and Gynecology, 171,* 1365–1372.

Leverenz, J.B., & Raskind, M.A. (1998). Early amyloid deposition in the medial temporal lobe of young Down syndrome patients: A regional quantitative analysis. *Experimental Neurology, 150,* 296–304.

Liu, M., Ge, Y., Cabelof, D.C., Aboukameel, A., Heydari, A.R., Mohammad, R., et al. (2005). Structure and regulation of the murine reduced folate carrier gene. *The Journal of Biological Chemistry, 280,* 5588–5597.

Lobaugh, N.J., Kraskov, V., Rombough, V., Rovet, J., Bryson, S., Greenbaum, R., et al. (2001). Piracetam therapy does not enhance cognitive functioning in children with Down syndrome. *Archives of Pediatric and Adolescent Medicine, 155,* 442–448.

Lott, I.T. (2002). Down syndrome and Alzheimer's disease. In R. Pary (Ed.), *Psychiatric problems in older persons with developmental disabilities* (pp. 25–34). Kingston, NY: NADD.

Lott, I.T., & Head, E. (2005). Alzheimer disease and Down syndrome: Factors in pathogenesis. *Neurobiology of Aging, 26,* 383–389.

Lott, I.T., Osann, K., Doran, E., & Nelson, L.D. (2002). Down syndrome and Alzheimer disease: Response to donepezil. *Archives of Neurology, 59,* 1133–1136.

Lynch, M.P., Oller, D.K., Steffens, M.L., Levine, S.L., Basinger, D.L., & Umbel, V. (1995). Onset of speech-like vocalizations in infants with Down syndrome. *American Journal of Mental Retardation, 100,* 68–86.

Malone, F.D. (2005). Nuchal translucency-based Down syndrome screening: Barriers to implementation. *Seminars in Perinatology, 29,* 272–276.

Malone, F.D., Canick, J.A., Ball, R.H., Nyberg, D.A., Comstock, C.H., Bukowski, R., et al. for the First and Second-Trimester Evaluation of Risk (FASTER) Research Consortium. (2005). First-trimester or second-trimester screening, or both, for Down's syndrome. *The New England Journal of Medicine, 353,* 2001–2011.

Mann, D.M., & Esiri, M.M. (1989). The pattern of acquisition of plaques and tangles in the brains of patients under 50 years of age with Down's syndrome. *Journal of Neurological Science, 89,* 169–179.

Mao, R., Zielke, C.L., Zielke, H.R., & Pevsner, J. (2003). Global up-regulation of chromosome 21 gene expression in the developing Down syndrome brain. *Genomics, 81,* 457–467.

McCarron, M., Gill, M., McCallion, P., & Begley, C. (2005). Health co-morbidities in age-
  ing persons with Down syndrome and Alzheimer's dementia. *Journal of Intellectual
  Disability Research, 49,* 560–566.
McCoy, E. (1992). Endocrine function in Down syndrome. In I.T. Lott & E.E. McCoy
  (Eds.), *Down syndrome: Advances in medical care* (pp. 71–82). New York: Wiley-Liss.
McGuire, D.E., & Chicoine, B. (1996). Depressive disorders in adults with Down syn-
  drome. *Habilitative Mental Healthcare Newsletter 15,* 26–27.
Menendez, M. (2005). Down syndrome, Alzheimer's disease and seizures. *Brain Develop-
  ment, 27,* 246–252.
Morris, J.K., Mutton, D.E., & Alberman, E. (2005). Recurrences of free trisomy 21: Analy-
  sis of data from the National Down Syndrome Cytogenetic Register. *Prenatal Diagnosis,
  25,* 1120–1128.
Mrak, R.E., & Griffin, W.S. (2004). Trisomy 21 and the brain. *Journal of Neuropathology and
  Experimental Neurology, 63,* 679–685.
Myers, B.A., & Pueschel, S.M. (1991). Psychiatric disorders in persons with Down syndrome. *Journal of Nervous and Mental Disease, 179,* 609–613.
Nam, J.-W., Shin, K.-R., Han, J., Lee, Y., Kim, V.N., & Zhang, B.-T. (2005). Human
  microRNA prediction through a probabilistic co-learning model of sequence and struc-
  ture. *Nucleic Acids Research, 33,* 3570–3581.
Nelson, L.D., Orme, D., Osann, K., & Lott, I.T. (2001). Neurological changes and emotional
  functioning in adults with Down syndrome. *Journal of Intellectual Disability Research, 45,*
  450–456.
Nicolaides, K.H., Azar, G., Byrne, D., Mansur, C., & Marks, K. (1992). Fetal nuchal translucency: Ultrasound screening for chromosomal defects in first trimester of pregnancy.
  The British Medical Journal, 304, 867–869.
Nixon, R.A. (2005). Endosome function and dysfunction in Alzheimer's disease and other
  neurodegenerative diseases. *Neurobiology of Aging, 26,* 373–382.
O'Doherty, A., Ruf, S., Mulligan, C., Hildreth, V., Errington, M.L., Cooke, S., et al. (2005).
  An aneuploid mouse strain carrying human chromosome 21 with Down syndrome
  phenotypes. *Science, 309,* 2033–2037.
Ogilvie, C.M., Donaghue, C., Fox, S.P., Docherty, Z., & Mann, K. (2005). Rapid prenatal
  diagnosis of aneuploidy using quantitative fluorescence-PCR (QF-PCR). *Journal of His-
  tochemistry and Cytochemistry, 53,* 285–288.
Olson, L.E., Richtsmeier, J.T., Leszl, J., & Reeves, R.H. (2004). A chromosome 21 critical
  region does not cause specific Down syndrome phenotypes. *Science, 306,* 687–690.
Olson, L.E., Roper, R.J., Baxter, L.L., Carlson, E.J., Epstein, C.J., & Reeves, R.H. (2004).
  Down syndrome mouse models Ts65Dn, Ts1Cje, and Ms1Cje/Ts65Dn exhibit variable
  severity of cerebellar phenotypes. *Developmental Dynamics, 230,* 581–589.
Patterson, D., & Costa, A.C.S. (2005). Down syndrome and genetics: A case of linked his-
  tories. *Nature Reviews Genetics, 6,* 137–147.
Pennington, B.F., Moon, J., Edgin, J., Stedron, J., & Nadel, L. (2003). The neuropsychology
  of Down syndrome: Evidence for hippocampal dysfunction. *Child Development, 74,* 76–93.
Pinette, M.G., Wax, J., Blackstone, J., Cartin, A., & McCrann, D. (2004). Timing of early
  amniocentesis and a function of membrane fusion. *Journal of Clinical Ultrasound, 43,* 8–11.
Pinter, J.D., Eliez, S., Schmitt, J.E., Capone, G.T., & Reiss, A.L. (2001). Neuroanatomy of
  Down's syndrome: A high-resolution MRI study. *American Journal of Psychiatry, 158,*
  1659–1665.
Prasher, V.P. (1995). Prevalence of psychiatric disorders in adults with Down syndrome.
  European Journal of Psychiatry, 9, 77–82.
Prasher, V.P., Huxley, A., & Haque, M.S. (2002). A 24-week, double blind, placebo-
  controlled trial of donepezil in patients with Down syndrome and Alzheimer's disease—
  pilot study. *International Journal of Geriatric Psychiatry, 17,* 270–278.
Pueschel, S.M., Anneren, G., Durlach, R., Flores, J., Sustrova, M., & Verma, I.C. (1995).
  Guidelines for optimal medical care of persons with Down syndrome: International
  League of Societies for Persons with Mental Handicap (ILSMH). *Acta Paediatrica, 84,*
  823–827.
Raafat, M., Brayton, J.B., Apgar, V., & Borgaonkar, D.S. (1975). A new approach to pre-
  natal diagnosis using trophoblast cells in maternal blood. *Birth Defects Original Article
  Series, 11,* 295–302.

Richtsmeier, J.T., Zumwalt, A., Carlson, E.J., Epstein, C.J., & Reeves, R.H. (2002). Cranio-facial phenotypes in segmentally trisomic mouse models for Down syndrome. *American Journal of Medical Genetics, 107,* 317–324.

Roizen, N.J., & Patterson, D. (2003). Down's syndrome. *Lancet, 361,* 1281–1289.

Roper, R.J., Baxter, L.L., Saran, N.G., Klinedinst, D.K., Beachy, P.A., & Reeves, R.H. (2006). Defective cerebellar response to mitogenic Hedgehog signaling in Down's syndrome mice. *Proceedings of the National Academy of Sciences of the United States of America, 103,* 1452–1456.

Rouvelet-Lecrux, A., Hannequin, D., Raux, G., Le Meur, N., Laquerriere, A., Vital, A., et al. (2006). APP locus duplication causes autosomal dominant early-onset Alzheimer disease with cerebral amyloid angiopathy. *Nature Genetics, 38,* 24–26.

Rutter, M. (2005). Incidence of autism spectrum disorders: Changes over time and their meaning. *Acta Paediatrica, 94,* 2–15.

Salman, M. (2002). Systematic review of the effect of therapeutic dietary supplements and drugs on cognitive function in subjects with Down syndrome. *European Journal of Paediatric Neurology, 6,* 213–219.

Shapiro, B.L. (1983). Down syndrome: A disruption of homeostasis. *American Journal of Medical Genetics, 14,* 241–269.

Shapiro, B.L. (1997). Whither Down syndrome critical regions? *Human Genetics, 99,* 421–423.

Shott, S.R., Amin, R., Chini, B., Heubi, C., Hotze, S., & Akers, R. (2006). Obstructive sleep apnea: Should all children with Down syndrome be tested? *Archives of Otolaryngology and Head and Neck Surgery, 132,* 432–436.

Simoni, G., Brambati, B., Danesino, C., Rossella, F., Terzoli, G.L., Ferrari, M., et al. (1983). Efficient direct chromosome analyses and enzyme determinations from chorionic villi samples in the first trimester of pregnancy. *Human Genetics, 63,* 349–357.

Simpson, J.L. (2005). Choosing the best prenatal screening protocol. *The New England Journal of Medicine, 353,* 2068–2070.

Stasko, M.R., & Costa, A.C.S. (2004). Experimental parameters affecting the Morris water maze performance of a mouse model of Down syndrome. *Behavioural Brain Research, 154,* 1–17.

Steele, M.W., & Breg, W.R. (1966). Chromosome analysis of human amniotic fluid cells. *Lancet, 1,* 383–385.

Sterling, E. (1992). Oral and dental considerations in Down syndrome. In I.T. Lott & E.E. McCoy (Eds.), *Down syndrome: Advances in medical care* (pp. 135–146). New York: Wiley-Liss.

Sun, X., Wang, Y., Qing, H., Christensen, M.A., Liu, Y., Zhou, W., et al. (2005). Distinct transcriptional regulation and function of the human BACE2 and BACE1 genes. *The FASEB Journal, 19,* 739–749.

Tepper, V., & Verso, M.L. (1964). The detection of foetal cells in the maternal circulation. *Medical Journal of Australia, 42,* 585–589.

Tyrrell, J., Cosgrave, M., McCarron, M., McPherson, J., Calvert, J., Kelly, A., et al. (2001). Dementia in people with Down's syndrome. *International Journal of Geriatric Psychiatry, 16,* 1168–1174.

Van Dyke, D.C., Harper, D.C., & Dyken, M.E. (1998). Alzheimer's disease and Down syndrome. *Down Syndrome Quarterly, 1998,* 3–11.

Wagner, D., Schunck, R., & Isebarth, H. (1964). Detection of trophoblast cells in the circulating blood of women with normal and complicated pregnancy. *Gynaecologica, 158,* 174–192.

Wald, N.J., Rodeck, C., Hackshaw, A.K., & Rudnicka, A. (2005). SURUSS in perspective. *Seminars in Perinatology, 29,* 225–235.

Warburton, D., Dallaire, L., Thangavelu, M., Ross, L., Levin, B., & Kline, J. (2004). Trisomy recurrence: A reconsideration based on North American data. *American Journal of Human Genetics, 75,* 376–385.

Webb, D.K. (2005). Optimizing therapy for myeloid disorders of Down syndrome. *British Journal of Haematology, 131,* 3–7.

Whetstine, J.R., Flatley, R.M., & Matherly, R.H. (2002). The human reduced folate carrier gene is ubiquitously and differentially expressed in normal tissues: Identification of seven non-coding exons and characterization of a novel promoter. *Biochemical Journal, 367,* 629–640.

White, N.S., Alkire, M.T., & Haier, R.J. (2003). A voxel-based morphometric study of non-demented adults with Down syndrome. *NeuroImage, 20,* 393–403.

Wisniewski, K.E. (1990). Down syndrome children often have brain with maturation delay, retardation of growth, and cortical dysgenesis. *American Journal of Medical Genetics Supplement, 7,* 274–281.

Wisniewski, K.E., Wisniewski, H.M., & Wen, G.Y. (1985). Occurrence of neuropathological changes and dementia of Alzheimer's disease in Down's syndrome. *Annals of Neurology, 17,* 278–282.

Zheng, H., Jiang, M., Trumbauer, M.E., Sirinathsinghji, D., Hopkins, R., Smith, D.W., et al. (1995). Beta-amyloid precursor protein-deficient mice show reactive gliosis and decreased locomotor activity. *Cell, 81,* 525–531.

CHAPTER 2

Etiology, Diagnosis, and Development in Fragile X Syndrome

RANDI J. HAGERMAN

*F*ragile X refers to a family of medical and developmental problems related to an expansion of the trinucleotide (CGG) repeats on the front end of the fragile X mental retardation 1 (FMR1) gene. This chapter reviews the genetics, diagnostic issues, neurobiology, clinical phenotype, neuroimaging, and medical conditions associated with fragile X. Involvement in some premutation carriers is also reviewed. The treatment of both the medical and behavioral problems are discussed, including psychopharmacological interventions. The chapter is written to guide the health care provider and the family on optimal interventions.

GENETICS OF FRAGILE X SYNDROME

The FMR1 gene, which was sequenced in 1991 by an international consortium (Verkerk et al., 1991), is located on the bottom end of the X chromosome at Xq27.3. Individuals in the typical population have 5–44 CGG repeats in the FMR1 gene, whereas carriers of the premutation have 55–200 repeats. Individuals with a repeat size between 45 and 54 are in the gray zone of instability. Most people who are affected by fragile X syndrome (FXS) have more than 200 repeats, which is considered a *full mutation* (Hagerman, 2002b; Maddalena et al., 2001). The premutation is unstable when a female passes it to her offspring. The risk of passing on a full mutation increases with greater repeat sizes in premutation carriers, leading to a 100% risk when an allele with more than 100 CGG repeats is being passed on. A full mutation usually causes intellectual disability (ID) in males and learning disabilities in females, although a broad spectrum of involvement occurs in both sexes. FXS is the most common inherited cause of ID known, although Down syndrome (DS) is the most common genetic disorder causing ID. DS is not usually inherited from generation to generation, as is FXS, unless a translocation involving chromosome 21 is present.

This work was supported by grants from the National Institute of Child Health and Human Development, including HD 36071 and HD 02274; the Centers for Disease Control and Prevention Collaborative Agreement Number U10/CCU925123; and the M.I.N.D. Institute at UC Davis Medical Center.

Thank you to Michele Ono for her assistance in completing the manuscript.

Usually a full mutation leads to methylation (placement of CH_3 groups on the backbone of the DNA) of the FMR1 gene. The methylation decreases the production of messenger RNA (mRNA), a copy of the gene that is normally converted into the protein product of the gene, the FMR1 protein (FMRP). Therefore, individuals who have a full mutation make little or no FMR1-mRNA and FMRP. It is the lack or deficiency of FMRP that causes FXS (Tassone et al., 1999). FXS is also possible if a deletion exists involving the FMR1 gene, if a point mutation occurs in FMR1 that renders the gene nonfunctional (De Boulle et al., 1993), or if an individual with the premutation has significantly lowered levels of FMRP, as described in the following paragraphs (Aziz et al., 2003; Goodlin-Jones, Tassone, Gane, & Hagerman, 2004; Tassone, Hagerman, Taylor, Mills, et al., 2000).

Males are usually more affected by FXS than females because males only have one X chromosome. When their only X has the full mutation, little or no FMRP is produced. In contrast, females have two X chromosomes, although one of their X chromosomes will be inactivated in every cell; therefore, if the X chromosome that carries the full mutation is inactivated in the majority of the female's cells, there will be less involvement compared with a male with the full mutation because the normal X is producing FMRP (Tassone et al., 1999).

Most research indicates that the level of FMRP detected in the blood correlates with the level of intellectual impairment of individuals with FXS (Bailey, Hatton, Tassone, Skinner, & Taylor, 2001; Loesch et al., 2003; Loesch, Huggins, & Hagerman, 2004; Tassone et al., 1999). Females with a favorable activation ratio (the majority of their cells have the normal X chromosome as the active X chromosome) will have a higher IQ score than females with a low activation ratio (Tassone et al., 1999). Males with FXS can produce a significant level of FMRP two different ways. One way is to have a full mutation that is partially or fully unmethylated, and the other is to have a significant percentage of cells with the premutation in addition to cells with the full mutation (a mosaic pattern on DNA testing). The cells with the premutation or without methylation will produce FMRP. The greater the percentage of cells with the premutation or without methylation, the larger the production of FMRP, and the higher the IQ score (Loesch et al., 2004; Tassone et al., 1999).

Approximately 15% of males with FXS have an IQ score higher than 70 and are described as high-functioning males without ID (Hagerman, Hull, et al., 1994). Approximately 75% of females with FXS have an IQ score higher than 70; however, the majority of females with FXS have learning disabilities, including impairments in language, executive function, and attention (Bennetto & Pennington, 2002; Bennetto, Pennington, Taylor, & Hagerman, 2001; Cornish, Sudhalter, & Turk, 2004; Cornish, Turk, et al., 2004).

Individuals with the premutation usually have a normal level of FMRP, but their level of FMR1-mRNA is elevated from 2 to 10 times normal (Kenneson, Zhang, Hagedorn, & Warren, 2001; Tassone, Hagerman, Taylor, Gane, et al., 2000). This unique molecular finding in premutation carriers is not seen in those with the full mutation unless they have a high level of mosaicism. The elevation of mRNA in premutation carriers is thought to be responsible for phenotypic features that are present in adult premutation carriers, including premature ovarian failure (POF) in 20% of females and fragile X–associated tremor/ataxia syndrome (FXTAS), an aging syndrome in some carriers (Hagerman & Hagerman, 2004).

The involvement in premutation carriers can include cognitive, behavioral, and neurological changes. These effects are related to toxicity of the elevated mRNA leading to dysregulation of a number of proteins (e.g., lamin A/C, αB-crystallin, myelin basic protein) important for neuronal function (Garcia Arocena et al., 2005; Iwahashi et al., 2006) and formation of intranuclear inclusions in neurons and astrocytes (Greco et al., 2002; Greco et al., 2006; Hagerman & Hagerman, 2004). This dysregulation of proteins leads to neuronal cell death, brain atrophy, and white matter disease. The clinical symptoms of FXTAS involve tremors, ataxia, neuropathy, and cognitive impairments after age 50 years in approximately 30% of male carriers but rarely in female carriers (Hagerman, Greco, et al., 2001; Hagerman, Leehey, et al., 2001; Jacquemont et al., 2003; Jacquemont et al., 2004). Psychiatric symptoms in carriers, such as anxiety, also appear to be related to an mRNA toxicity effect (Bacalman et al., 2006; Hessl et al., 2005). The RNA toxicity in carriers has substantially expanded the phenotypic involvement and prevalence of individuals affected by fragile X, well beyond those with FXS.

Evidence exists that the RNA toxicity effect in premutation carriers can lead to attention-deficit/hyperactivity disorder (ADHD) and social impairments in children and young adults, particularly males (Aziz et al., 2003; Cornish et al., 2005; Farzin et al., 2006; Goodlin-Jones et al., 2004). On occasion individuals with the premutation will have a deficit of FMRP that can lead to FXS with both physical and cognitive features of the disorder, including prominent ears, ID, and/or autism (Aziz et al., 2003; Goodlin-Jones et al., 2004; Hagerman, Ono, & Hagerman, 2005; Tassone, Hagerman, Taylor, Mills, et al., 2000). In some individuals there may be a combination of problems (an impairment of FMRP and an elevation of FMR1-mRNA), which causes these individuals to be at risk for both cognitive impairments and late-onset neurological problems (e.g., FXTAS).

PREVALENCE

FXS is responsible for 2%–3% of all forms of ID (Sherman, 2002). FXS also represents approximately 30% of all forms of X-linked ID; therefore, when two brothers have ID, there is a 30% chance that the cause is FXS. The FMR1 mutation occurs in 2%–6% of cases of autism of unknown etiology (Estecio, Fett-Conte, Varella-Garcia, Fridman, & Silva, 2002; Reddy, 2005; Wassink, Brzustowicz, Bartlett, & Szatmari, 2004). Thus, all individuals with ID or autism of unknown etiology should be tested for the FMR1 mutation.

Screening studies in individuals with developmental disabilities that have extrapolated back to the general population have demonstrated that approximately 1 in 3,600 males has the fragile X full mutation (Crawford, Acuna, & Sherman, 2001; Crawford et al., 2002; Turner, Webb, Wake, & Robinson, 1996). The prevalence of FXS in females has not been well studied because most females with FXS do not have ID. The prevalence of the premutation is much higher in females, however, with approximately 1 in 129–250 females and 1 in 600–800 males in the general population with the premutation (Beckett, Yu, & Long, 2005; Dombrowski et al., 2002; Rousseau, Rouillard, Morel, Khandjian, & Morgan, 1995). Although most individuals with the premutation have typical intellectual abilities (Bennetto & Pennington, 2002; Reiss, Freund, Abrams, Boehm, & Kazazian, 1993), learning disabilities, emotional problems, endocrine problems, or neurological involvement are common, as described previously, and further increases the impact of the FMR1 mutation on the general population (Hagerman & Hagerman, 2002; Hessl et al., 2005).

NEUROBIOLOGY

FMRP is an mRNA-binding protein that negatively regulates the translation of many mRNAs into proteins. Advances in neurobiology have demonstrated that mRNAs that are important for maturation of the dendrite and plasticity (changes) of the synapse are often regulated by FMRP (Darnell, Warren, & Darnell, 2004; Jin et al., 2004; Willemsen, Oostra, Bassell, & Dictenberg, 2004). When FMRP is absent, as in FXS, there is dysregulation of a number of neurotransmitter systems that affect the phenotype in FXS. For instance, there is upregulation of the metabotropic glutamate 5 (mGluR5) system in the hippocampus (Bear, Huber, & Warren, 2004; Huber, Roder, & Bear, 2001). Enhanced mGluR5 activity leads to enhanced long-term depression that weakens synaptic connections. The stimulation of mGluR5 receptors leads to internalization of AMPA receptors (a type of glutamate receptor) through a process that requires protein synthesis, and FMRP normally represses this process. The lack of FMRP in FXS leads to enhanced LTD and subsequent excessive internalization of AMPA receptors. Long, weak, and immature synaptic connections have been documented in the knockout mouse model of fragile X and in humans with FXS (Beckel-Mitchener & Greenough, 2004; Irwin et al., 2001; Willemsen et al., 2004). A variety of clinical features of FXS—including cognitive impairments, tactile hypersensitivity, poor eye contact, and seizures—are thought to be related to enhanced mGluR5 activity (Bear et al., 2004).

In 2005, evidence for enhanced long-term depression was also found in the synaptic connection of parallel fibers to Purkinje cells in the cerebellum in the knockout mouse, leading to attenuation of the cerebellar eyelid conditioning in the knockout mouse and in humans with FXS (Koekkoek et al., 2005). Cerebellar dysfunction in FXS is related to the motor impairments and perhaps other cognitive problems in FXS (Koekkoek et al., 2005; Mostofsky et al., 1998). The discovery of enhanced long-term depression and mGluR5 activity in fragile X has important treatment implications, including the use of mGluR5 antagonists and ampakines in individuals with FXS (Bear et al., 2004; Berry-Kravis et al., 2006; Dolen & Bear, 2005).

The gamma-aminobutyric acid (GABA) system is also affected by the FMRP impairment in FXS. The GABA system is an important inhibitory system in the central nervous system (CNS), and the GABA alpha (GABA$_A$) receptors are down regulated in FXS (D'Antuono, Merlo, & Avoli, 2003; El Idrissi et al., 2005; Kooy, 2003). This abnormality can lead to an imbalance of stimulatory and inhibitory systems in the CNS. For instance, cholinergic activation in the CNS normally depresses excitatory responses by increasing GABA release from interneuron terminals. In the fragile X knockout mouse model, however, there is decreased GABA$_A$ receptor mediated inhibition (D'Antuono et al., 2003) leading to hyperexcitability of the knockout mouse (Chen, Bedair, McKay, Bowers, & Mazure, 2001; Chen & Toth, 2001). Hyperexcitability also is seen in humans, both behaviorally and psychophysiologically, as described later in this chapter (Miller et al., 1999; Roberts, Boccia, Bailey, Hatton, & Skinner, 2001). Seizures, which occur in

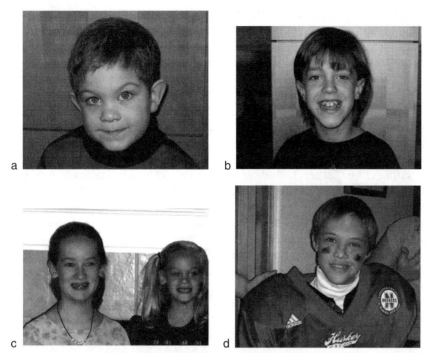

Figure 2.1.   a) Young boy with fragile X syndrome. Notice the slightly prominent ears. b) Ten-year-old boy with fragile X syndrome. DNA studies show that he is mosaic with both the premutation and full mutation. His features are minimal, including mildly prominent ears and a mildly long face. c) Two sisters with fragile X syndrome. Note the mildly prominent ears in the younger sister. d) Young boy with fragile X syndrome and Down syndrome in addition to an autism spectrum disorder. He is nonverbal and has had severe behavioral problems and hypotonia.

20% of individuals with fragile X (Musumeci et al., 1999), are thought to be related to a decrease of appropriate inhibition and excessive hyperexcitability in FXS. A variety of other physical and behavioral features may be related to the many mRNAs that are dysregulated by the absence of FMRP.

PHENOTYPIC INVOLVEMENT

Physical characteristics of FXS include an elongated face, long and prominent ears, high palate, flat feet, hyperextensible finger joints, and soft velvet-like skin (Hagerman, 2002b). These physical features become more prominent as the individual ages, particularly the long and prominent ears and the elongated face. Most children with FXS do not have dysmorphic features that are considered abnormal or unusual as do children with DS, so children with FXS are usually not recognized as having the syndrome by physical features alone (see Figure 2.1; Lachiewicz, Dawson, & Spiridigliozzi, 2000). These children are typically not diagnosed until after 3 years of age, leading to a delay in intervention (Bailey, Skinner, Hatton, & Roberts, 2000).

One of the most characteristic features among males with FXS is macroorchidism (large testicles). This feature, however, does not begin to appear for the majority of males until 8 years of age or later (as the child begins puberty; Lachiewicz & Dawson, 1994). By the end of puberty, approximately 90% of adolescent boys with FXS will have macroorchidism. The cause of the macroorchidism is not known. Men with FXS are typically fertile and can reproduce, but their sperm with the X chromosome will only carry the premutation (Reyniers et al., 1993). Therefore, daughters of an affected male with the full mutation or a male with the premutation will have the premutation. There have been rare exceptions to this rule, however, and Zeesman and colleagues (2004) have reported a female with a low-end full mutation who was born to a high-functioning male with a mosaic pattern in his FMR1-DNA.

Most of the physical problems in FXS are related to a connective tissue dysplasia associated with abnormal elastin fibers (Hagerman, 2002b; Waldstein et al., 1987). FMRP likely regulates the translation of proteins involved with the formation of connective tissue. A number of medical problems are associated with loose connective tissue, including occasional joint dislocations, hernias, and recurrent otitis media. Recurrent otitis media can negatively affect the development of early expressive and receptive language skills; thus, vigorous treatment of recurrent otitis with pressure equalization (PE) tubes or prophylactic antibiotics is recommended (Hagerman, 2002a).

Other medical problems associated with FXS include strabismus, occurring in 8%–30% of affected individuals (Hatton, Buckley, Lachiewicz, & Roberts, 1998; King, Hagerman, & Houghton, 1995); mitral valve prolapse and/or dilation at the base of the aorta, occurring in approximately 50% of adults; and gastroesophageal reflux (GER), which is seen in the majority of individuals in infancy (Hagerman, 2002b). A large head and hypotonia are also typically seen in infancy.

Seizures

Approximately 20% of males with FXS have seizures (Berry-Kravis, 2002; Incorpora, Sorge, Sorge, & Pavone, 2002; Musumeci et al., 1999; Sabaratnam, Vroegop, & Gangadharan, 2001). Seizures are more common in males than females with FXS, with only a few reports describing seizures in females (Berry-Kravis, 2002; Singh, Sutherland, & Manson, 1999). Berry-Kravis and colleagues (2006) reviewed the seizure frequency in 23 females with FXS and found only 1 (3%) with seizures. She had a pattern of central-temporal or rolandic spike wave discharges that are typical of benign focal epilepsy of childhood (BFEC). This pattern is also seen in the majority of males with FXS (Berry-Kravis, 2002; Musumeci et al., 1999). Individuals with FXS and BFEC with central temporal spikes are likely to grow out of their seizures after childhood (Berry-Kravis, 2002; Musumeci et al., 1999). Most individuals have complex partial seizures (CPS), but approximately 25% have generalized tonic-clonic seizures and are more likely to have multifocal spikes on electroencephalogram (EEG) than those with CPS (Berry-Kravis, 2002). Although most individuals with FXS and seizures respond well to either carbamazepine or divalproex (anticonvulsants) in childhood, about 15% have generalized seizures that are poorly controlled and persist into adulthood (Berry-Kravis, 2002; Incorpora et al., 2002; Musumeci et al., 1999).

Behavioral Phenotype

Infants with FXS typically have good eye contact and respond appropriately to social interaction. Commonly, however, infants suffer from frequent vomiting, which is related to GER, and some infants have an exaggerated startle response and irritability that likely relates to hypersensitivity to sensory stimuli. Psychophysiological studies have demonstrated an enhanced sympathetic response to sensory stimuli (Miller et al., 1999) and decreased parasympathetic tone, particularly with transitions (Roberts et al., 2001). Sometime in the second year, significant tactile defensiveness and poor eye contact become apparent. Self-injurious behavior, including hand biting and head hitting, develops approximately around age 30 months (Symons, Clark, Hatton, Skinner, & Bailey, 2003).

A toddler study conducted in 2005 demonstrated the early onset of inhibitory impairments in oculomotor control in boys with FXS as young as 14 months (Scerif et al., 2005). These toddlers were not able to inhibit prosaccade movements (shifting of the eyes) to a peripheral stimulus that anticipated a subsequent target as well as typically developing toddlers. In addition, the typical age-related changes to both prosaccade and antisaccade eye movements directed to a target did not develop in the toddlers with FXS. In another study of toddlers with FXS, impairments were seen in inhibition of manual responses compared with controls (Scerif, Cornish, Wilding, Driver, & Karmiloff-Smith, 2004).

Psychophysiology studies have demonstrated decreased prepulse inhibition in children with fragile X (Frankland et al., 2004). Some researchers hypothesize that abnormalities in inhibitory control are related to frontal-subcortical impairments. These impairments are also related to executive function problems, ADHD, and impulse control issues that have been commonly reported in children and adults with FXS (Cornish, Munir, & Cross, 2001; Hatton et al., 2002; Loesch et al., 2003; Munir, Cornish, & Wilding, 2000; Sobesky et al., 1996). Hyperactivity and ADHD are seen in approximately 80% of males with FXS and in approximately 30% of females with the full mutation (Hagerman et al., 1992). Females with the full mutation who do not have ADHD usually have executive function impairments even when their IQ scores are in the normal range (Cornish, Sudhalter, et al., 2004; Cornish, Swainson, et al., 2004; Sobesky et al., 1996).

Impulsivity is also related to aggression in individuals with FXS (R.J. Hagerman, 2002b). Most aggression is not premeditated but is usually precipitated by excessive stimuli or hyperarousal leading to anxiety and subsequent impulsive behavior, such as hitting. Fluctuations in mood are also common; thus, abrupt anger outbursts are seen in about 30% of adolescents and young adults with FXS (Hagerman, 2002b).

ADHD may be related to the hyperarousal that is present with sensory stimuli. In one study of children with FXS, when the degree of ADHD improved with the use of stimulants, the degree of hyperarousal decreased as measured by the electrodermal response to sensory stimuli (Hagerman, Miller, et al., 2002). Stimulants can also be used to treat aggression, as described in the Treatment section in this chapter.

Anxiety is common in both males and females with FXS (Freund, Reiss, & Abrams, 1993; Hagerman, 2002b; Hessl et al., 2001). Anxiety is often easier to recognize in girls with FXS because they can present with shyness and social anxiety, whereas boys have a variety of behavior problems, including hyperactivity and aggression, which may hide the anxiety. Anxiety sometimes can be so severe in girls that selective mutism (talking only in some environments but not in others) is present (R. J. Hagerman, Hills, Scharfenaker, & Lewis, 1999). This presentation is more common in young females who do not demonstrate ADHD, perhaps because impulsive vocalizations are a deterrent to selective mutism.

Hessl and colleagues (2004) have proposed that anxiety is related to hypothalamic-pituitary-adrenal (HPA) axis dysfunction in FXS. Several lines of evidence exist for this hypothesis, including studies demonstrating elevated cortisol release after stressors in boys with FXS (Hessl et al., 2002; Wisbeck et al., 2000). The glucocorticoid receptor mRNA is regulated by FMRP (Miyashiro et al., 2003), so absence of FMRP may lead to significant dysregulation of the HPA axis in FXS. Annexin, a protein modulator of the glucocorticoid receptor, is also dysregulated in FXS (Sun, Cohen, & Kaufmann, 2001). In a study by Hessl and colleagues (2001) of children with FXS, the degree of anxiety correlated with the level of FMRP in girls, but not in boys.

Autism

Autism occurs in approximately 25%–33% of males and in approximately 5%–15% of females with FXS (Bailey, Hatton, Skinner, & Mesibov, 2001; Bailey, Hatton, Tassone, et al., 2001; Hagerman, 2002b; Kaufmann et al., 2004; Loesch et al., 2006; Rogers, Wehner, & Hagerman, 2001). The presence of autism is associated with a lower IQ score and an impairment in adaptive behavior in children with FXS compared with those with FXS without autism and those with autism without FXS (Bailey, Hatton, Tassone, et al., 2001; Hatton et al., 2003; Kaufmann et al., 2004; Loesch et al., 2006; Rogers et al., 2001). Although initial studies did not demonstrate a correlation between FMRP levels and autism (Bailey, Hatton, Tassone, et al., 2001), subsequent studies showed this relationship. When the IQ score is controlled, however, the relationship between autism and FMRP disappears (Loesch et al., 2006).

Children who have autism and FXS have more severe receptive and expressive language impairments then children with FXS alone (Philofsky, Hepburn, Hayes, Hagerman, & Rogers, 2004). The presence of autism is not necessarily related to the severity of hand flapping, poor eye contact, and hand biting, but it represents severe social and communication impairments leading to the behavioral phenotype of autism (Kau et al., 2004; Kaufmann et al., 2004). A continuum of severity of autism in fragile X occurs, and it can be measured by the Autism Diagnostic Observation Schedule (ADOS; Lord, Rutter, DiLavore, & Risi, 1999). Although as many as 30% of individuals with FXS have autism, heterogeneity within this category exists, so some individuals have complete disinterest in social interactions and others have a mild interest that is affected by severe anxiety and social withdrawal to stimuli. An additional 20% of males with FXS have more interest in social interactions but meet criteria for pervasive developmental disorder-not otherwise specified (PDD-NOS; Harris et al., 2004).

Autism in FXS is likely due to the additive effect of dysfunction in several genes whose translation is regulated by FMRP. Approximately 50% of males are not on the autism spectrum disorder (ASD) continuum and can interact relatively well in social situations. Many children with FXS have social impairments but also an interest and sincerity in social interactions that endears them to their peers. For example, one young man with FXS at a local high school was the only student to receive a standing ovation from his classmates at graduation. Similarly, a few male teens with FXS and autism or ASD from different states have been voted homecoming kings by their high school classmates. Although they each met criteria for ASD on multiple measures—including the ADOS, the Autism

Diagnostic Interview–Revised (ADI-R; Lord, Rutter, & Le Couteur, 1994), and the *Diagnostic and Statistical Manual of Mental Disorders* (*DSM-IV*; American Psychiatric Association, 1994)—their personalities were endearing in some ways to their classmates. Another common trait among individuals with FXS is a great sense of humor. These strengths in personality combined with tenacity for routines, even for work, can be beneficial in both vocational and academic settings.

Using the ADI-R as the only criteria may overdiagnose autism because the impairments seen at ages 3 and 4 years may improve by middle childhood with therapy and treatment (Harris et al., 2004). When assessing autism, it is important to use multiple measures including a clinical assessment and the ADOS.

NEUROIMAGING

Unique structural and functional brain changes occur in both children and adults with FXS compared with age- and IQ score-matched controls. The posterior cerebellar vermis is smaller in both males and females with FXS, and the hippocampus, caudate, lateral ventricles, and fourth ventricles are larger (Eliez, Blasey, Freund, Hastie, & Reiss, 2001; Hessl et al., 2004; Kates, Folley, Lanham, Capone, & Kaufman, 2002; Reiss, Aylward, Freund, Joshi, & Bryan, 1991; Reiss, Lee, & Freund, 1994). In addition, Reiss and colleagues (1994) have demonstrated an age-related decline in the superior temporal gyrus in both males and females with FXS, suggesting that FMRP is important throughout life. These structural changes relate to the neuropsychological impairments reported in FXS. Mostofsky and colleagues (1998) have demonstrated that the size of the posterior cerebellar vermis in females with FXS inversely correlates with full scale IQ score, verbal IQ score, performance IQ score, visual-spatial abilities on block design, visual-spatial and motor and memory abilities, and executive function abilities. The size of the caudate and lateral ventricles are inversely correlated with IQ score in both males and females with FXS, whereas control participants had the opposite relationship—a larger caudate predicted a higher IQ score (Reiss, Abrams, Greenlaw, Freund, & Denckla, 1995).

Functional MRI studies have been informative of dynamic brain processing impairments in females with FXS. Several studies have demonstrated an impairment in the recruitment of the neural network needed to solve problems, including math calculations (Rivera, Menon, White, Glaser, & Reiss, 2002), visual-spatial working memory tasks (Kwon et al., 2001), and a cognitive interference task (the counting Stroop; Tamm, Menon, Johnston, Hessl, & Reiss, 2002). These studies have also demonstrated that the FMRP level correlated with the activation impairment, suggesting a causal relationship. The neuroanatomical changes in FXS, specifically long, thin, and immature or weak synaptic connections, seen in human and animal studies (Beckel-Mitchener & Greenough, 2004; Irwin et al., 2001; Irwin, Galvez, & Greenough, 2000; Willemsen et al., 2004), fit with an inability to strongly activate an appropriate neural network to problem solve. Such neuroimaging studies can be used for future treatment trials.

TREATMENT

Treatment is available for all children and adults with FXS, even though no cure is available. Treatment involves a multimodality approach from multiple professionals including speech-language pathologists; occupational therapists; psychologists; special education teachers; assistive technology experts; and a variety of physicians, including pediatricians, psychiatrists, neurologists, ophthalmologists, orthopedists, obstetricians, and otolaryngologists. Many of the chapters in this book focus on language, motor, behavior, and educational interventions in children with FXS. This section focuses on the medical and psychopharmacological interventions. It is important to remember, however, that synergistic benefits are likely to occur when therapies are combined with medical interventions. For instance, treatment of persistent fluid in the middle ear that resolves a hearing loss could affect how an individual responds and progresses during speech and language therapy. Use of a stimulant to improve attention and concentration may also facilitate academic progress, computer use, and motor coordination. On the other hand, side effects from medication use may also have deleterious effects on development. For example, a high dose of stimulant medication can lead to decreased language use, and clonidine or atypical antipsychotics can cause excessive sedation. Therefore, careful medical monitoring is essential whenever medications are used.

The quality of the home environment, including parental responsivity, the learning materials available for the child, and the physical surroundings, has a significant impact on the cognitive abilities (Dyer-Friedman et al., 2002), the presence of autism (Hessl et al., 2001), and the adaptive skills of a child with FXS (Glaser et al., 2003). It is, therefore, important for clinicians to encourage the best environment and educate the family regarding how to optimally respond to a child with FXS. When significant behavioral problems exist that are difficult for the family to handle, referral to a psychologist who can provide ongoing therapy to the child and his or her family is valuable, and guidance for therapy can be found in Braden (2000) and Epstein, Riley, and Sobesky (2002). A behavioral intervention program to help with sleep disturbances in children with FXS has been shown to be efficacious (Weiskop, Richdale, & Matthews, 2005).

Medical Interventions

In infancy and early childhood, recurrent acute otitis media infection can be a frequent medical complication of FXS (Hagerman, Altshul-Stark, & McBogg, 1987). Antibiotic treatment is necessary for infections (American Academy of Pediatrics and American Academy of Family Physicians, 2004). When persistent fluid becomes a problem due to otitis media, placement of PE tubes would drain the fluid and eliminate the conductive hearing loss associated with recurrent infections (American Academy of Pediatrics, 2004). Having normal hearing is important for language development. Use of prophylactic antibiotics may also be helpful to decrease the frequency of infections. An otolaryngologist may also be involved in treating recurrent sinusitis, a problem for approximately 25% of children with FXS (Hagerman, 2002b). In severe cases, sinus surgery may be needed to facilitate drainage and eliminate recurrent infections.

GER is seen in approximately 30% of infants with FXS. Infants with GER present with recurrent emesis in the first weeks or months of life (Hagerman, 2002b). Often, thickening the child's food and seating him or her upright after feeding will adequately treat this problem; however, on occasion, medication—or in rare circumstances surgery, including a Nissen procedure or Thal fundoplication (procedure that tightens the junction between the esophagus and stomach)—is needed (Hagerman, 2002a). Hernias occur in approximately 15% of young children with FXS, including a direct or indirect inguinal hernia, which requires surgery, or an umbilical hernia, which typically does not require surgical repair (Hagerman, 2002b).

For treatment of flat feet or recurrent joint dislocations, orthopedic intervention is rarely needed. Ligamentous laxity related to the connective tissue dysplasia is typically the cause of these problems. A shoe insert, a pair of straight last shoes, or an orthopedic appliance is usually used for severely flat feet, but often a regular shoe with ankle support is sufficient.

Orthodontic work is sometimes needed because of a high palate and dental crowding. Braces and palate expanders are often used to correct these problems. On occasion, individuals with FXS have a delayed loss of primary (baby) teeth. More commonly, dental surgery is needed to treat caries because extreme oral tactile sensitivity and severe anxiety often interfere with appropriate care in a dentist's office.

Routine care for children with FXS includes an ophthalmological or optometric examination before age 4 years. Strabismus occurs in 8%–30% of children with FXS, and refraction errors are common (Hatton et al., 1998; King et al., 1995; Maino, Schlange, Maino, & Caden, 1990; Maino, Wesson, Schlange, Cibis, & Maino, 1991). It is important that children with FXS undergo treatment for strabismus, such as wearing an eye patch or glasses or using eye drops, to avoid amblyopia, a more permanent visual loss.

Connective tissue dysplasia may lead to excessive ureter dilation with recurrent infections and GER. Therefore, recurrent infections should be evaluated with a voiding cystourethrogram (a study of urine flow to rule out obstruction) or other radiological evaluation. Hypertension is also relatively common in adolescents and adults with FXS, so blood pressure should be routinely followed in clinic visits, especially if medications that increase blood pressure are used (Hagerman, 2002a).

Mitral valve prolapse (MVP) and/or aortic root dilation requires periodic cardiology follow up. If the MVP is significant or associated with regurgitation, antibiotic prophylaxis with dental procedures or surgical procedures associated with bacterial contamination, such as gastrointestinal surgery, is recommended to avoid subacute bacterial endocarditis (Ferrieri et al., 2002; Hagerman, 2002a). Typically, the aortic dilation stabilizes over time, and mitral regurgitation is minimal. Rarely have individuals with FXS died suddenly; however, when they have, it has been presumed that they died from a cardiac arrhythmia related to MVP (Hagerman, 2002b). All adults with FXS should have a cardiology evaluation, including an echocardiogram and ECG, to evaluate the existence and severity of MVP, aortic root dilation, and possible arrhythmias.

Treatment of Seizures

The treatment of frequent seizures in early childhood can often have a positive effect on development and behavior in children with FXS. This is particularly important if the seizures are common and interfere with the normal processing of stimuli, including language or social interactions. Sometimes seizures are not recognized because staring spells can be considered behavior problems or inattentiveness. Individuals that have a history of regression in developmental abilities, particularly if autism or ASD is present, should have an EEG. Usually children with FXS who have seizures respond well to anticonvulsants, including divalproex or carbamazepine (Berry-Kravis, 2002; Musumeci et al., 1999). The use of phenobarbital should be avoided in children with FXS because it can worsen hyperactivity. Newer anticonvulsants, including levetiracetam (Keppra), oxcarbazepine (Trileptal), and topiramate (Topamax), are associated with fewer side effects than most older anticonvulsants and have been effective in many individuals with FXS; however, controlled studies have not been completed with participants with FXS (French et al., 2004). Lamotrigine (Lamictal) has also been effective in many individuals with FXS, but it holds a significant risk for rash, and even Stevens-Johnson syndrome, if it is combined with valproate to treat seizures. Most anticonvulsants—except gabapentin (Neurontin), which often causes an increase in behavior problems—can also help with mood stabilization (Hagerman, 2002a).

Psychopharmacology

There are a variety of medications used to treat behavior problems in children and adults with FXS. The most common behavior problem in children is ADHD.

Treatment of Attention-Deficit/Hyperactivity Disorder

Hyperactivity is often noted in preschool children (3 years of age or younger) with FXS. Behavioral interventions with significant structure and positive reinforcement either verbally (e.g., praise) or through the use of reinforcers (e.g., stickers) should always be used when treating hyperactivity (Braden, 2000; Epstein et al., 2002). Sensory integration occupational therapy can also be helpful, although controlled studies demonstrating efficacy are needed. Environmental overstimulation can exacerbate hyperarousal and hyperactivity, and an occupational therapist can teach parents and teachers of children with FXS calming techniques to improve these behaviors (Scharfenaker, O'Connor, Stackhouse, & Noble, 2002). One controlled trial has demonstrated efficacy in using stimulants for treatment of ADHD in FXS (Hagerman, Murphy, & Wittenberger, 1988). Stimulants have also been shown to decrease sympathetic hyperarousal in an electrodermal study with children with FXS (Hagerman et al., 2002). Stimulants, however, can often increase irritability in children with FXS younger than 5 years of age; thus, an alternative, such as clonidine (Catapres) or guanfacine (Tenex), can be tried between 3 and 5 years. These medications are adrenergic agonists, which decrease blood pressure, but they have an overall calming effect on hyperarousal. The response rate to clonidine in children with FXS is approximately 60% (Amaria, Billeisen, & Hagerman, 2001; Berry-Kravis & Potanos, 2003; Hagerman, Riddle, Roberts, Brease, & Fulton, 1995). Clonidine or guanfacine can also be used to help with sleep disturbances when administered at night because sedation is a significant side effect (Hagerman et al., 1995). Because of this side effect, a very low dose should be used in young children. An ECG is recommended in a follow-up visit, especially if these medications are used with stimulants because prolongation of cardiac conduction can sometimes occur (Hagerman, 2002a).

When a child with FXS and ADHD turns 5 years old, consideration of a long-acting stimulant is recommended. Although Concerta, a once-daily osmotic controlled release capsule formulation of methylphenidate (Wilens et al., 2003), may work best, many children are not able to swallow pills or capsules at this age. The use of a preparation that can be opened and sprinkled on food that is swallowed without chewing (e.g., applesauce) is commonly needed. Such preparations include Metadate CD and Ritalin LA, both of which come in capsules containing small granules. Adderall XR, a mixture of four different dextroamphetamine and levoamphetamine salts, is another long-acting stimulant that can be opened and sprinkled. There have been no comparison studies to determine relative efficacy among the long-acting preparations in individuals with FXS. All stimulants can decrease appetite and increase blood pressure and heart rate; thus, growth parameters and vitals should be completed by the primary care health provider two to four times per year. If there is sleep disruption at night with stimulants, then shorter-acting preparations at a decreased dose should be tried.

Stimulants can improve ADHD symptoms and also aggressive tendencies, particularly aggression related to impulsivity (Connor, Glatt, Lopez, Jackson, & Melloni, 2002). If stimulants are not helpful for impulsive aggressive behavior, other medications such as clonidine (described previously) or atypical antipsychotics (described in a later section) are usually helpful.

Atomoxetine (Strattera), which is a nonstimulant preparation that blocks the re-uptake of norepinephrine at the synapse, is an alternative to stimulants (Michelson et al., 2001; Perwien et al., 2004). The results of atomoxetine are similar to imipramine or desipramine, other alternative treatments for ADHD, but imipramine and desipramine are tricyclics, which can slow cardiac conduction, particularly in overdose. Atomoxetine can often be helpful for both ADHD and anxiety, but it typically is not as consistently helpful for ADHD as the stimulants.

Pharmacotherapy for Anxiety

The selective serotonin reuptake inhibitors (SSRIs) are the mainstay of anxiety treatment for individuals with FXS. Only rates of response (approximately 70%), however, have been studied in individuals with FXS (Berry-Kravis & Potanos, 2004; Hagerman, Fulton, et al., 1994); controlled trials have not been conducted. Anxiety can also be a common problem in carriers of the premutation, particularly mothers of children with FXS (Franke et al., 1998; Hessl et al., 2005; Sobesky, Porter, Pennington, & Hagerman, 1995). SSRI agents typically work well to treat this problem and should be considered, especially if the mother has a sleep disturbance related to her anxiety (Hagerman, 1999; Hagerman, Fulton, et al., 1994). The SSRIs can be added to other medication and are typically combined with stimulants in children with FXS (Amaria et al., 2001). Some of the SSRIs, especially fluoxetine (Prozac), can interfere with the metabolism of other medications such as anticonvulsants. Citalopram (Celexa), escitalopram (Lexapro), and sertraline (Zoloft) are SSRIs that have the least interference with anticonvulsants (Hagerman, 2002a). In approximately 20% of individuals with FXS, significant activation may occur, with the SSRIs leading to hyperactivity, manic behavior, or aggression (Hagerman, Fulton, et al., 1994). These behavioral responses may not occur until 2–4 months after beginning the medication. Fluoxetine has the most activation and citalopram has the least; thus, lowering the dose, switching to citalopram, or discontinuing this type of medication should be tried if activation occurs. Use of a mood stabilizer, such as an atypical antipsychotic (described in the next section), can also be helpful.

SSRIs are called *antidepressant medication*, although they are rarely used for this purpose in individuals with FXS. SSRIs also help obsessive-compulsive behavior, which is common in FXS and related to perseverative behavior. Often obsessive rituals will improve with SSRIs, and the irritability, even tantrum behavior, associated with inflexible thinking typically improves when an individual is taking an SSRI. On occasion the activation of an SSRI will increase speech, although these agents will not create speech when the child is nonverbal (Hagerman, 2002a). Fluoxetine has been shown to be helpful in preschool children with autism because it improves language and socialization (DeLong, Ritch, & Burch, 2002; DeLong, Teague, & McSwain Kamran, 1998). Therefore, if a child has both autism and FXS, fluoxetine or another SSRI can be considered to boost language and socialization.

Use of Atypical Antipsychotics

Atypical antipsychotics can be helpful in the treatment of aggression, mood instability, severe hyperactivity, and psychotic thinking in children and adults with FXS. The first atypical antipsychotic that was widely used in FXS was risperidone (Risperdal). McCracken and colleagues (2002) showed that risperidone helps decrease aggression, stereotypies, and agitation in 60% of children with autism (without FXS). Aman and colleagues (2002) demonstrated that risperidone improved disruptive behavior in children with cognitive impairments, and this trial included children with FXS along with other disorders. The main side effect of risperidone is obesity; thus, it should be avoided in children who demonstrate the Prader-Willi phenotype (obesity and hyperphagia) associated with severe hyperphagia in FXS (de Vries et al., 1993; de Vries & Niermeijer, 1994; Nowicki et al., 2007; Schrander-Stumple et al., 1994). Unusual motor movements (tardive dyskinesias) are rare side effects of risperidone but should be monitored along with liver function studies.

Although risperidone can be very effective in children with FXS, a newer atypical antipsychotic, aripiprazole (Abilify), has shown remarkable effects, according to anecdotal reports (please visit the medication bulletin board at http://www.fragilex.org for more information). Aripiprazole does not cause significant weight gain like risperidone, and it has a partial agonist effect at dopamine D2 receptors; thus, aripiprazole can help significantly with attention and concentration, and it can have remarkable mood stabilizing effects in children with FXS. Judging by aripiprazole's initial popularity, it will likely become more frequently used for children and adults with FXS than risperidone; however, it is expensive and requires justification for most insurance companies to cover its use.

New Interventions

The future holds promise from advances in molecular and neurobiology for new agents specific for individuals with FXS. Because of enhanced long-term depression and evidence of reduced AMPA receptors in the knockout mouse (Li, Pelletier, Perez Velazquez, & Carlen, 2002), the use of ampakines that are positive AMPA receptor modulators should be useful in FXS. A controlled trial of an investigational ampakine, CX516, that has been helpful in other conditions, including dementia and schizophrenia (Goff et al., 2001; Lynch, 2002), was not helpful in adults with FXS (Berry-Kravis et al., 2006). Although this medication was well tolerated without significant side effects, CX516 produced no positive cognitive or behavioral effects compared with placebo in adults with FXS (Berry-Kravis et al., 2006). CX516 is a relatively weak ampakine; perhaps a stronger ampakine will be helpful in the future.

Another future approach to FXS intervention is the use of mGluR5 antagonists that can reverse enhanced long-term depression in FXS. mGluR5 antagonists have been used in the knockout mouse and reduced the audiogenic seizure phenotype in this mouse (Bauchwitz, Yan, & Rammal, 2004). mGluR5 antagonists have also been used in the fragile X fruit fly to reverse the abnormal courtship behavior and neuronal overgrowth found in this *Drosophila* model of FXS (McBride et al., 2005). McBride and colleagues also used lithium in this *Drosophila* model and found the same beneficial effect as MPEP. Although the mGluR5 antagonists are not yet available for clinical use, lithium is available. Lithium down-regulates the mGluR5 pathway by blocking turnover of inositol triphosphate (Bauer, Alda, Priller, & Young, 2003). In the 1990s, lithium was helpful for treating aggression and mood instability in individuals with FXS (Hagerman, 1996). Lithium, however, has not been studied regarding cognitive and neurological benefits in fragile X, so controlled trials are needed.

Newer mGluR5 antagonists such as fenobam (Porter et al., 2005) are being investigated, and controlled trials in FXS will likely be initiated. The future is hopeful for new treatments in FXS; thus, enhanced efforts are warranted to identify a greater number of those at risk for fragile X.

CONCLUSIONS

The FMR1 mutation can cause FXS when a significant impairment of FMRP occurs. In addition, involvement in premutation carriers may include premature ovarian failure, ADHD, emotional problems, and late onset of tremor and ataxia or FXTAS. It is essential to screen for FXS with FMR1-DNA testing in all individuals with ID or autism of unknown etiology. Subsequent genetic counseling and family studies are likely to reveal different types of involvement from the premutation or full mutation. Treatment is also essential for all children and most adults with FXS, and a multimodality approach, as described in this chapter and elsewhere in this book, can be remarkably helpful for individuals with FXS and their families.

REFERENCES

Aman, M.G., De Smedt, G., Derivan, A., Lyons, B., Findling, R.L., Hagerman, R.J., et al. (2002). Double-blind, placebo-controlled study of risperidone for the treatment of disruptive behaviors in children with subaverage intelligence. *American Journal of Psychiatry, 159,* 1337–1346.

Amaria, R.N., Billeisen, L.L., & Hagerman, R.J. (2001). Medication use in fragile X syndrome. *Mental Health Aspects of Developmental Disabilities, 4*(4), 143–147.

American Academy of Pediatrics. (2004). Otitis media with effusion. *Pediatrics, 113*(5), 1412–1429.

American Academy of Pediatrics and American Academy of Family Physicians. (2004). Diagnosis and management of acute otitis media. *Pediatrics, 113,* 1451–1465.

American Psychiatric Association. (1994). *Diagnostic and statistical manual of mental disorders* (4th ed.). Washington, DC: Author.

Aziz, M., Stathopulu, E., Callias, M., Taylor, C., Turk, J., Oostra, B., et al. (2003). Clinical features of boys with fragile X premutations & intermediate alleles. *American Journal of Medical Genetics, 121B*(1), 119–127.

Bacalman, S., Farzin, F., Bourgeois, J., Cogswell, J., Goodlin-Jones, B., Gane, L., et al. (2006). Psychiatric phenotype of the fragile X-associated tremor/ataxia syndrome (FXTAS) in males: Newly described fronto-subcortical dementia. *Journal of Clinical Psychiatry, 67*(1), 87–94.

Bailey, D.B., Jr., Hatton, D.D., Skinner, M., & Mesibov, G.B. (2001). Autistic behavior, FMR1 protein, and developmental trajectories in young males with fragile X syndrome. *Journal of Autism and Developmental Disorders, 31*(2), 165–174.

Bailey, D.B., Jr., Hatton, D.D., Tassone, F., Skinner, M., & Taylor, A.K. (2001). Variability in FMRP and early development in males with fragile X syndrome. *American Journal on Mental Retardation, 106*(1), 16–27.

Bailey, D.B., Jr., Skinner, D., Hatton, D., & Roberts, J. (2000). Family experiences and factors associated with the diagnosis of fragile X syndrome. *Journal of Developmental and Behavioral Pediatrics, 21*(5), 315–321.

Bauchwitz, R.P., Yan, Q., & Rammal, M. (2004, October). *Modulation of mGluR5 activity in vivo can ameliorate phenotypic markers of fragile X syndrome in mice.* Paper presented at the meeting of the Society for Neuroscience, San Diego, CA.

Bauer, M., Alda, M., Priller, J., & Young, L.T. (2003). Implications of the neuroprotective effects of lithium for the treatment of bipolar and neurodegenerative disorders. *Pharmacopsychiatry, 36*(Suppl.3), S250–254.

Bear, M.F., Huber, K.M., & Warren, S.T. (2004). The mGluR theory of fragile X mental retardation. *Trends in Neurosciences, 27*(7), 370–377.

Beckel-Mitchener, A., & Greenough, W.T. (2004). Correlates across the structural, functional, and molecular phenotypes of fragile X syndrome. *Mental Retardation and Developmental Disabilities Research Reviews, 10,* 53–59.

Beckett, L., Yu, Q., & Long, A.N. (2005). *The impact of fragile X: Prevalence, numbers affected, and economic impact.* Paper presented at the National Fragile X Awareness Day Research Seminar, Sacramento, CA.

Bennetto, L., & Pennington, B.F. (2002). Neuropsychology. In R.J. Hagerman & P.J. Hagerman (Eds.), *Fragile X syndrome: Diagnosis, treatment, and research* (3rd ed., pp. 206–248). Baltimore: The Johns Hopkins University Press.

Bennetto, L., Pennington, B.F., Taylor, A., & Hagerman, R.J. (2001). Profile of cognitive functioning in women with the fragile X mutation. *Neuropsychology, 15*(2), 290–299.

Berry-Kravis, E. (2002). Epilepsy in fragile X syndrome. *Developmental Medicine and Child Neurology, 44*(11), 724–728.

Berry-Kravis, E., Krause, S.E., Block, S.S., Guter, S., Wuu, J., Leurgans, S., et al. (2006). Effect of CX516, an AMPA-modulating compound, on cognition and behavior in fragile X syndrome: A controlled trial. *Journal of Child and Adolescent Psychopharmacology, 16*(5), 525–540.

Berry-Kravis, E., & Potanos, K. (2003). Clinical response to psychopharmacology for behavior in fragile X syndrome. *Annals of Neurology, 54,* S144.

Berry-Kravis, E., & Potanos, K. (2004). Psychopharmacology in fragile X syndrome—present and future. *Mental Retardation and Developmental Disabilities Research Reviews, 10*(1), 42–48.

Braden, M.L. (2000). *Fragile, handle with care: More about fragile X syndrome, adolescents and adults.* Dillon, CO: Spectra Publishing Co.

Chen, L., & Toth, M. (2001). Fragile X mice develop sensory hyperreactivity to auditory stimuli. *Neuroscience, 103*(4), 1043–1050.

Chen, N.C., Bedair, H.S., McKay, B., Bowers, M.B., Jr., & Mazure, C. (2001). Clozapine in the treatment of aggression in an adolescent with autistic disorder. *Journal of Clinical Psychiatry, 62*(6), 479–480.

Connor, D.F., Glatt, S.J., Lopez, I.D., Jackson, D., & Melloni, R.H., Jr. (2002). Psychopharmacology and aggression. I: A meta-analysis of stimulant effects on overt/covert aggression-related behaviors in ADHD. *Journal of the American Academy of Child & Adolescent Psychiatry, 41*(3), 253–261.

Cornish, K., Swainson, R., Cunnington, R., Wilding, J., Morris, P., & Jackson, G. (2004). Do women with fragile X syndrome have problems in switching attention: Preliminary findings from ERP and fMRI. *Brain and Cognition, 54*(3), 235–239.

Cornish, K.M., Kogan, C., Turk, J., Manly, T., James, N., Mills, A., et al. (2005). The emerging fragile X premutation phenotype: Evidence from the domain of social cognition. *Brain and Cognition, 57*(1), 53–60.

Cornish, K.M., Munir, F., & Cross, G. (2001). Differential impact of the FMR-1 full mutation on memory and attention functioning: A neuropsychological perspective. *Journal of Cognitive Neuroscience, 13*(1), 144–150.

Cornish, K.M., Sudhalter, V., & Turk, J. (2004). Attention and language in fragile X. *Mental Retardation and Developmental Disabilities Research Reviews, 10,* 11–16.

Cornish, K.M., Turk, J., Wilding, J., Sudhalter, V., Munir, F., Kooy, F., et al. (2004). Annotation: Deconstructing the attention deficit in fragile X syndrome: A developmental neuropsychological approach. *Journal of Child Psychology and Psychiatry and Allied Disciplines, 45*(6), 1042–1053.

Crawford, D.C., Acuna, J.M., & Sherman, S.L. (2001). FMR1 and the fragile X syndrome: Human genome epidemiology review. *Genetics in Medicine, 3*(5), 359–371.

Crawford, D.C., Meadows, K.L., Newman, J.L., Taft, L.F., Scott, E., Leslie, M., et al. (2002). Prevalence of the fragile X syndrome in African-Americans. *American Journal of Medical Genetics, 110*(3), 226–233.

D'Antuono, M., Merlo, D., & Avoli, M. (2003). Involvement of cholinergic and gabaergic systems in the fragile X knockout mice. *Neuroscience, 119*(1), 9–13.

Darnell, J.C., Warren, S.T., & Darnell, R.B. (2004). The fragile X mental retardation protein, FMRP, recognizes G-quartets. *Mental Retardation and Developmental Disabilities Research Reviews, 10*(1), 49–52.

De Boulle, K., Verkerk, A.J., Reyniers, E., Vits, L., Hendrickx, J., Van Roy, B., et al. (1993). A point mutation in the FMR-1 gene associated with fragile X mental retardation. *Nature Genetics, 3*(1), 31–35.

de Vries, B.B., Fryns, J.P., Butler, M.G., Canziani, F., Wesby-van Swaay, E., vanHemel, J.O., et al. (1993). Clinical and molecular studies in fragile X patients with a Prader-Willi-like phenotype. *Journal of Medical Genetics, 30,* 761–766.

de Vries, B.B., & Niermeijer, M.F. (1994). The Prader-Willi-like phenotype in fragile X patients: A designation facilitating clinical (and molecular) differential diagnosis. *Journal of Medical Genetics, 31*(10), 820.

DeLong, G.R., Ritch, C.R., & Burch, S. (2002). Fluoxetine response in children with autistic spectrum disorders: Correlation with familial major affective disorder and intellectual achievement. *Developmental Medicine and Child Neurology, 44,* 652–659.

DeLong, G.R., Teague, L.A., & McSwain Kamran, M. (1998). Effects of fluoxetine treatment in young children with idiopathic autism. *Developmental Medicine and Child Neurology, 40*(8), 551–562.

Dolen, G., & Bear, M.F. (2005). Courting a cure for fragile X. *Neuron, 45*(5), 642–644.

Dombrowski, C., Levesque, M.L., Morel, M.L., Rouillard, P., Morgan, K., & Rousseau, F. (2002). Premutation and intermediate-size FMR1 alleles in 10 572 males from the general population: Loss of an AGG interruption is a late event in the generation of fragile X syndrome alleles. *Human Molecular Genetics, 11*(4), 371–378.

Dyer-Friedman, J., Glaser, B., Hessl, D., Johnston, C., Huffman, L.C., Taylor, A., et al. (2002). Genetic and environmental influences on the cognitive outcomes of children with fragile X syndrome. *Journal of the American Academy of Child and Adolescent Psychiatry, 41*(3), 237–244.

El Idrissi, A., Ding, X.H., Scalia, J., Trenkner, E., Brown, W.T., & Dobkin, C. (2005). Decreased GABA(A) receptor expression in the seizure-prone fragile X mouse. *Neuroscience Letters, 377*(3), 141–146.

Eliez, S., Blasey, C., Freund, L.S., Hastie, T., & Reiss, A. (2001). Brain anatomy, gender and IQ in children and adolescents with fragile X syndrome. *Brain, 124*(Pt 8), 1610–1618.

Epstein, J., Riley, K., & Sobesky, W. (2002). The treatment of emotional and behavioral problems. In R.J. Hagerman & P.J. Hagerman (Eds.), *Fragile X syndrome: Diagnosis, treatment, and research* (3rd ed., pp. 339–362). Baltimore: The Johns Hopkins University Press.

Estecio, M., Fett-Conte, A.C., Varella-Garcia, M., Fridman, C., & Silva, A.E. (2002). Molecular and cytogenetic analyses on Brazilian youths with pervasive developmental disorders. *Journal of Autism and Developmental Disorders, 32*(1), 35–41.

Farzin, F., Perry, H., Hessl, D., Loesch, D., Cohen, J., Bacalman, S., et al. (2006). Autism spectrum disorders and attention deficit/hyperactivity disorder in boys with the fragile X premutation. *Journal of Developmental and Behavioral Pediatrics, 27*(2), 137–114.

Ferrieri, P., Gewitz, M.H., Gerber, M.A., Newburger, J.W., Dajani, A.S., Shulman, S.T., et al. (2002). Unique features of infective endocarditis in childhood. *Pediatrics, 109*(5), 931–943.

Franke, P., Leboyer, M., Gansicke, M., Weiffenbach, O., Biancalana, V., Cornillet-Lefebre, P., et al. (1998). Genotype-phenotype relationship in female carriers of the premutation and full mutation of FMR-1. *Psychiatry Research, 80*(2), 113–127.

Frankland, P.W., Wang, Y., Rosner, B., Shimizu, T., Balleine, B.W., Dykens, E.M., et al. (2004). Sensorimotor gating abnormalities in young males with fragile X syndrome and FMR1-knockout mice. *Molecular Psychiatry, 9*(4), 417–425.

French, J.A., Kanner, A.M., Bautista, J., Abou-Khalil, B., Browne, T., Harden, C.L., et al. (2004). Efficacy and tolerability of the new antiepileptic drugs I: Treatment of new onset epilepsy: Report of the Therapeutics and Technology Assessment Subcommittee and Quality Standards Subcommittee of the American Academy of Neurology and the American Epilepsy Society. *Neurology, 62*(8), 1252–1260.

Freund, L.S., Reiss, A.L., & Abrams, M.T. (1993). Psychiatric disorders associated with fragile X in the young female. *Pediatrics, 91*(2), 321–329.

Garcia Arocena, D., Iwahashi, C.K., Won, N., Beilina, A., Ludwig, A.L., Schwartz, P.H., et al. (2005). Induction of inclusion formation and disruption of lamin A/C structure by premutation CGG-repeat RNA in human cultured neural cells. *Human Molecular Genetics, 14*(23), 1–11.

Glaser, B., Hessl, D., Dyer-Friedman, J., Johnston, C., Wisbeck, J., Taylor, A., et al. (2003). Biological and environmental contributions to adaptive behavior in fragile X syndrome. *American Journal of Medical Genetics, Part A, 117*(1), 21–29.

Goff, D.C., Leahy, L., Berman, I., Posever, T., Herz, L., Leon, A.C., et al. (2001). A placebo-controlled pilot study of the ampakine CX516 added to clozapine in schizophrenia. *Journal of Clinical Psychopharmacology, 21*(5), 484–487.

Goodlin-Jones, B., Tassone, F., Gane, L.W., & Hagerman, R.J. (2004). Autistic spectrum disorder and the fragile X premutation. *Journal of Developmental and Behavioral Pediatrics, 25*(6), 392–398.

Greco, C., Berman, R.F., Martin, R.M., Tassone, F., Schwartz, P.H., Chang, A., et al. (2006). Neuropathology of fragile X-associated tremor/ataxia syndrome (FXTAS). *Brain, 129,* 243–255.

Greco, C., Hagerman, R.J., Tassone, F., Chudley, A., Del Bigio, M.R., Jacquemont, S., et al. (2002). Neuronal intranuclear inclusions in a new cerebellar tremor/ataxia syndrome among fragile X carriers. *Brain, 125*(8), 1760–1771.

Hagerman, P.J., & Hagerman, R.J. (2004). The fragile-X premutation: A maturing perspective. *American Journal of Human Genetics, 74*(5), 805–816.

Hagerman, R.J. (1996). Physical and behavioral phenotype. In R.J. Hagerman & A. Cronister (Eds.), *Fragile X syndrome: Diagnosis, treatment and research* (2nd ed., pp. 3–87). Baltimore: The Johns Hopkins University Press.

Hagerman, R.J. (1999). Fragile X syndrome. In *Neurodevelopmental disorders: Diagnosis and treatment* (pp. 61–132). New York: Oxford University Press.

Hagerman, R.J. (2002a). Medical follow-up and pharmacotherapy. In R.J. Hagerman & P.J. Hagerman (Eds.), *Fragile X syndrome: Diagnosis, treatment and research* (3rd ed., pp. 287–338). Baltimore: The Johns Hopkins University Press.

Hagerman, R.J. (2002b). Physical and behavioral phenotype. In R.J. Hagerman & P.J. Hagerman (Eds.), *Fragile X syndrome: Diagnosis, treatment and research* (3rd ed., pp. 3–109). Baltimore: The Johns Hopkins University Press.

Hagerman, R.J., Altshul-Stark, D., & McBogg, P. (1987). Recurrent otitis media in boys with the fragile X syndrome. *American Journal of Diseases of Children, 141,* 184–187.

Hagerman, R.J., Fulton, M.J., Leaman, A., Riddle, J., Hagerman, P.J., & Sobesky, W. (1994). Fluoxetine therapy in fragile X syndrome. *Developmental Brain Dysfunction, 7,* 155–164.

Hagerman, R.J., Greco, C., Chudley, A., Leehey, M., Tassone, F., Grigsby, J., et al. (2001). Neuropathology and neurodegenerative features in some older male premutation carriers of fragile X syndrome. *American Journal of Human Genetics, 69*(4 Suppl.), 177.

Hagerman, R.J., & Hagerman, P.J. (2002). The fragile X premutation: Into the phenotypic fold. *Current Opinion in Genetics and Development, 12,* 278–283.

Hagerman, R.J., Hills, J., Scharfenaker, S., & Lewis, H. (1999). Fragile X syndrome and selective mutism. *American Journal of Medical Genetics, 83,* 313–317.

Hagerman, R.J., Hull, C.E., Safanda, J.F., Carpenter, I., Staley, L.W., O'Connor, R.A., et al. (1994). High functioning fragile X males: Demonstration of an unmethylated fully expanded FMR-1 mutation associated with protein expression. *American Journal of Medical Genetics, 51*(4), 298–308.

Hagerman, R.J., Jackson, C., Amiri, K., Silverman, A.C., O'Connor, R., & Sobesky, W. (1992). Girls with fragile X syndrome: Physical and neurocognitive status and outcome. *Pediatrics, 89*(3), 395–400.

Hagerman, R.J., Leehey, M., Heinrichs, W., Tassone, F., Wilson, R., Hills, J., et al. (2001). Intention tremor, parkinsonism, and generalized brain atrophy in male carriers of fragile X. *Neurology, 57,* 127–130.

Hagerman, R.J., Miller, L.J., McGrath-Clarke, J., Riley, K., Goldson, E., Harris, S.W., et al. (2002). Influence of stimulants on electrodermal studies in fragile X syndrome. *Microscopy Research and Technique, 57*(3), 168–173.

Hagerman, R.J., Murphy, M.A., & Wittenberger, M.D. (1988). A controlled trial of stimulant medication in children with the fragile X syndrome. *American Journal of Medical Genetics, 30*(1–2), 377–392.

Hagerman, R.J., Ono, M.Y., & Hagerman, P.J. (2005). Recent advances in fragile X: A model for autism and neurodegeneration. *Current Opinion in Psychiatry, 18,* 490–496.

Hagerman, R.J., Riddle, J.E., Roberts, L.S., Brease, K., & Fulton, M. (1995). A survey of the efficacy of clonidine in fragile X syndrome. *Developmental Brain Dysfunction, 8,* 336–344.

Harris, S.W., Goodlin-Jones, B., Nowicki, S., Beran, S., Hessl, D., Tassone, F., et al. (2004). *ADOS-G profiles in males with fragile X syndrome.* Paper presented at the 54th Annual Meeting of the American Society of Human Genetics, October 26–30, Toronto, Ontario, Canada.

Hatton, D., Hooper, S.R., Bailey, D.B., Skinner, M.L., Sullivan, K.M., & Wheeler, A. (2002). Problem behavior in boys with fragile X syndrome. *American Journal of Medical Genetics, 108*(2), 105–116.

Hatton, D.D., Buckley, E.G., Lachiewicz, A., & Roberts, J. (1998). Ocular status of young boys with fragile X syndrome: A prospective study. *Journal of the American Association for Pediatric Ophthalmology and Strabismus, 2*(5), 298–301.

Hatton, D.D., Wheeler, A.C., Skinner, M.L., Bailey, D.B., Sullivan, K.M., Roberts, J.E., et al. (2003). Adaptive behavior in children with fragile X syndrome. *American Journal on Mental Retardation, 108*(6), 373–390.

Hessl, D., Dyer-Friedman, J., Glaser, B., Wisbeck, J., Barajas, R.G., Taylor, A., et al. (2001). The influence of environmental and genetic factors on behavior problems and autistic symptoms in boys and girls with fragile X syndrome. *Pediatrics, 108*(5), e88.

Hessl, D., Glaser, B., Dyer-Friedman, J., Blasey, C., Gunnar, M., Hastie, T., et al. (2002). Cortisol and behavior in fragile X syndrome. *Psychoneuroendocrinology, 27,* 855–872.

Hessl, D., Rivera, S.M., & Reiss, A.L. (2004). The neuroanatomy and neuroendocrinology of fragile X syndrome. *Mental Retardation and Developmental Disabilities Research Reviews, 10*(1), 17–24.

Hessl, D., Tassone, F., Loesch, D.Z., Berry-Kravis, E., Leehey, M.A., Gane, L.W., et al. (2005). Abnormal elevation of FMR1 mRNA is associated with psychological symptoms in individuals with the fragile X premutation. *American Journal of Medical Genetics, Part B: Neuropsychiatric Genetics, 139*(1), 115–121.

Huber, K.M., Roder, J.C., & Bear, M.F. (2001). Chemical induction of mGluR5- and protein synthesis-dependent long-term depression in hippocampal area CA1. *Journal of Neurophysiology, 86*(1), 321–325.

Incorpora, G., Sorge, G., Sorge, A., & Pavone, L. (2002). Epilepsy in fragile X syndrome. *Brain and Development, 24*(8), 766–769.

Irwin, S.A., Galvez, R., & Greenough, W.T. (2000). Dendritic spine structural anomalies in fragile-X mental retardation syndrome. *Cerebral Cortex, 10,* 1038–1044.

Irwin, S.A., Patel, B., Idupulapati, M., Harris, J.B., Crisostomo, R.A., Larsen, B.P., et al. (2001). Abnormal dendritic spine characteristics in the temporal and visual cortices of patients with fragile-X syndrome: A quantitative examination. *American Journal of Medical Genetics, 98*(2), 161–167.

Iwahashi, C.K., Yasui, D.H., An, H.-J., Greco, C.M., Tassone, F., Nannen, K., et al. (2006). Protein composition of the intranuclear inclusions of FXTAS. *Brain, 129,* 256–271.

Jacquemont, S., Hagerman, R.J., Leehey, M., Grigsby, J., Zhang, L., Brunberg, J.A., et al. (2003). Fragile X premutation tremor/ataxia syndrome: Molecular, clinical, and neuroimaging correlates. *American Journal of Human Genetics, 72,* 869–878.

Jacquemont, S., Hagerman, R.J., Leehey, M.A., Hall, D.A., Levine, R.A., Brunberg, J.A., et al. (2004). Penetrance of the fragile X-associated tremor/ataxia syndrome in a premutation carrier population. *Journal of American Medical Association, 291*(4), 460–469.

Jin, P., Zarnescu, D.C., Ceman, S., Nakamoto, M., Mowrey, J., Jongens, T.A., et al. (2004). Biochemical and genetic interaction between the fragile X mental retardation protein and the microRNA pathway. *Nature Neuroscience, 7*(2), 113–117.

Kates, W.R., Folley, B.S., Lanham, D.C., Capone, G.T., & Kaufman, W.E. (2002). Cerebral growth in fragile X syndrome: Review and comparison with Down syndrome. *Microscopy Research and Technique, 57,* 159–167.

Kau, A.S.M., Tierney, E., Bukelis, I., Stump, M.H., Kates, W.R., Trescher, W.H., et al. (2004). Social behavior profile in young males with fragile X syndrome: Characteristics and specificity. *American Journal of Medical Genetics, 126A,* 9–17.

Kaufmann, W.E., Cortell, R., Kau, A.S., Bukelis, I., Tierney, E., Gray, R.M., et al. (2004). Autism spectrum disorder in fragile X syndrome: Communication, social interaction, and specific behaviors. *American Journal of Medical Genetics, 129A*(3), 225–234.

Kenneson, A., Zhang, F., Hagedorn, C.H., & Warren, S.T. (2001). Reduced FMRP and increased FMR1 transcription is proportionally associated with CGG repeat number in intermediate-length and premutation carriers. *Human Molecular Genetics, 10,* 1449–1454.

King, R.A., Hagerman, R.J., & Houghton, M. (1995). Ocular findings in fragile X syndrome. *Developmental Brain Dysfunction, 8,* 223–229.

Koekkoek, S.K., Yamaguchi, K., Milojkovic, B.A., Dortland, B.R., Ruigrok, T.J., Maex, R., et al. (2005). Deletion of FMR1 in Purkinje cells enhances parallel fiber LTD, enlarges spines, and attenuates cerebellar eyelid conditioning in fragile X syndrome. *Neuron, 47*(3), 339–352.

Kooy, R.F. (2003). Of mice and the fragile X syndrome. *Trends in Genetics, 19*(3), 148–154.

Kwon, H., Menon, V., Eliez, S., Warsofsky, I.S., White, C.D., Dyer-Friedman, J., et al. (2001). Functional neuroanatomy of visuospatial working memory in fragile X syndrome: Relation to behavioral and molecular measures. *American Journal of Psychiatry, 158*(7), 1040–1051.

Lachiewicz, A.M., & Dawson, D.V. (1994). Do young boys with fragile X syndrome have macroorchidism? *Pediatrics, 93*(6 Pt 1), 992–995.

Lachiewicz, A.M., Dawson, D.V., & Spiridigliozzi, G.A. (2000). Physical characteristics of young boys with fragile X syndrome: Reasons for difficulties in making a diagnosis in young males. *American Journal of Medical Genetics, 92*(4), 229–236.

Li, J., Pelletier, M.R., Perez Velazquez, J.L., & Carlen, P.L. (2002). Reduced cortical synaptic plasticity and GluR1 expression associated with fragile X mental retardation protein deficiency. *Molecular and Cellular Neurosciences, 19*(2), 138–151.

Loesch, D.Z., Bui, M.Q., Dissanayake, C., Clifford, S., Gould, E., Bulhak-Paterson, D., et al. (2006). Molecular and cognitive predictors of the continuum of autistic behaviors in fragile X. *Neuroscience and Biobehavioral Reviews, 31,* 315–326.

Loesch, D.Z., Bui, M.Q., Grigsby, J., Butler, E., Epstein, J., Huggins, R.M., et al. (2003). Effect of the fragile X status categories and the FMRP levels on executive functioning in fragile X males and females. *Neuropsychology, 17*(4), 646–657.

Loesch, D.Z., Huggins, R.M., & Hagerman, R.J. (2004). Phenotypic variation and FMRP levels in fragile X. *Mental Retardation and Developmental Disabilities Research Reviews, 10*(1), 31–41.

Lord, C., Rutter, M., DiLavore, P.C., & Risi, S. (1999). *Autism Diagnostic Observation Schedule.* Los Angeles, CA: Western Psychological Services.

Lord, C., Rutter, M., & Le Couteur, A. (1994). Autism Diagnostic Interview–Revised: A revised version of a diagnostic interview for caregivers of individuals with possible pervasive developmental disorders. *Journal of Autism and Developmental Disorders, 24*(5), 659–685.

Lynch, G. (2002). Memory enhancement: The search for mechanism-based drugs. *Nature Neuroscience, 5 Suppl,* 1035–1038.

Maddalena, A., Richards, C.S., McGinniss, M.J., Brothman, A., Desnick, R.J., Grier, R.E., et al. (2001). Technical standards and guidelines for fragile X: The first of a series of disease—specific supplements to the Standards and Guidelines for Clinical Genetics Laboratories of the American College of Medical Genetics. Quality Assurance Subcommittee of the Laboratory Practice Committee. *Genetics in Medicine, 3*(3), 200–205.

Maino, D.M., Schlange, D., Maino, J.H., & Caden, B. (1990). Ocular anomalies in fragile X syndrome. *Journal of the American Optometric Association, 61*(4), 316–323.

Maino, D.M., Wesson, M., Schlange, D., Cibis, G., & Maino, J.H. (1991). Optometric findings in the fragile X syndrome. *Optometry and Vision Science, 68*(8), 634–640.

McBride, S.M., Choi, C.H., Wang, Y., Liebelt, D., Braunstein, E., Ferreiro, D., et al. (2005). Pharmacological rescue of synaptic plasticity, courtship behavior, and mushroom body defects in a Drosophila model of fragile X syndrome. *Neuron, 45*(5), 753–764.

McCracken, J.T., McGough, J., Shah, B., Cronin, P., Hong, D., Aman, M.G., et al. (2002). Risperidone in children with autism and serious behavioral problems. *The New England Journal of Medicine, 347*(5), 314–321.

Michelson, D., Faries, D., Wernicke, J., Kelsey, D., Kendrick, K., Sallee, F.R., et al. (2001). Atomoxetine in the treatment of children and adolescents with attention-deficit/hyperactivity disorder: A randomized, placebo-controlled, dose-response study. *Pediatrics, 108*(5), E83.

Miller, L.J., McIntosh, D.N., McGrath, J., Shyu, V., Lampe, M., Taylor, A.K., et al. (1999). Electrodermal responses to sensory stimuli in individuals with fragile X syndrome: A preliminary report. *American Journal of Medical Genetics, 83,* 268–279.

Miyashiro, K.Y., Beckel-Mitchener, A., Purk, T.P., Becker, K.G., Barret, T., Liu, L., et al. (2003). RNA cargoes associating with FMRP reveal deficits in cellular functioning in Fmr1 null mice. *Neuron, 37*(3), 417–431.

Mostofsky, S.H., Mazzocco, M.M., Aakalu, G., Warsofsky, I.S., Denckla, M.B., & Reiss, A.L. (1998). Decreased cerebellar posterior vermis size in fragile X syndrome: Correlation with neurocognitive performance. *Neurology, 50*(1), 121–130.

Munir, F., Cornish, K.M., & Wilding, J. (2000). A neuropsychological profile of attention deficits in young males with fragile X syndrome. *Neuropsychologia, 38,* 1261–1270.

Musumeci, S.A., Hagerman, R.J., Ferri, R., Bosco, P., Dalla Bernardina, B., Tassinari, C.A., et al. (1999). Epilepsy and EEG findings in males with fragile X syndrome. *Epilepsia, 40*(8), 1092–1099.

Nowicki, S.T., Tassone, F., Ono, M.Y., Ferranti, J., Croquette, M.F., Goodlin-Jones, B., et al. (2007). The Prader-Willi phenotype of fragile X syndrome. *Journal of Developmental and Behavioral Pediatrics, 28,* 133–138.

Perwien, A.R., Faries, D.E., Kratochvil, C.J., Sumner, C.R., Kelsey, D.K., & Allen, A.J. (2004). Improvement in health-related quality of life in children with ADHD: An analysis of placebo controlled studies of atomoxetine. *Journal of Developmental and Behavioral Pediatrics, 25*(4), 264–271.

Philofsky, A., Hepburn, S.L., Hayes, A., Hagerman, R.J., & Rogers, S.J. (2004). Linguistic and cognitive functioning and autism symptoms in young children with fragile X syndrome. *American Journal on Mental Retardation, 109*(3), 208–218.

Porter, R.H., Jaeschke, G., Spooren, W., Ballard, T.M., Buttelmann, B., Kolczewski, S., et al. (2005). Fenobam: A clinically validated nonbenzodiazepine anxiolytic is a potent, selective, and noncompetitive mGlu5 receptor antagonist with inverse agonist activity. *Journal of Pharmacology and Experimental Therapeutics, 315*(2), 711–721.

Reddy, K.S. (2005). Cytogenetic abnormalities and fragile-X syndrome in Autism Spectrum Disorder. *BMC Medical Genetics, 6*(1), 3.

Reiss, A.L., Abrams, M.T., Greenlaw, R., Freund, L., & Denckla, M.B. (1995). Neurodevelopmental effects of the FMR1 full mutation in humans. *Nature Medicine, 1*(2), 159–167.

Reiss, A.L., Aylward, E., Freund, L.S., Joshi, P.K., & Bryan, R.N. (1991). Neuroanatomy of fragile X syndrome: The posterior fossa. *Annals of Neurology, 29*(1), 26–32.

Reiss, A.L., Freund, L., Abrams, M.T., Boehm, C., & Kazazian, H. (1993). Neurobehavioral effects of the fragile X premutation in adult women: A controlled study. *American Journal of Human Genetics, 52*(5), 884–894.

Reiss, A.L., Lee, J., & Freund, L. (1994). Neuroanatomy of fragile X syndrome: The temporal lobe. *Neurology, 44*(7), 1317–1324.

Reyniers, E., Vits, L., De Boulle, K., Van Roy, B., Van Velzen, D., de Graaff, E., et al. (1993). The full mutation in the FMR-1 gene of male fragile X patients is absent in their sperm. *Nature Genetics, 4*(2), 143–146.

Rivera, S.M., Menon, V., White, C.D., Glaser, B., & Reiss, A.L. (2002). Functional brain activation during arithmetic processing in females with fragile X syndrome is related to FMR1 protein expression. *Human Brain Mapping, 16*, 206–218.

Roberts, J.E., Boccia, M.L., Bailey, D.B., Hatton, D., & Skinner, M. (2001). Cardiovascular indices of physiological arousal in boys with fragile X syndrome. *Developmental Psychobiology, 39*(2), 107–123.

Rogers, S.J., Wehner, E.A., & Hagerman, R.J. (2001). The behavioral phenotype in fragile X: Symptoms of autism in very young children with fragile X syndrome, idiopathic autism, and other developmental disorders. *Journal of Developmental and Behavioral Pediatrics, 22*(6), 409–417.

Rousseau, F., Rouillard, P., Morel, M.L., Khandjian, E.W., & Morgan, K. (1995). Prevalence of carriers of premutation-size alleles of the FMRI gene-and implications for the population genetics of the fragile X syndrome. *American Journal of Human Genetics, 57*(5), 1006–1018.

Sabaratnam, M., Vroegop, P.G., & Gangadharan, S.K. (2001). Epilepsy and EEG findings in 18 males with fragile X syndrome. *Seizure, 10*(1), 60–63.

Scerif, G., Cornish, K., Wilding, J., Driver, J., & Karmiloff-Smith, A. (2004). Visual search in typically developing toddlers and toddlers with fragile X or Williams syndrome. *Developmental Science, 7*(1), 116–130.

Scerif, G., Karmiloff-Smith, A., Campos, R., Elsabbagh, M., Driver, J., & Cornish, K. (2005). To look or not to look? Typical and atypical development of oculomotor control. *Journal of Cognitive Neuroscience, 17*(4), 591–604.

Scharfenaker, S., O'Connor, R., Stackhouse, T., & Noble, L. (2002). An integrated approach to intervention. In R.J. Hagerman & P.J. Hagerman (Eds.), *Fragile X syndrome: Diagnosis, treatment and research* (3rd ed., pp. 363–427). Baltimore: The Johns Hopkins University Press.

Schrander-Stumple, C., Gerver, W.-T., Meyer, H., Engelen, J., Mulder, H., & Fryns, J.-P. (1994). Prader-Willi-like phenotype in fragile X syndrome. *Clinical Genetics, 45*, 175–180.

Sherman, S. (2002). Epidemiology. In R.J. Hagerman & P.J. Hagerman (Eds.), *Fragile X syndrome: Diagnosis, treatment and research* (3rd ed., pp. 136–168). Baltimore: The Johns Hopkins University Press.

Singh, R., Sutherland, G.R., & Manson, J. (1999). Partial seizures with focal epileptogenic electroencephalographic patterns in three related female patients with fragile-X syndrome. *Journal of Child Neurology, 14*(2), 108–112.

Sobesky, W.E., Porter, D., Pennington, B.F., & Hagerman, R.J. (1995). Dimensions of shyness in fragile X females. *Developmental Brain Dysfunction, 8*, 280–292.

Sobesky, W.E., Taylor, A.K., Pennington, B.F., Bennetto, L., Porter, D., Riddle, J., et al. (1996). Molecular-clinical correlations in females with fragile X. *American Journal of Medical Genetics, 64*(2), 340–345.

Sun, H.T., Cohen, S., & Kaufmann, W.E. (2001). Annexin-1 is abnormally expressed in fragile X syndrome: Two-dimensional electrophoresis study in lymphocytes. *American Journal of Medical Genetics, 103*(1), 81–90.

Symons, F.J., Clark, R.D., Hatton, D.D., Skinner, M., & Bailey, D.B., Jr. (2003). Self-injurious behavior in young boys with fragile X syndrome. *American Journal of Medical Genetics, Part A, 118*(2), 115–121.

Tamm, L., Menon, V., Johnston, C.K., Hessl, D.R., & Reiss, A.L. (2002). fMRI study of cognitive interference processing in females with fragile X syndrome. *Journal of Cognitive Neuroscience, 14*(2), 160–171.

Tassone, F., Hagerman, R.J., Iklé, D.N., Dyer, P.N., Lampe, M., Willemsen, R., et al. (1999). FMRP expression as a potential prognostic indicator in fragile X syndrome. *American Journal of Medical Genetics, 84*(3), 250–261.

Tassone, F., Hagerman, R.J., Taylor, A.K., Gane, L.W., Godfrey, T.E., & Hagerman, P.J. (2000). Elevated levels of FMR1 mRNA in carrier males: A new mechanism of involvement in fragile X syndrome. *American Journal of Human Genetics, 66*, 6–15.

Tassone, F., Hagerman, R.J., Taylor, A.K., Mills, J.B., Harris, S.W., Gane, L.W., et al. (2000). Clinical involvement and protein expression in individuals with the FMR1 premutation. *American Journal of Medical Genetics, 91*, 144–152.

Turner, G., Webb, T., Wake, S., & Robinson, H. (1996). Prevalence of fragile X syndrome. *American Journal of Medical Genetics, 64*(1), 196–197.

Verkerk, A.J., Pieretti, M., Sutcliffe, J.S., Fu, Y.H., Kuhl, D.P., Pizzuti, A., et al. (1991). Identification of a gene (FMR-1) containing a CGG repeat coincident with a breakpoint cluster region exhibiting length variation in fragile X syndrome. *Cell, 65*(5), 905–914.

Waldstein, G., Mierau, G., Ahmad, R., Thibodeau, S.N., Hagerman, R.J., & Caldwell, S. (1987). Fragile X syndrome: Skin elastin abnormalities. *Birth Defects: Original Article Series, 23*, 103–114.

Wassink, T.H., Brzustowicz, L.M., Bartlett, C.W., & Szatmari, P. (2004). The search for autism disease genes. *Mental Retardation and Developmental Disabilities Research Reviews, 10*(4), 272–283.

Weiskop, S., Richdale, A., & Matthews, J. (2005). Behavioural treatment to reduce sleep problems in children with autism or fragile X syndrome. *Developmental Medicine and Child Neurology, 47*(2), 94–104.

Wilens, T., Pelham, W., Stein, M., Conners, C.K., Abikoff, H., Atkins, M., et al. (2003). ADHD treatment with once-daily OROS methylphenidate: Interim 12-month results from a long-term open-label study. *Journal of the American Academy of Child and Adolescent Psychiatry, 42*(4), 424–433.

Willemsen, R., Oostra, B.A., Bassell, G.J., & Dictenberg, J. (2004). The fragile X syndrome: From molecular genetics to neurobiology. *Mental Retardation and Developmental Disabilities Research Reviews, 10*(1), 60–67.

Wisbeck, J.M., Huffman, L.C., Freund, L., Gunnar, M., Davis, E.P., & Reiss, A.L. (2000). Cortisol and social stressors in children with fragile X: A pilot study. *Journal of Developmental and Behavioral Pediatrics, 21*, 278–282.

Zeesman, S., Zwaigenbaum, L., Whelan, D.T., Hagerman, R.J., Tassone, F., & Taylor, S.A. (2004). Paternal transmission of fragile X syndrome. *American Journal of Medical Genetics, 129A*(2), 184–189.

Speech and Language Profiles in Down Syndrome and Fragile X Syndrome

Assessment and Intervention Implications

Communication and Language Development in Infants and Toddlers with Down Syndrome or Fragile X Syndrome

AUDRA STERLING AND STEVEN F. WARREN

D elayed and disordered speech and language development are among the hallmark features of both Down syndrome (DS) and fragile X syndrome (FXS; Abbeduto & Hagerman, 1997; Dodd, 1975; Kumin, 1996). These delays and disorders are usually apparent early in development. For example, concern about delayed language development has been identified by parents of children eventually diagnosed with FXS as the source of their first serious concerns about their children (Roberts, Hatton, & Bailey, 2001). Because DS is normally diagnosed before or at birth, parents of children with DS are likely to expect delays in communication and language development. This early knowledge can provide parents of children with DS with a distinct advantage in terms of starting intervention as early as possible. Although DS and FXS share many similarities in language development, each has unique phenotypic differences that are relevant to assessment and especially to intervention.

This chapter focuses on communication and language development in infants and toddlers with DS or FXS from birth to age 3 years. By their third birthdays, most children with DS and most boys and some girls with FXS will still be in the early stages of language development, and some will not yet be speaking. Consequently, we concentrate primarily on prelinguistic communication development up through the single-word stage of expressive language development. The next chapter focuses primarily on language development in preschool and school-age children.

Communication development begins at birth for all children. This chapter summarizes what is known to date about the prelinguistic period in children with DS or FXS and addresses topics such as oral-motor development, phonological development, sign language and gestures, joint attention, and imitation—all of

The first author wishes to acknowledge the traineeship support of NIDCD Grant T32 DC000052. The second author wishes to acknowledge the support for his research of NICHD Grants P30 HD02528 and NICHD P30 HD003110 and NIDCD Grant R01 HD44868.

which lead to a child's first words. The research literature on these issues is much more extensive for children with DS relative to children with FXS. But new research with young children with FXS is beginning to change this imbalance. After characterizing development in infants and toddlers with DS or FXS, this chapter discusses the potential impact these characteristics can have on interactions with parents and other caregivers, as well as implications for assessment and intervention.

CHARACTERISTICS OF EARLY COMMUNICATION AND LANGUAGE DEVELOPMENT

We address several of the major topics involved in early language and communication development for children with DS or FXS in the following sections.

Hearing Development

Hearing children progress through a number of stages during the first 2 years of life. Evidence has verified that fetuses begin to hear during the third trimester and that newborns can already discriminate the sound of their mother's voice (Hepper, 2002). Typically developing infants from birth to 3 months react to loud sounds and smile when spoken to. Around 3–6 months, they look upward or turn to new sounds and begin to enjoy rattles and toys that make noise; by 6–10 months, they respond to their own name and look at things or pictures if someone is talking about them. Some studies report that frequent otitis media and mild hearing loss in the first year of life are linked with lower scores on tests of speech production, as well as receptive and expressive language (Roberts, Burchinal, & Zeisel, 2002; Rovers et al., 2000), although there is some controversy with this finding (Paradise, 1998; Roberts et al., 2004). Otitis media affects both typically developing children and children with developmental disabilities, such as DS or FXS.

Down Syndrome

Children with DS are reported to have frequent cases of ear infections and fluctuating hearing loss in the first few years of life (Roberts & Medley, 1995; Schwartz & Schwartz, 1978). Lynch, Oller, Steffens, and Levine (1995) found that 6 of the 13 infants with DS in their study had a hearing loss of 25–40 dB, most likely the result of otitis media. The research on hearing development in young children with DS has focused almost exclusively on the impact of otitis media.

Fragile X Syndrome

No evidence indicates that hearing does not develop normally in children with FXS, with the exception of otitis media and the disruption of hearing during these periods of time. In a study of boys with FXS, Hagerman and Falkenstein (1987) found that prior to age 5, 63% of the children in their study had six or more ear infections. Simko, Hornstein, Soukup, and Bagamery (1989) also found a high incidence of recurrent otitis media in young boys with FXS (45% of 20 children with FXS). Research to date with children with FXS has focused on otitis media and not necessarily on hearing development.

Summary

It is difficult to say if hearing develops in children with DS or FXS in the same way as it does in typically developing children. Persistent otitis media, resulting in a documented hearing loss in infants with DS, is a common occurrence. Recurrent otitis media often affects both children with DS and children with FXS in early childhood. It is important to note that the literature on the impact of otitis media is somewhat contradictory (Roberts et al., 2004). Roberts and colleagues (2004) suggested that the studies that did find significant results might not have used reliable methodology, including poor timing of data collection and faulty otitis media documentation procedures. Consequently, it remains unclear whether and to what extent a history of recurrent otitis media affects language development in children with DS or FXS.

Oral-Motor Development

Typically developing infants proceed through a number of oral-motor developmental phases. At birth, infants have a number of reflexes that guide their oral-motor skills, including rooting, tongue protrusion, and suckling. These reflexes are replaced during the first few months of infancy by mature sucking, tongue lateralization, and the ability to bite and chew solid foods. The muscle tone in an infant's jaw, tongue, lips, and cheeks continues to develop, allowing for advanced eating and eventually speech (Hall, 2001). Few typically developing children deal with the oral-motor difficulties that both children with DS or FXS face.

Down Syndrome

Children with DS have motor impairments that generally affect the development of speech. These impairments include low muscle tone in the tongue, lips, and cheeks, resulting in less firm and precise production of speech sounds (Kumin, 1996; Spender et al., 1995; Spender et al., 1996). As a result, children with DS have difficulty in speech production and intelligibility stemming at least in part from difficulty with muscle timing and coordination. Children with DS tend to have a high, narrow, arched palate; enlarged tonsils and adenoids; and a small mouth and jaw area in comparison with the size of the tongue (Kumin, 1996; Strome & Strome, 1992). These physical characteristics combined with low muscle tone contribute to the difficulty children with DS have in producing the precise sounds and sound combinations required for intelligible speech. Some children with DS have problems with intelligibility throughout their lives (Kumin, 1994).

Fragile X Syndrome

Children with FXS also have a number of oral-motor problems, including a high, narrow, arched palate (Hagerman, 1996); oral tactile defensiveness and drooling (Scharfenaker, Hickman, & Braden, 1996); and cleft palate in 5% of children (Partington, 1984). Children with FXS can also show many of the characteristics of childhood apraxia of speech (Hanson, Jackson, & Hagerman, 1986).

Summary

Both children with DS or FXS suffer from a number of oral-motor problems that can affect speech production and intelligibility. Oral-motor development problems do persist for some children.

Phonological Development

Phonological development in infants progresses through a number of stages during the first year of life. Typically developing infants generally begin with cooing around 2–3 months, then make the transition to vocal play, then babbling. An early sign of meaningful speech is the onset of canonical babbling, which begins around 6 or 7 months. This type of babbling is composed of alternating consonants and vowels. Reduplicated babbling, consisting of multisyllabic utterances (e.g., bababa, dadada), becomes increasingly common during the latter part of this phase. First words typically overlap with the late canonical babbling stage (Stoel-Gammon, 1997).

Down Syndrome

In terms of *early* phonological development, infants with DS do not appear to be delayed. Dodd (1972) reported no differences between 10 infants with DS and 10 typically developing infants in the development of speech sounds at 9 and 13 months. Although the two groups differed significantly on their Bayley Scales of Infant Development (Bayley, 1969) scores, they did not differ on the number and variety of consonants and vowels produced, time spent vocalizing, and number and length of utterances.

Smith and Oller (1981) also reported that the age of onset of reduplicated babbling in 10 infants with DS did not differ from that in 8 typically developing infants in a longitudinal design. The typically developing infants began using reduplicated babbling at 8 months, and the infants with DS began doing so at 8.4 months. Smith and Oller also found that both groups demonstrated a similar developmental profile for place of articulation in terms of babbling, with both groups using back consonants in the first 6 months of life and then shifting to front consonants between 7 and 9 months. Smith and Oller concluded that the development of early prelinguistic vocalizations is not delayed in infants with DS.

Lynch and colleagues (1995) found that the average age of onset of canonical babbling for infants with DS was 9 months, which is about 2 months later than for typically developing infants. It was also noted that once canonical babbling began, it was not as consistent compared with the typically developing infant group. This latter finding, however, can be accounted for by impairments within the motor domain and does not refute the findings of early babbling development (Stoel-Gammon, 1997).

There is a consensus across studies that the onset of meaningful speech and linguistic development in children with DS is delayed. Smith (1984) compared 10 typically developing infants with 10 infants with DS and found that the typically developing infants said their first words on average 6 months before infants with DS and were also more intelligible. The typically developing children had an average of 50% interpretable utterances by 18 months, whereas the children with DS had an average of only 5% interpretable utterances at 30 months, which was approximately 9 months after they spoke their first words. The delays seen in phonological development seem to persist even after the children are speaking.

Fragile X Syndrome

Little research exists on phonological development in children younger than 3 years with FXS. It does appear that young children with FXS have problems in intelligibility, as well as omission or distortion of certain vowel and consonant sounds, based on the fact that older children with FXS have these problems (Abbeduto & Hagerman, 1997). Although a prospective study of phonological development in children with FXS has yet to be reported, it is likely that these problems would be evident within the first 3 years of life. Roberts, Mirrett, Anderson, Burchinal, and Neebe (2002) studied 22 older children with FXS. The children in this study ranged in age from 21–77 months, with a mean age of 49.2 months. The authors used the Communication and Symbolic Behavior Scales™ (CSBS™; Wetherby & Prizant, 1993) and examined the vocal communication subscale (i.e., use of vocalizations, different consonants). The children seemed to have a relative strength in vocalizations and verbalizations compared with gesturing, reciprocity, and symbolic behavior. Roberts and colleagues also found a correlation between the children's vocalizations and their use of gestures and communicative function.

Summary

Children with DS do not seem to show a delay in terms of early phonological development. They proceed through the same stages of development as typically developing infants in terms of onset of canonical babbling and place of articulation of early vocalizations. As children with DS get older, however, a clear delay emerges. Problems with intelligibility arise once children with DS begin speaking and persist well past 3 years of age. Children with FXS also have problems with intelligibility, in addition to a number of other phonological delays. Children with FXS appear to have a relative strength in phonological development compared with use of gestures and so forth, but phonological development is delayed. To date, however, there have been few studies that have examined phonological development in very young children with FXS because diagnosis often does not occur until after a delay in language development.

Sign Language and Gestures

The development of gestures in typically developing children marks an important step in nonverbal communication development. The development of gestures, such as pointing, typically begins around 12 months (Bates, 1976) and allows young children to direct the attention of people around them (Mundy, Kasari, Sigman, & Ruskin, 1995). Researchers have looked at the intentional use of gestures in young children because these early skills are thought to reflect important cognitive processes, such as coordinational attention, representational thought, and the ability to plan action sequences (Bates, Benigni, Bretherton, Camaioni, & Volterra, 1979; McEvoy, Rogers, & Pennington, 1993).

Down Syndrome

Sign language has been found to help reduce frustration and challenging behaviors in children with speech delays (Remington & Clarke, 1996). Miller (1992) observed the development of signs and spoken language in a group of 44 young children with DS. He found that by 17 months' mental age, the children's vocabulary contained twice as many signed as spoken words. At 26 months' mental age, however, there was an increase in spoken language, and the number of signed words declined.

Caselli and colleagues (1998) examined the use of gestures and the emergence of spoken words in a group of 40 Italian children with DS ranging in age from 10 to 49 months, using the Italian version (Caselli & Casadio, 1995) of the MacArthur-Bates Communicative Development Inventories (CDIs; Fenson et al., 1992). They compared the children in the study to the normative data collected by the authors for the CDI. The children with DS used significantly more gestures compared with the control group. This difference, however, was apparent only once both groups of children had a lexical comprehension level of more than 100 words. Children with DS used more gestures, particularly when using pretend gestures (e.g., playing with dolls) and symbolic communication gestures (e.g., "gone," "hot," "be quiet"). Caselli and colleagues suggested that the children in their study seemed to have a "specialization" in nonverbal communication, possibly due to the fact that they had been exposed to gestures more than the control groups.

Mundy, Sigman, Kasari, and Yirmiya (1988) looked at the emergence of nonverbal communication skills in a group of 30 young children with DS ranging in age from 18 to 48 months. They found that these children used gestures such as reaching and pointing at a marginally significant decreased rate when requesting an object compared with the typically developing control group. They suggested that this could be due to young children with DS lacking sufficient interest in objects relative to social partners (Kasari, Mundy, Yirmiya, & Sigman, 1990).

Fragile X Syndrome

The literature on language development in children with FXS to date has focused primarily on school-age children. Roberts, Mirrett, and colleagues (2002) studied 22 children with FXS ranging in age from 21 to 77 months, although all of the children were developmentally younger than 28 months (mean chronological age 49.2 months). They reported a significant delay in both conventional gestures (e.g., pushing unwanted objects away) and distal gestures (e.g., pointing at an object located across the room).

Summary

Nonverbal communication appears to be a relative strength for young children with DS. Sign language is commonly used when children are very young, but once spoken language starts to catch up, the use of signs declines. Although children with DS are relatively good at using gestures, they do not use gestures as frequently as their typically developing peers when requesting an object. Children with FXS are probably delayed in the use of gestures, specifically conventional and distal gestures, although more research is needed to confirm this.

Joint Attention

The development of joint attention has a major influence on early language development. Joint attention refers to an infant's ability to engage a social partner in his or her focus of attention, typically involving gaze coordination between the partner and object of interest (Tager-Flusberg & Sullivan, 1998). Joint attention allows infants to reference objects in a social context, imitate others, communicate with gestures, and regulate emotions (Adamson & Russell, 1999). Instances of joint attention allow the social partner to interact with the child at a point when the partner's language input may have optimal impact on learning (McCathren, Yoder, & Warren, 1995). Tomasello and Farrar (1986) found a positive correlation between the vocabulary size of typically developing children at 21 months and the mother's ability to maintain her child's focus of attention by referencing toys with which the child was actively engaged. Numerous studies have reported a relationship between a delayed onset of joint attention and delayed communication development in young children with developmental disabilities, including children with DS (Mundy et al., 1988; Smith & Tetzchner, 1986).

Down Syndrome

Although young children with DS are often characterized as being very social (Gibbs & Thorpe, 1983; Wishart & Johnston, 1990), they do exhibit some problems with joint attention, particularly in infancy. One difficulty for infants with DS pertains to eye contact. Reciprocal eye contact is not only delayed, but its development is also specifically impaired (Berger & Cunningham, 1981, 1983). Berger and Cunningham found that infants with DS increased eye contact with their caregivers at a much slower rate, reaching a peak 7–10 weeks after their typically developing peers. In addition, once mutual eye contact was established, infants with DS tended to maintain these high levels of eye contact much longer than typically developing infants. Berger (1990) argued that this trend indicates a low level of visual exploration in infants with DS. Kasari and colleagues (1990) reported a similar finding in 30 young children with DS (mean age of 22.9 months). The children in this study not only looked more often to the experimenter's face compared with a group of typically developing children of the same mental age, but they also looked away from the interaction more often and looked less often at the nonfocal toys. The authors noted that this deficiency in exploring and assessing their environment could possibly hinder the ability of children with DS to acquire language skills.

Mundy and colleagues (1988) examined social interaction skills in a group of 30 children with DS. The children were divided into two groups based on mental age scores, with the mean age of 22.9 months (*SD* = 6 months) for the group with lower mental age scores and 43 months (*SD* = 12.1 months) for the group with higher mental age scores. They found that children with DS had more social interaction behaviors, such as initiating turn-taking routines or throwing toys while smiling at the adult in the room, but were requesting objects significantly less often compared with their typically developing peers. The children with DS demonstrated impairments when requesting assistance with objects or requesting objects but did not have difficulties requesting an experimenter to repeat a physical interaction game. Mundy and colleagues suggest that perhaps children with

DS prefer to engage in social interactions, even to the point of neglecting object-requesting behaviors.

Fragile X Syndrome

At present very little research exists on the development of joint attention in young children with FXS. Using the CSBS™, Roberts, Mirrett, and colleagues (2002) found that the young boys with FXS that they observed had a number of strengths and weaknesses in terms of joint attention. They examined 22 children with FXS ranging in age from 21 to 77 months. The young boys demonstrated relative strengths in social affective signaling, gaze shifts, and using both gestures and vocalizations in conjunction; however, they demonstrated weaknesses in repair strategies, positive affect, and both conventional and distal gestures.

In addition to the findings just described, Murphy and Abbeduto (2005) noted a number of phenotypical characteristics of children with FXS that may make achieving joint attention problematic. For example, individuals with FXS have problems with hyperarousal, including stimulation behaviors such as rocking and hand flapping. Self-directed aggression is also not uncommon in children with FXS. This in turn creates an obstacle for joint attention, because it requires the coordination of the dyad's behaviors. Similarly, attention is impaired and hyperactivity is often noted in children with FXS (Hagerman, 1996). Murphy and Abbeduto hypothesize that children with FXS may avoid social interactions in order to avoid hyperarousal, which in time may cause their caregivers to become less attentive to occasions for joint attention.

Summary

Children with DS have a number of difficulties relating to joint attention. Young children with DS demonstrate low levels of visual exploration, making it challenging for them to explore and learn about their surroundings. Children with DS do not seem to have difficulties with social interaction behaviors, but they do demonstrate impairments in requesting objects. Young boys with FXS seem to have strengths and weaknesses that could both enhance and also inhibit joint attention. In addition to these characteristics, the phenotype of FXS includes a number of behaviors that are hypothesized to create barriers to joint attention. These strengths and weaknesses have not been examined in children younger than two, however, and the research has involved only males.

Imitation

As imitation develops, it comes to serve several functions for infants and toddlers. These functions provide a means of turn taking and communication with a partner and allow infants and toddlers to share emotions and to acquire the form, meaning, and function of new words (Rogers, Hepburn, Stackhouse, & Wehner, 2003; Speidel & Nelson, 1989). At first, imitation involves facial expressions, body movements, and vocalizations, both by children and caregivers (Meltzoff & Gopnik, 1993; Nadel, Guerini, Peze, & Rivet, 1999). These early forms of imitation can serve as a primitive form of social interaction in which the caregiver imitates the child, who in turn imitates the caregiver (Rogers et al., 2003). As the infant continues to develop, imitation takes on different roles, including early peer interactions, and serves as a way to share mutual experiences of activities, emotions, and thought (Nadel & Peze, 1993; Stern, 1985; Uzgiris, 1999).

Presence of Autism

A complicating factor in the development of some young children with FXS is the co-occurrence of autism. It is estimated that approximately 15%–25% of individuals (mostly males but some females) with FXS meet the diagnostic criteria for autism (Bailey et al., 1998; Dykens & Volkmar, 1997). However, 50%–90% of males with FXS are reported to show some of the symptoms of autism, including hand biting, hand flapping, perseveration in speech, tactile defensiveness, and poor eye contact (Bailey et al., 1998; Feinstein & Reiss, 1998). Males with both FXS and autism typically have more severe language and social impairments, as well as lower IQ scores, compared with children with FXS without autism (Bailey et al., 1998). Rogers, Wehner, and Hagerman (2001) examined the presence of autism in 24 children (23 boys, 1 girl) with FXS between the ages of 21 and 48 months. Eight of the children in the study had both autism and FXS, whereas the remaining 16, including the one girl, had FXS only. Rogers and colleagues also recruited a group of children with autism but no FXS. The authors found that the children with both FXS and autism scored lower on measures of both expressive and receptive language compared with the children who had FXS but not autism and the children who had autism but not FXS. In short, the co-occurrence of FXS and autism almost inevitably means that communication and social skills will be more severely impaired from early in development onward.

Down Syndrome

Imitation has been reported to be a relative strength in children with DS (Hodapp et al., 1992; Rast & Meltzoff, 1995). Wright, Lewis, and Collis (2006) examined imitation in a group with 18 children with DS between the ages of 11 and 43 months and compared them with 18 typically developing children matched on developmental age. The authors found that the children with DS used imitation more frequently in both object search and play compared with the typically developing children. The children with DS were also more likely to imitate this counter-functional play (using a toy brush on a truck instead of a doll) compared with the typically developing children. Wright and colleagues suggested that these findings support the notion that children with DS use social cues and imitation to solve problems or in play more readily than typically developing children.

Fragile X Syndrome

Rogers and colleagues (2003) examined the development of imitation skills in a group of 18 children with FXS. They looked at imitation skills in young children with autism, children with FXS, and children with similar developmental delays. The mean age of the children with FXS was 34 months, and the mean nonverbal and verbal mental ages were 21 months and 18 months, respectively. The children with FXS showed a weakness in imitation compared with the group of children with developmental delays. On closer inspection, the authors found that the children with FXS who did not have autism actually had imitation scores similar to the group of children with developmental delays, whereas the children with both FXS and autism had more significant delays and looked much like the group of children with autism.

Summary

Imitation is a relative strength for children with DS, at least during this period in development. Some evidence exists that children with DS retain imitation as a learning strategy longer than their typically developing peers (Sokolov, 1992), which may become problematic during the later stages of language development, when alternative learning strategies become more useful (Speidel & Nelson, 1989). Children with FXS, particularly children with both FXS and autism, show more substantial impairments in imitation early on, and these may persist.

Lexical Development: Expressive Language

Typically developing children usually speak their first word sometime around the end of their first year, although many children do not say their first word until 18 months or later. During this time, there is quite a bit of overlap with canonical babbling. First words are typically nouns, consisting of names for people and objects. Around the second year, children typically experience a vocabulary burst. Bloom (1993) reported that children typically demonstrate their increasing vocabulary at around 19 months and that shortly thereafter they begin combining two words.

Down Syndrome

Young children with DS exhibit delays in the onset of expressive language. The mean age at which children with DS produce their first spoken word is 18 months (Gillham, 1979), although there is quite a bit of variability within this finding. Stray-Gunderson (1986) found a range from 9 months to 7 years for production of the first word. Children with DS typically begin combining two words at approximately 30 months, varying anywhere from 18 to 60 months (Gillham, 1979). Their first words are similar in function to the first words of typically developing children, consisting primarily of names for people or animals (Cardoso-Martins, Mervis, & Mervis, 1985). Kumin, Goodman, and Councill (1991) reported that children with DS are often able to sign words that are indicative of expressive referential vocabulary before 12 months of age. So although children with DS might not be using spoken language before the age of 18 months, they are often able to communicate before the end of their first year.

Kumin, Councill, and Goodman (1999) examined the growth of expressive vocabulary in a sample of 130 children with DS between the ages of 1 and 5 years. They used the CDIs (Fenson et al., 1992) to obtain a parent report of vocabulary, including both signs and speech. The 1-year-olds in their study were reported by their parents to have a mean of 13.9 words, although the range was quite large (2–53 words). The authors reported a steady increase in expressive vocabulary at each age. The mean number of words that parents reported that their child used by 2 years of age was 54.9, and by 3 years of age the average was 168.3 words. Kumin and colleagues also reported a shift from signed to spoken language between 3 and 4 years of age.

Kumin and colleagues (1999) looked at two-word combinations in the same group of young children with DS. Most of the children in the study were not combining words at age 2; however, by 3 years of age, 69% of the children had started combining words. Typically, children begin combining words anywhere from 19–24 months of age (Nelson, 1983).

Fragile X Syndrome

Young children with FXS also exhibit delays in the onset of expressive language. Roberts, Hatton, and Bailey (2001) reported an average age of 28 months for first spoken words in a group of 26 young boys with FXS ranging in age from 9 to 88 months. The authors obtained their data from a parent interview at the onset of the study. Parents reported more of a delay in expressive compared with receptive language skills. Parents were given The ABILITIES Index (Simeonsson & Bailey, 1991), which asked them to describe how their child was functioning on several domains. Parents indicated a suspected delay in both receptive and expressive language by 12 months of age; however, they began to rank expressive communication as more of a problem compared with receptive communication, particularly by 30 months. In addition, a subgroup of boys with both FXS and autism was observed; these children were either completely nonverbal or extremely limited in their expressive abilities (a few single words).

Roberts, Mirrett, and Burchinal (2001) examined expressive language development in 39 older boys with FXS ranging in age from 20 to 86 months, with a mean age of 57.3 months. The authors used the Reynell Developmental Language Scales (Reynell; Reynell & Gruber, 1990). The boys with FXS were acquiring expressive language at approximately one third of the rate expected for typically developing children. In addition, the boys acquired expressive language skills more slowly than receptive language skills.

Summary

Both children with DS or FXS are delayed in the emergence of spoken language. Children with DS on average produce their first spoken word at 18 months and begin combining words around 30 months. Research has shown, however, that children with DS are able to communicate with the use of sign language well before they begin using spoken language. One study on boys with FXS reported an average age of 28 months for first spoken words and found expressive language develops significantly slower compared with typically developing children, even when the children are older. Children with both FXS and autism are typically more severely affected, and spoken language can be greatly affected.

Lexical Development: Receptive Language

Receptive language is defined as what a child understands when listening to speech. Comprehension generally develops before production. Infants begin to recognize familiar names and objects, including their own name, and then they begin to understand verbal input and commands. Benedict (1979) reported that the onset of comprehension in very young children preceded production by nearly 4 months. The children she followed were able to acquire 10 words in comprehension, compared with 4 words productively. By 13 months, the average child in her study could comprehend approximately 50 words but had not yet said his or her first word.

Down Syndrome

Expressive language development is significantly delayed compared with receptive language in children with DS (Kumin et al., 1991; Miller, 1987). Miller (1992) examined how production and comprehension were related to mental age in a group of 43 children with DS between the ages of 11 and 58 months. He found that most of the children showed a profile of comprehension commensurate with mental age, but production was delayed. Miller noted not only that comprehension skills surpassed production skills consistently but also that the gap widened with increasing chronological age.

Fragile X Syndrome

Research on receptive language in very young children with FXS is fairly limited. Roberts, Mirrett, and colleagues (2002) looked at comprehension scores on the Reynell in their study involving 22 boys with FXS. The boys ranged in age from 21 to 77 months, with a mean age of 49.2 months at the first time point. The mean comprehension developmental age on the Reynell scale was 22.2 months, compared with a mean production developmental age of 21.6 months. One year later, the boys were at a mean comprehension developmental age of 30.7 months, compared with 28 months for production. Interestingly, the children's scores on the CSBS™ predicted their receptive language skills at the follow-up visit 1 year later. As stated previously, Roberts, Mirrett, and Burchinal (2001) found that receptive language developed at a faster rate than expressive language. The authors also found that as the children got older, the gap began to widen between receptive and expressive language.

Summary

For both children with DS or FXS, receptive language is more advanced than production. This gap tends to widen as children with DS get older. Research on children with FXS suggests that they develop relatively better comprehension skills compared with children with DS, but only a few children with FXS younger than age 2 have been studied to date.

Overall Summary of Speech and Language Development in Children with Down Syndrome or Fragile X Syndrome

Children with both DS or FXS display a variety of communication impairments. Children with both syndromes have oral-motor problems that contribute to language delays, although the impact of otitis media is unclear. Children with DS seem to have a relative strength in nonverbal requesting skills, as well as imitation, whereas males with both FXS and autism have a significant delay in terms of imitation skills. The very early stages of phonological development do not seem to be impaired for infants with DS. As development progresses, however, most young children with DS do fall behind their typically developing peers, beginning with canonical babbling and extending through spoken words. Expressive language is much more delayed compared with receptive language in children with DS. Male children with FXS have demonstrated a significant delay in the emergence of first spoken words, and children with both FXS and autism are sometimes still nonverbal even at 3 years of age or older. The work on early language development in FXS is still in its very early stages, particularly the work on acquisition of phonology and receptive language skills. One interesting point to note is the lack of research on language development of girls with FXS. The literature to date has focused primarily on boys. The research on young children with DS does not report differences between boys and girls, and this gender distinction seems to be important only in terms of FXS.

IMPACT OF YOUNG CHILDREN WITH DOWN SYNDROME OR FRAGILE X SYNDROME ON CAREGIVER BEHAVIOR

Communication and language development is a cumulative process that occurs roughly 12–14 hours per day, day after day, for many years. This process is affected by both environmental and biological variables. Among environmental variables, caregivers obviously provide an important source of input for young children. This input may be affected both by the aspects of the caregiver (e.g., education level, stress levels, preferred parenting style) and by how easily children initiate and engage in interaction and how quickly they acquire language. The process is bidirectional, with the caregiver affecting the child and the child affecting the caregiver. In disorders that are primarily biological in origin, the environment plays an important, cumulative role in development over time (Warren, 2004). This section examines ways in which having children with DS or FXS may affect parenting styles during the first few years of life.

Parenting style can have a profound impact on the development of young children. For example, parental responsivity has been found to affect children's cognitive, emotional, and language development (Landry, Smith, Miller-Loncar, & Swank, 1998; Landry, Smith, Swank, Assel, & Vellet, 2001). Generally speaking, a parent who is highly responsive to his or her young child frequently engages in a style of behavior that maintains the child's focus of attention, expands on the child's initiations with comments and questions, and only occasionally redirects the child to a new topic. Compelling evidence exists that children who experience sustained highly responsive parenting from birth to 3 years tend to score significantly higher on cognitive tests, achieve language milestones earlier, and develop better social skills, although this work does not include children with DS and other developmental disabilities (Calkins, Smith, Gill, & Johnson, 1998; Landry et al., 2001; Landry, Garner, Swank, & Baldwin, 1996). It may be difficult, however, for a parent to employ a highly responsive parenting style with a child who rarely initiates or who frequently engages in inappropriate behaviors.

Effects of Down Syndrome on Caregiver Behavior

In addition to language and cognitive delays, children with DS can have various behavioral issues that can affect parenting style and that in turn can be affected by parenting responses over time. Although children with DS have been characterized as being affectionate and relatively easy in temperament, some children with DS are noted for lacking task persistence (Hupp & Abbeduto, 1991) and for being stubborn, inattentive, and mildly oppositional, particularly in high-demand situations (Ganiban, Wagner, & Cicchetti, 1990; Gibson, 1978). Children with DS tend to have lower rates of maladaptive behaviors than children with autism (Dykens & Kasari, 1997). Nevertheless, the attributes of children with DS most likely to affect parenting style on an ongoing basis are passivity, relatively low initiation rates, difficulty maintaining a focus of attention, and low task persistence. Each of these characteristics alone or in combination could increase the difficulty of employing a highly responsive parenting style (Girolametto, Weitzman, & Clements-Baartman, 1998) and cumulatively could result over time in further delays in cognitive and language development.

Slonims, Cox, and McConachie (2006) compared 46 mother–child dyads—half of whom included typically developing children, the other half of whom included children with DS—on a number of social-interaction behaviors when the children were 8 and 20 weeks of age. At 8 weeks of age, infants with DS were already significantly less communicative and lively than the typically developing infants, but there were no overt differences in the behaviors of the mothers. At 20 weeks of age, however, the mothers of the children with DS had become more remote and less sensitive to their infants. The analysis suggested that these changes were driven by the child's behavior.

Tannock (1988) examined parenting style in mothers who had children with DS compared with mothers with typically developing children at the same developmental level. She specifically measured how often the mothers used response (e.g., commands, questions), topic (e.g., introducing something to which the child is not actively attending), and turn-taking controls. She found that mothers of children with DS tended to take more frequent and longer turns compared with the mothers of the typically developing children. The mothers of children with DS used these various controls to support and encourage participation during their interactions. They also used topic control more frequently compared with controls.

Crawley and Spiker (1983) examined maternal parenting style within a sample of 18 mothers of 2-year-old children with DS. They focused on the individual differences in mother–child interaction patterns and predicted that the differences in patterns of interactions would be related to the competence levels of the children, measured by the Bayley Mental Development Index (MDI; Bayley, 1969). Directiveness was found to be unrelated to MDI scores or the other maternal qualities evaluated. Mood and stimulation values were correlated with the children's MDI scores, whereas sensitivity and elaborativeness were not related to MDI scores. Although this study did not use a control group of typically developing children, the results do suggest that perhaps several variables (e.g., mood, stimulation value) may be related to cognitive development in children with DS.

Roach, Barratt, Miller, and Leavitt (1998) also examined maternal parenting style within a play-based context. Their primary focus was on directive, supportive, and nondirective behaviors of 28 mothers of children with DS between the ages of 16 and 30 months (mental age range 10–17 months) compared with mothers of developmentally and chronologically matched typically developing children. They found that mothers of children with DS were significantly more vocally directive compared with mothers of developmentally and chronologically matched children. Vocal directives were defined as any vocalization in which the mother requested an action or object from the child. The mothers of the children with DS tended to shoulder more of the responsibility of the interaction compared with the other mothers in the study. The authors suggested that perhaps the reason for these findings was that the children with DS in general were less active during the parent–child play session when compared with the other children.

The studies reviewed are representative of a larger body of literature (e.g., Berger & Cunningham, 1981; Cicchetti & Sroufe, 1976; Kasari et al., 1990; Knieps, Walden, & Baxter, 1994), which indicates that, from early on, children with DS present a substantial challenge to the ability of parents to employ the kind of highly responsive parenting style that has been linked to optimal cognitive and language development. A directive parenting style, however, does not necessarily equate to an unresponsive parenting style (McCathren et al., 1995) and probably reflects a natural adaptation of parents to their children's struggles with attentional focus and engagement (Cardoso-Martins & Mervis, 1985; Crawley & Spiker, 1983; Marfo, 1990). Directives that follow a child's attention lead and occur within routine interactions can help the child make the link between words, objects, and events (Barnes, Gutfreund, Satterly, & Wells, 1983).

Effects of Fragile X Syndrome on Caregiver Behavior

As with children with DS, children with FXS can behave in ways that make highly responsive parenting a challenge. Many children with FXS are hyperactive. They often have a limited attention span, and they may be hypersensitive to auditory, visual, or tactile stimuli (Baumgardner, Reiss, Freund, & Abrams, 1995). It is not uncommon for males with FXS to display self-injurious and repetitive or autism-like behaviors, such as hand biting, hand flapping, poor eye contact, and shyness. For some children, these behaviors may be present as early as the second or third year of life (Hagerman, 1996). Poor joint attention in children with FXS may, over time, cause parents to become inattentive and nonresponsive in their interactions with their children (Murphy & Abbeduto, 2005). Disrupted social interactions may then cumulatively affect communication and language development because a child not only receives less language input but also less optimal language input.

Maternal Characteristics that Affect Responsivity

Maternal variables that are known to have an effect on responsivity include low educational attainment (i.e., less than a high school education), mild intellectual disability, substance abuse, and depression (Hooper, Burchinal, Roberts, Zeisel, & Neebe, 1998; Miller, Miceli, Whitman, & Borkowski, 1996; Osofsky & Thompson, 2000; Rutter & Quinton, 1984). Although carriers of FXS do not typically have lower IQ scores than noncarriers, carriers of FXS are at risk for a range of subtle to severe problems that could hinder their interactions with their children with FXS. Women who are carriers may have subtle cognitive impairments in attention, verbal memory, and executive function (Freund, Reiss, & Abrams, 1993; Sobesky, Hull, & Hagerman, 1994). In addition, female carriers are more prone to depression and social anxiety and are often characterized as more affectively labile (Sobesky et al., 1994; Thompson, Rogeness, McClure, Clayton, & Johnson, 1996). These risk factors can be associated with lower responsivity, particularly the influence of maternal mental health on parent–child interactions (Goldsmith & Rogoff, 1995; Osofsky & Thompson, 2000).

It is important to note the genetic distinction between biological mothers of children with FXS and mothers of children with DS. Although both disorders are genetic in origin, mothers of children with FXS pass the gene directly to their children and as carriers may directly experience its effects at the premutation or full-mutation level. Mothers of children with FXS may struggle with the disorder in a very personal way, via their own mental health (Sobesky et al., 1994). Nevertheless, both groups of women experience a higher level of stress compared with mothers of typically developing children (Hodapp, Ly, Fidler, & Ricci, 2001; Roach, Orsmond, & Barratt, 1999).

Studies are now beginning to examine the role of maternal responsivity in the development of young children with FXS (Brady, Sterling, Warren, Fleming, & Marquis, 2006; Sterling, Brady, Warren, Fleming, & Marquis, 2006). Preliminary results indicate that there is a strong positive relationship between a highly responsive parenting style and cognitive and language development in young children with FXS, even when the children's cognitive development levels are controlled for. The presence of autism in children with FXS substantially impedes the employment of a highly responsive parenting style, just as it generally does for parents of children with autism without FXS. Preliminary data also suggest that mothers with the full mutation of FXS are more likely to have a less responsive, more directive parenting style than mothers with the premutation.

IMPLICATIONS FOR ASSESSMENT AND INTERVENTION

Our review indicates a number of ways in which young children with DS differ from young children with FXS in terms of early communication and language development. Nevertheless, the general needs in terms of assessment and intervention are remarkably similar in these two groups. First, virtually all young children with DS and all boys and many girls with FXS may benefit from intervention as early as possible. Valuable intervention may be provided in the first year of life for children with DS. In the absence of newborn screening, children with FXS are not likely to be specifically diagnosed until they are nearing their second birthday, sometimes later. Young boys with FXS, however, typically show sufficient developmental delays to qualify for early intervention services sometime during their second year of life, usually several months before they are actually diagnosed. The early and general nature of the communication-related delays in children with DS and boys and some girls with FXS has several specific implications for intervention.

Need for Prelinguistic Intervention

If children are still prelinguistic (e.g., use fewer than 10 nonimitative words or signs, understand fewer than 75 words receptively, make fewer than two intentional communication acts per minute), prelinguistic milieu teaching should initially be implemented under the direction of a speech-language pathologist (Warren et al., 2006). Once a child's communication level moves beyond these criteria, expressive vocabulary should be targeted using milieu language intervention techniques. These interventions are discussed in more detail in Chapter 7 in this book and in other publications (e.g., McCauley & Fey, 2006).

Need for Parent Training and Support

Direct child intervention should be supplemented with training and support aimed at helping parents create and maintain a highly responsive communication environment for their children throughout the day to the greatest extent possible (Girolametto & Weitzman, 2006). Many parents will already naturally engage in such a style, which is characterized by following their children's attentional lead, frequent conversational turn taking, and many comments and questions about their children's focus of attention (Richman, Miller, & LeVine, 1992). Other parents may be less experienced with this style of interaction. Nevertheless, nearly all parents can benefit from a training program that helps them achieve and maintain this style as naturally and effortlessly as possible. Speech-language pathologists trained in It Takes Two to Talk—The Hanen Program for Parents (see http://www.hanen.org) are often able to provide such a program in as few as eight 1-hour sessions. This approach is also discussed in Chapter 7 in this book and in other publications (e.g., Girolametto & Weitzman, 2006).

Need for Early Sign Instruction

Young children with DS as well as boys and some girls with FXS may benefit initially from learning a small number of highly functional signs (e.g., signs for "more," "mommy," and "daddy"; signs for favorite toys and foods). Early sign instruction is already used with many young children with DS. Although very little published research exists on the effects of early sign training with children with DS, there is no indication that acquiring signs interferes with learning to talk, and signs may even help children be more effective communicators prior to the onset of spoken language (Hopmann & Devenny, 1993).

Use of Augmentative and Alternative Communication Approaches

If a child with DS or FXS has not begun to speak by age 3, serious consideration should be given to implementing an augmentative and alternative communication approach, as these children may still learn to speak later in childhood. For more information on augmentative and alternative communication, please see Chapter 11.

Targeting Specific Areas of Skill Weakness

Children with DS or FXS have individual strengths and weaknesses. Specific areas of weakness may reflect a child's underlying phenotype or could simply reflect unique characteristics of the individual child. In any case, such weaknesses should be addressed via individualized family and/or child education plans, such as those systematically provided by early intervention programs. For example, an inability to imitate may impede communication and language development and disrupt intervention efforts. Similarly, the ability of a child to engage in joint attention with another individual is a pivotal skill in communication development. These types of pivotal skills should be taught to the extent possible in the context of everyday routines and interactions, just like other skills. The effectiveness of these efforts, however, may be improved by specifically focusing some intervention time directly on these areas in order to accelerate the effectiveness of more general intervention efforts.

FUTURE RESEARCH DIRECTIONS

We obviously know far more about early communication and language development of children with DS compared with children with FXS. The relatively high prevalence of DS coupled with fact that children with DS are identified before or at birth has facilitated a large amount of basic descriptive research since the 1970s. Nevertheless, much of what we do know about children with DS is based on studies with relatively small samples. Furthermore, some central issues exist that have received little investigation. Two of these issues are worth additional comment. First, although we know that children with DS have a specific profile of strengths and weaknesses, we do not know how these strengths and weaknesses interact to impede or enhance development. For example, does the relative weakness in short-term working memory displayed by children with DS support an overreliance on imitation in social interaction? Sokolov's (1992) study of linguistic imitation in 48 children with DS suggested that this may be the case and that this relative strength could actually complicate later language development. This and other dynamic interactions between relative strengths and weaknesses in pivotal abilities have been rarely studied even though they may hold the key to developing more effective interventions.

Second, recent research has shown that 8-week-old infants with DS are significantly less communicative and lively than typically developing infants and that by 20 weeks this was clearly affecting mother–child interaction (Slonims et al., 2006). We do not know, however, how much these patterns of mother–child interaction themselves contribute to delays and differences in communication and language development. Further research on mother–child interactions is important because it may hold the key to more effective interventions that seek to optimize the language learning environment as early as possible for children with DS.

Future research needs relative to children with FXS are more basic in nature. Because FXS is relatively rare, and newborn diagnoses are extremely rare, there has not yet been a single substantial prospective study of early communication and language development in children with FXS. Furthermore, most of the research that does exist with toddlers and older children has focused on creating mostly general profiles of development. Thus, research with children with FXS is still in its foundational stages, and our picture of this developmental period is spotty at best. It is difficult to see how this can change in the absence of research that corresponds with newborn screening efforts conducted in specific states, or clusters of states, or large cities. If, however, a large number of newborns could be screened for FXS, this picture could become much clearer over the next 5–10 years.

CONCLUSION

Both children with DS and children with FXS show delays in the development of communication skills. It seems that children with DS have a profile of strengths and weaknesses. Not enough research exists to date to make this same statement for children with FXS, particularly in very young children with FXS, although the growing body of research has allowed some insight into the challenges these young children face. The impact of parenting is of great importance, especially during this time period. Mothers of children with DS or FXS must cope with unique parenting challenges, especially mothers who are themselves carriers of the FXS gene. As knowledge of the phenotypes of these disorders increases, and as children are identified at earlier ages, researchers will be able to target interventions for parents and children starting at very young ages.

REFERENCES

Abbeduto, L., & Hagerman, R.J. (1997). Language and communication in fragile X syndrome. *Mental Retardation and Developmental Disabilities Research Reviews, 3,* 313–322.

Adamson, L.B., & Russell, C.L. (1999). Emotion regulation and the emergence of joint attention. In P. Rochat (Ed.), *Early social cognition: Understanding others in the first months of life* (pp. 281–297). Mahwah, NJ: Lawrence Erlbaum Associates.

Bailey, D.B., Mesibov, G.B., Hatton, D.D., Clark, R.D., Roberts, J.E., & Mayhew, L. (1998). Autistic behavior in young boys with fragile X syndrome. *Journal of Autism and Developmental Disorders, 28,* 499–508.

Barnes, S., Gutfreund, M., Satterly, D., & Wells, G. (1983). Characteristics of adult speech which predict children's language development. *Journal of Child Language, 10,* 65–84.

Bates, E. (1976). *Language and context.* New York: Academic Press.

Bates, E., Benigni, L., Bretherton, I., Camaioni, L., & Volterra, V. (1979). *The emergence of symbols: Cognition and communication in infancy.* New York: Academic Press.

Baumgardner, T.L., Reiss, A.L., Freund, L.S., & Abrams, M.T. (1995). Specifications of the neurobehavioral associations in males with fragile X syndrome. *Pediatrics, 95,* 744–752.

Bayley, N. (1969). *Bayley Scales of Infant Development: Birth to Two Years.* San Antonio, TX: The Psychological Corporation.

Benedict, H. (1979). Early lexical development: Comprehension and production. *Journal of Child Language, 6,* 183–200.

Berger, J. (1990). Interactions between parents and their infants with Down syndrome. In D. Cicchetti & M. Beeghly (Eds.), *Children with Down syndrome: A developmental perspective* (pp. 101–146). New York: Cambridge University Press.

Berger, J., & Cunningham, C. (1981). The development of eye contact between mothers and normal versus Down's syndrome infants. *Developmental Psychology, 17,* 678–689.

Berger, J., & Cunningham, C. (1983). The development of early vocal behaviors and interactions in Down syndrome and non-handicapped infant-mother pairs. *Developmental Psychology, 19,* 322–331.

Bloom, L. (1993). *The transition from infancy to language: Acquiring the power of expression.* New York: Cambridge University Press.

Brady, N., Sterling, A., Warren, S.F., Fleming, K., & Marquis, J. (2006, March). *How does maternal responsivity relate to communication skills in young children with fragile X syndrome?* Poster session presented at the Gatlinburg Conference on Research and Theory in Intellectual and Developmental Disabilities, San Diego, CA.

Calkins, S.D., Smith, C.L., Gill, K.L., & Johnson, M.C. (1998). Maternal interactive style across contexts: Relations to emotional, behavioral, and physiological regulation during toddlerhood. *Social Development, 7,* 350–369.

Cardoso-Martins, C., & Mervis, C.B. (1985). Maternal speech to prelinguistic children with Down syndrome. *American Journal of Mental Deficiency, 5,* 451–458.

Cardoso-Martins, C., Mervis, C.B., & Mervis, C.A. (1985). Early vocabulary acquisition by children with Down syndrome. *American Journal of Mental Deficiency, 90,* 177–184.

Caselli, M.C., & Casadio, P. (1995). *Il primo vocabolario del bambino.* Milano: Franco Angeli.

Caselli, M.C., Vicari, S., Longobardi, E., Lami, L., Pizzoli, C., & Stella, G. (1998). Gestures and words in early development of children with Down syndrome. *Journal of Speech, Language, and Hearing Research, 41,* 1125–1135.

Cicchetti, D., & Sroufe, L.A. (1976). The relationship between affective and cognitive development in Down's syndrome infants. *Child Development, 47,* 920–929.

Crawley, S.B., & Spiker, D. (1983). Mother-child interactions involving two-year-olds with Down syndrome: A look at individual differences. *Child Development, 54*, 1312–1323.

Dodd, B. (1975). Recognition and reproduction of words by Down's syndrome and non-Down's syndrome retarded children. *American Journal of Mental Deficiency, 80*, 306–311.

Dodd, B.J. (1972). Comparison of babbling patterns in normal and Down syndrome infants. *Journal of Mental Deficiency Research, 16*, 35–40.

Dykens, E.M., & Kasari, C. (1997). Maladaptive behavior in children with Prader-Willi syndrome, Down syndrome, and non-specific mental retardation. *American Journal on Mental Retardation, 102*, 228–237.

Dykens, E., & Volkmar, F. (1997). Medical conditions associated with autism. In D. Cohen & F. Volkmar (Eds.), *Handbook of autism and pervasive developmental disorders* (pp. 388–410). New York: Wiley.

Feinstein, C., & Reiss, A.L. (1998). Autism: The point of view from fragile X studies. *Journal of Autism and Developmental Disorders, 28*, 393–405.

Fenson, L., Dale, P.S., Reznick, J.S., Thal, D., Bates, E., Hartung, J.P., et al. (1992). *The MacArthur-Bates Communicative Development Inventories: User's guide and technical manual*. Baltimore: Paul H. Brookes Publishing Co.

Freund, L.S. Reiss, A.L., & Abrams, M.T. (1993). Psychiatric disorders associated with fragile X in the young female. *Pediatrics, 91*, 321–329.

Ganiban, J., Wagner, S., & Cicchetti, D. (1990). Temperament and Down syndrome. In D. Cicchetti & M. Beeghly (Eds.), *Children with Down syndrome: A developmental perspective* (pp. 63–100). New York: Cambridge University Press.

Gibbs, M.V., & Thorpe, J.G. (1983). Personality stereotype of noninstitutionalized Down syndrome children. *American Journal of Mental Deficiency, 87*, 601–605.

Gibson, D. (1978). *Down's syndrome: The psychology of mongolism*. Cambridge: Cambridge University Press.

Gillham, B. (1979). *The First Words Language Programme: A basic language programme for mentally handicapped children*. London: George Allen & Unwin.

Girolametto, L., & Weitzman, E. (2006). It Takes Two to Talk—The Hanen Program for Parents: Early language intervention through caregiver training. In S.F. Warren & M.E. Fey (Series Eds.) & R.J. McCauley & M.E. Fey (Vol. Eds.), *Communication and language intervention series: Treatment of language disorders in children* (pp. 77–103). Baltimore: Paul H. Brookes Publishing Co.

Girolametto, L., Weitzman, E., & Clements-Baartman, J. (1998). Vocabulary intervention for children with Down syndrome: Parent training using focused stimulation. *Infant-Toddler Intervention, 8*, 109–125.

Goldsmith, D.F., & Rogoff, B. (1995). Sensitivity and teaching by dysphoric and nondysphoric women in structured versus unstructured situations. *Developmental Psychology, 31*, 388–394.

Hagerman, R.J. (1996). Physical and behavioral phenotype. In R.J. Hagerman & A. Cronister (Eds.), *Fragile X syndrome: Diagnosis, treatment, and research* (2nd ed., pp. 3–87). Baltimore: The Johns Hopkins University Press.

Hagerman, R.J., & Falkenstein, A.R. (1987). An association between recurrent otitis media in infancy and later hyperactivity. *Clinical Pediatrics, 26*, 253–257.

Hall, K.D. (2001). *Pediatric dysphagia: Resource guide*. San Diego: Singular, Thompson Learning.

Hanson, D.M., Jackson, A.W., & Hagerman, P.J. (1986). Speech disturbances (cluttering) in mildly impaired males with the Martin-Bell/fragile X syndrome. *American Journal of Medical Genetics, 23*, 195–206.

Hepper, P.G. (2002). Prenatal development. In A. Slater & M. Lewis (Eds.), *Introduction to infant development* (pp. 39–60). Oxford: Oxford University Press.

Hodapp, R.M., Leckman, J.F., Dykens, E.M., Sparrow, S.S., Zelinsky, D.G., & Ort, S.I. (1992). K-ABC profiles in children with fragile X syndrome, Down syndrome and non-specific mental retardation. *American Journal of Mental Retardation, 97*, 39–46.

Hodapp, R.M., Ly, T.M., Fidler, D.J., & Ricci, L.A. (2001). Less stress, more rewarding: Parenting children with Down syndrome. *Parenting: Science and Practice, 1*, 317–337.

Hooper, S., Burchinal, M., Roberts, E.J., Zeisel, S., & Neebe, E. (1998). Social and family risk factors for infant development at one year: An application of the cumulative risk model. *Journal of Applied Developmental Psychology, 19*, 85–96.

Hopmann, M.R., & Devenny, D.A. (1993). The use of signs by children with Down syndrome. *Down Syndrome Today, 2*(2), 22–23.

Hupp, S.C., & Abbeduto, L. (1991). Persistence as an indicator of mastery motivation in young children with cognitive delays. *Journal of Early Intervention, 15,* 219–225.

Kasari, C., Mundy, P., Yirmiya, N., & Sigman, M. (1990). Affect and attention in children with Down syndrome. *American Journal on Mental Retardation, 95,* 55–67.

Knieps, L., Walden, T.A., & Baxter, A. (1994). Affective expressions of toddlers with and without Down syndrome in a social referencing context. *American Journal on Mental Retardation, 99,* 301–312.

Kumin, L. (1994). Intelligibility of speech in children with Down syndrome in natural settings: Parents' perspective. *Perceptual and Motor Skills, 78,* 307–313.

Kumin, L. (1996). Speech and language skills in children with Down syndrome. *Mental Retardation and Developmental Disabilities, 2,* 109–115.

Kumin, L., Councill, C., & Goodman, M. (1999). Expressive vocabulary in young children with Down syndrome: From research to treatment. *Infant-Toddler Intervention, 9,* 87–100.

Kumin, L., Goodman, M., & Councill, C. (1991). Comprehensive communication intervention for school-aged children with Down syndrome. *Infant-Toddler Intervention, 1,* 275–296.

Landry, S.H., Garner, P.W., Swank, P.R., & Baldwin, C.D. (1996). Effects of maternal scaffolding during joint toy play with preterm and full-term infants. *Merrill-Palmer Quarterly, 42,* 177–199.

Landry, S.H., Smith, K.E., Miller-Loncar, C.L., & Swank, P.R. (1998). The relation of change in maternal interactive styles to the developing social competence of full-term and preterm children. *Child Development, 69,* 105–123.

Landry, S.H., Smith, K.E., Swank, P.R., Assel, M.A., & Vellet, S. (2001). Does early responsive parenting have a special importance for children's development or is consistency across early childhood necessary? *Developmental Psychology, 37,* 387–403.

Lynch, M.P., Oller, D.K., Steffens, M.L., & Levine, S.L. (1995). Onset of speech-like vocalizations in infants with Down syndrome. *American Journal on Mental Retardation, 100,* 68–86.

Marfo, K. (1990). Maternal directiveness in interactions with mentally handicapped children: An analytical commentary. *Journal of Child Psychology and Psychiatry, 31,* 531–549.

McCathren, R.B., Yoder, P.J., & Warren, S.F. (1995). The role of directives in early language intervention. *Journal of Early Intervention, 19,* 91–101.

McCauley, R.J., & Fey, M.E. (Vol. Eds.) & Warren, S.F., & Fey, M.E. (Series Eds.). (2006). *Communication and language intervention series: Treatment of language disorders in children.* Baltimore: Paul H. Brookes Publishing Co.

McEvoy, R., Rogers, S., & Pennington, B. (1993). Executive function and social communication deficits in young autistic children. *Journal of Child Psychology and Psychiatry, 34,* 563–578.

Meltzoff, A., & Gopnik, A. (1993). The role of imitation in understanding persons and developing a theory of mind. In S. Baron-Cohen, H. Tager-Flusberg, & D.J. Cohen (Eds.), *Understanding other minds* (pp. 335–366). Oxford: Oxford University Press.

Miller, C.L., Miceli, P.J., Whitman, T.L., & Borkowski, J.G. (1996). Cognitive readiness to parent and intellectual-emotional development in children of adolescent mothers. *Developmental Psychology, 32,* 533–541.

Miller, J.F. (1987). Language and communication characteristics of children with Down syndrome. In S. Pueschel (Ed.), *New perspectives in Down syndrome* (pp. 232–262). Baltimore: Paul H. Brookes Publishing Co.

Miller, J.F. (1992). Development of speech and language in children with Down syndrome. In I.T. Lott & E.E. McCoy (Eds.), *Down syndrome: Advances in medical care* (pp. 39–50). New York: Wiley-Liss, Inc.

Mundy, P., Kasari, C., Sigman, M., & Ruskin, E. (1995). Nonverbal communication and early language acquisition in children with Down syndrome and in normally developing children. *Journal of Speech and Hearing Research, 38,* 157–167.

Mundy, P., Sigman, M., Kasari, C., & Yirmiya, N. (1988). Nonverbal communication skills in Down syndrome children. *Child Development, 59,* 235–249.

Murphy, M.M., & Abbeduto, L. (2005). Indirect genetic effects and the early language development of children with genetic mental retardation syndromes: The role of joint attention. *Infants & Young Children, 18,* 47–59.

Nadel, J., Guerini, C., Peze, A., & Rivet, C. (1999). The evolving nature of imitation as a format for communication. In J. Nadel & G. Butterworth (Eds.), *Imitation in infancy* (pp. 209–234). Cambridge, England: Cambridge University Press.

Nadel, J., & Peze, A. (1993). What makes immediate imitation communicative in toddlers and autistic children? In J. Nadel & L. Camaioni (Eds.), *New perspectives in early communication development* (pp. 139–156). London: Routledge.

Nelson, K. (1983). Structure and strategy in learning to talk. *Monographs of the Society for Research in Child Development, 38,* 1–2.

Osofsky, J.D., & Thompson, M.D. (2000). Adaptive and maladaptive parenting: Perspectives on risk and protective factors. In J.P. Shonkoff & S.J. Meisels (Eds.), *Handbook of early childhood intervention* (pp. 54–75). New York: Cambridge University Press.

Paradise, J.L. (1998). Otitis media and child development: Should we worry? *Pediatrics Infectious Disease Journal, 17,* 1076–1083.

Partington, M.W. (1984). The fragile X syndrome: Preliminary data on growth and development in males. *American Journal of Medical Genetics, 17,* 175–194.

Rast, M., & Meltzoff, A.N. (1995). Memory and representation in young children with Down syndrome: Exploring deferred imitation and object permanence. *Development and Psychopathology, 7,* 393–407.

Remington, B., & Clarke, S. (1996). Alternative and augmentative systems of communication for children with Down's syndrome. In J. Rondal, J. Perera, & L. Nadel (Eds.), *Down syndrome: psychological, psychobiological, and socio-educational perspectives* (pp. 129–143). London: Whurr.

Reynell, J.K., & Gruber, C.P. (1990). *Reynell Developmental Language Scales.* Los Angeles: Western Psychological Services.

Richman, A.L., Miller, P.M., & LeVine, R.A. (1992). Cultural and educational variations in maternal responsiveness. *Developmental Psychology, 28*(4), 614–621.

Roach, M.A., Barratt, M.S., Miller, J.F., & Leavitt, L.A. (1998). The structure of mother–child play: Young children with Down syndrome and typically developing children. *Developmental Psychology, 34,* 77–87.

Roach, M.A., Orsmond, G.I., & Barratt, M.S. (1999). Mothers and fathers of children with Down syndrome: Parental stress and involvement in childcare. *American Journal on Mental Retardation, 104,* 422–436.

Roberts, J.E., Burchinal, M.R., & Zeisel, S.A. (2002). Otitis media in early childhood relation to children's school-age language and academic skills. *Pediatrics, 110,* 1–11.

Roberts, J.E., Hatton, D.D., & Bailey, D.B. (2001). Development and behavior of male toddlers with fragile X syndrome. *Journal of Early Intervention, 24,* 207–223.

Roberts, J.E., Hunter, L., Gravel, J., Rosenfeld, R., Berman, S., Haggard, M., et al. (2004). Otitis media, hearing loss, and language learning: Controversies and current research. *Developmental Pediatrics, 25,* 110–122.

Roberts, J.E., & Medley, L. (1995). Otitis media and speech-language sequelae in young children: Current issues in management. *American Journal of Speech-Language Pathology, 4,* 15–24.

Roberts, J.E., Mirrett, P., Anderson, K., Burchinal, M., & Neebe, E. (2002). Early communication, symbolic behavior, and social profiles of young males with fragile X syndrome. *American Journal of Speech Language Pathology, 11,* 295–304.

Roberts, J.E., Mirrett, P., & Burchinal, M. (2001). Receptive and expressive communication development of young males with fragile X syndrome. *American Journal on Mental Retardation, 106,* 216–230.

Rogers, S.J., Hepburn, S.L., Stackhouse, T., & Wehner, E. (2003). Imitation performance in toddlers with autism and those with other developmental disorders. *Journal of Child Psychology and Psychiatry, 44,* 763–781.

Rogers, S.J., Wehner, E.A., & Hagerman, R. (2001). The behavioral phenotype in fragile X: Symptoms of autism in very young children with fragile X syndrome, idiopathic autism, and other developmental disorders. *Developmental and Behavioral Pediatrics, 22,* 409–417.

Rovers, M.M., Straatman, H., Ingels, K., van der Wilt, G.J., van den Broek, P., & Zielhuis, G.A. (2000). The effect of ventilation tubes on hearing development in infants with otitis media with effusion: A randomized trial. *Pediatrics, 106*, e42.

Rutter, M., & Quinton, D. (1984). Parental psychiatric disorders: Effects on children. *Psychological Medicine, 14*, 853–880.

Scharfenaker, S., Hickman, L., & Braden, M. (1996). An integrated approach to intervention. In R.J. Hagerman & A. Cronister (Eds.), *Fragile X syndrome: Diagnosis, treatment, and research* (2nd ed., pp. 327–372). Baltimore: The Johns Hopkins University Press.

Schwartz, D.M., & Schwartz, R.H. (1978). Acoustic impedance and otoscopic findings in young children with Down's syndrome. *Archives of Otolaryngology, 104*, 652–656.

Simeonsson, R.J., & Bailey, D.B. (1991). *The ABILITIES Index.* Chapel Hill: University of North Carolina.

Simko, A., Hornstein, L., Soukup, S., & Bagamery, N. (1989). Fragile X syndrome: Recognition in young children. *Pediatrics, 83*, 547–552.

Slonims, V., Cox, A., & McConachie, H. (2006). Analysis of mother-infant interaction in infants with Down syndrome and typically developing infants. *American Journal on Mental Retardation, 111*(4), 273–289.

Smith, B.L. (1984). Implications of infant vocalizations for assessing phonological disorders. In N.J. Lass (Ed.), *Speech and language: Advances in basic research* (Vol. 11, pp. 169–194). New York: Academic Press.

Smith, B.L., & Oller, D.K. (1981). A comparative study of pre-meaningful vocalizations produced by normally developing and Down's syndrome infants. *Journal of Speech and Hearing Disorders, 46*, 46–51.

Smith, L., & Tetzchner, S. (1986). Communicative, sensorimotor, and language skills of young children with Down syndrome. *American Journal of Mental Deficiency, 91*, 57–66.

Sobesky, W.E., Hull, C.E., & Hagerman, R.J. (1994). Symptoms of schizotypal personality disorder in fragile X women. *Journal of the American Academy of Child and Adolescent Psychiatry, 33*, 247–255.

Sokolov, J.L. (1992). Linguistic imitation in children with Down syndrome. *American Journal of Mental Retardation, 97*, 209–221.

Speidel, G.E., & Nelson, K.E. (Eds.). (1989). *The many faces of imitation in language learning.* New York: Springer-Verlag.

Spender, Q., Dennis, J., Stein, A., Cave, D., Percy, E., & Reilly, S. (1995). Impaired oral-motor function with Down's syndrome: A study of three twin pairs. *European Journal of Disorders of Communication, 30*, 77–87.

Spender, Q., Stein, A., Dennis, J., Reilly, S., Percy, E., & Cave, D. (1996). An exploration of feeding difficulties in children with DS. *Developmental Medicine and Child Neurology, 38*, 681–694.

Sterling, A., Brady, N., Warren, S.F., Fleming, K., & Marquis, J. (2006, March). *What factors influence maternal responsivity of young children with fragile X syndrome (FXS)?* Poster session presented at the Gatlinburg Conference on Research and Theory in Intellectual and Developmental Disabilities, San Diego, CA.

Stern, D.N. (1985). *The interpersonal world of the human infant.* New York: Basic Books.

Stoel-Gammon, C. (1997). Phonological development in Down syndrome. *Mental Retardation and Developmental Disabilities Research Reviews, 3*, 300–306.

Stray-Gunderson, K. (1986). *Babies with Down syndrome: A new parents guide.* Rockville, MD: Woodbine House.

Strome, S.E., & Strome, M. (1992). Down syndrome: An otolaryngologic perspective. *Journal of Otolaryngology, 21*, 394–397.

Tager-Flusberg, H., & Sullivan, K. (1998). Early language development in children with mental retardation. In J.A. Burack, R.M. Hodapp, & E. Zigler (Eds.), *Handbook of mental retardation* (pp. 208–239). Cambridge, England: Cambridge University Press.

Tannock, R. (1988). Mothers' directiveness in their interactions with their children with and without Down syndrome. *American Journal of Mental Retardation, 93*, 154–165.

Thompson, N.M., Rogeness, G.A., McClure, E., Clayton, R., & Johnson, C. (1996). Influence of depression on cognitive functioning in fragile X females. *Psychiatry Research, 64*, 97–104.

Tomasello, M., & Farrar, M.J. (1986). Joint attention and early language. *Child Development, 57,* 1454–1463.

Uzgiris, I.C. (1999). Imitation as activity: Its developmental aspects. In J. Nadel & G. Butterworth (Eds.), *Imitation in infancy* (pp. 186–206). Cambridge, England: Cambridge University Press.

Warren, S.F. (2004). Intervention as experiment. In R. Rice and S. Warren (Eds.), *Developmental language disorders: From phenotypes to etiologies* (pp. 187–206). Mahwah, NJ: Lawrence Erlbaum Associates.

Warren, S.F., Bredin-Oja, S.L., Fairchild, M., Finestack, L.H., Fey, M.E., & Brady, N.C. (2006). Responsivity education: Prelinguistic milieu teaching. In S.F. Warren & M.E. Fey (Series Eds.) & R.J. McCauley & M.E. Fey (Vol. Eds.), *Communication and language intervention series: Treatment of language disorders in children* (pp. 47–103). Baltimore: Paul H. Brookes Publishing Co.

Wetherby, A.M., & Prizant, B.M. (1993). *Communication and Symbolic Behavior Scales™.* Baltimore: Paul H. Brookes Publishing Co.

Wishart, J.G., & Johnston, F.H. (1990). The effects of experience on attribution of a stereotyped personality to children with Down's syndrome. *Journal of Mental Deficiency Research, 34,* 409–420.

Wright, I., Lewis, V., & Collis, G.M. (2006). Imitation and representational development in young children with Down syndrome. *British Journal of Developmental Psychology, 24,* 429–450.

CHAPTER 4

Language of Preschool and School-Age Children with Down Syndrome and Fragile X Syndrome

JOANNE E. ROBERTS, ROBIN S. CHAPMAN,
GARY E. MARTIN, AND LAUREN MOSKOWITZ

C hildren with Down syndrome (DS) and children with fragile X syndrome (FXS) generally have language difficulties, although there is considerable variability among children (Abbeduto & Chapman, 2005; Rice, Warren, & Betz, 2005). DS is the most common genetic cause of intellectual disability (ID), and FXS is the most common inherited genetic cause of ID. Although language delays are common in both children with DS and children with FXS, the specific profile of language skills differs in the two populations, as do some of the potential mechanisms that explain language difficulties. An understanding of the similarities and differences in the language phenotype of individuals with DS and individuals with FXS, as well as the possible causes and contributory factors, will reveal important implications for language assessment and intervention for these populations.

This chapter discusses the development of language in children with DS and FXS during the preschool and school-age years. We begin by describing language development in typical populations during the preschool and school-age years. Findings in receptive and expressive language are cited, focusing on three domains of language—vocabulary, syntax, and pragmatics. The chapter explores whether children with DS and children with FXS have language difficulties that reflect a general language delay commensurate with the children's mental level (i.e., degree of ID) or a language profile specific to DS or FXS. Underlying mechanisms that may explain language difficulties are also explained. Focus is placed on language development during the preschool and school-age years, and strategies are suggested for language assessment and intervention, as well as for parent involvement for children with DS or FXS. Throughout the chapter, suggestions for future research are cited and discussed.

LANGUAGE OF TYPICALLY DEVELOPING PRESCHOOL AND SCHOOL-AGE CHILDREN

Examination of language acquisition in typically developing children provides insight into the language learning process and whether there are differences in the acquisition process for children with DS and children with FXS. A brief summary of language acquisition in vocabulary, syntax, and pragmatics in typically developing children follows. These domains are discussed in the contexts of language comprehension and production. *Language comprehension,* also called *receptive language,* refers to one's ability to understand the language of others. *Language production,* also called *expressive language,* usually refers to spoken language but also includes manual signs and written language, all of which convey messages to a listener using words and sentences. See Gleason (2005) and Paul (2007) for further details of typical language development.

Vocabulary

Vocabulary refers to the rules for meanings of words. A particular word has many characteristics that determine its meaning, and a child must learn the critical factors when acquiring the use of a word. Children's early words relate to the most meaningful people and things in their environment (e.g., "mommy," "daddy," "milk"). At approximately 18 months, children produce nearly 50 words, understand as many as 300, and begin to combine words into multiword utterances (e.g., "Baby cry," "Daddy eat pie"). By the age of 2 years, word knowledge dramatically increases, and words are used for many purposes such as to indicate location (e.g., "ball floor") or possession (e.g., "my car"). Approximately 500 words are produced and 1,000 words understood at $2^{1}/_{2}$–3 years of age. At 3–5 years, children use more complex concepts (e.g., quantity, spatial relationships) and begin talking about causality, mental states, and temporal relations. At approximately 5 years, they begin using more advanced conjunctions (e.g., "when," "because") and develop metalinguistic knowledge to identify grammatical versus ungrammatical utterances and to segment words into phonemes. By the age of 7 years, expressive vocabulary increases to a range of 3,000–12,000 words. Between the ages of 9 and 12 years, school and the ability to read facilitate new word learning, particularly in the acquisition of a literate lexicon or words that occur in school (e.g., *assume, examine, develop*), along with the use of abstract concepts such as definitions and figurative expressions (e.g., *She's a whirlwind*).

Syntax

Syntax refers to the rule system for putting words together to form phrases and sentences. Syntactic rules are gradually acquired as children begin to combine words. One-word utterances are usually present at approximately 12 months, two-word utterances at approximately 18 months, and three-word utterances at approximately 2 years. The 2- to $2^{1}/_{2}$-year-old may produce many two- and three-word utterances but will also continue to produce one-word utterances and may even occasionally use a six-word utterance. The child then begins to use different sentence types such as negatives (e.g., "She not little"), questions (e.g.,

"Mommy sleeping?"), and imperatives (e.g., "Gimme that!"), although early forms may not be grammatically correct. At approximately 3 years of age, a typically developing child begins to use complex sentence structures to join and embed clauses, (e.g., "Mommy says that the doggie's crying."). By the time a child reaches the age of 5 years, basic and complex syntactic structures are established, yet the refinement of complex sentence usage continues throughout the school years. The 7- to 9-year-old child begins to develop syntax for literate language, and by 12 years, he or she is able to use more complex syntax for logical relationships (e.g., "Dad sold the car because it was too small") and for academic settings and writing (e.g., "Insects balance the food chain for all animals").

Pragmatics

Pragmatics refers to the use of language for social interaction. Three different aspects of pragmatics are commonly examined: intentions, discourse, and narration. A person speaks with communicative intentions (e.g., to request an object, to protest something, to share information). *Discourse* refers to the conversational interaction between two or more individuals in which the individuals take turns to maintain or change a topic and repair or modify communication when it is unclear. Narration refers to the use of language for telling or recounting a story or experience. Early nonverbal turn-taking interactions between infants and their caregivers (e.g., when a caregiver comments on an infant's unintentional facial expressions or eye gaze) form the basis for later turn-taking in conversation. Between 9 and 12 months, infants begin to consistently and intentionally use gestures and vocalizations to communicate. The 2-year-old can request information, provide an answer to a question, and acknowledge the other speaker. Between 3 and 3½ years, the child maintains a conversational topic and provides new information regarding that topic. By 4 years, a child's language focuses not only on the immediate environment but also on events and people more distant in time, including topics from the past and potential topics in the future. The child can adjust language to the listeners' abilities and provide a narrative, which may jump from event to event without many temporal and causal relationships. By 5 years, most children can maintain a topic 80% of the time, and their narratives contain unifying schemes, although they may not indicate a resolution to that narrative. Between the ages of 7 and 9 years, a child can understand another person's point of view and provide conversational repairs by defining terms that are unclear to the listener. By 12 years, a child can make coherent transitions between topics and produce narratives that include referencing of thoughts and feelings about a story's events and resolution.

LANGUAGE OF PRESCHOOL AND
SCHOOL-AGE CHILDREN WITH DOWN SYNDROME

Expressive language difficulties are generally present from infancy in children with DS, and some of the phenotypic characteristics of language seen in DS, such as grammatical impairments, are present by 2–3 years of age (Fidler, 2005; Fidler, Hepburn & Rogers, 2006; Miller, 1988, 1995; for review, see Chapman & Hesketh, 2000). In a study of eighty 1- to 11-year-old children with DS, a significant weakness in communication relative to daily living and socialization skills was found in children's profiles (Dykens, Hodapp, & Evans, 2006). Toddlers with DS have also been found to show stronger social skills and weaker expressive language compared with groups of children of mixed developmental disabilities and typically developing children matched for mental age (Fidler et al., 2006). The proportion of children with DS showing expressive deficits increases at age 4 years, and the gap between expressive and receptive skills widens during school-age years (Chapman, Hesketh, & Kistler, 2002; Miller, 1995). Expressive syntax as measured by mean length of utterance (MLU), particularly grammatical morpheme acquisition, is delayed relative to syntax comprehension (Caselli et al., 1998; Chapman, Seung, Schwartz, & Kay-Raining Bird, 1998; Eadie, Fey, Douglas, & Parsons, 2002; Fowler, 1988). Among 4- to 7-year-old children with DS, morphosyntactic skills are weaker in both comprehension and production than lexical skills (Vicari, Caselli, & Tonucci, 2000).

Language Comprehension

Receptive Vocabulary

Although receptive vocabulary appears to be a relative strength in children with DS, findings are inconsistent as to whether receptive vocabulary is equivalent to mental age expectations. Review of early childhood data finds receptive vocabulary to be a strength. Lexical comprehension of children with DS kept pace with expectations based on mental age in early childhood (Miller, 1995), as reported by parents on the MacArthur Communicative Development Inventories (Fenson et al., 1992). Chapman, Schwartz, and Kay-Raining Bird (1991) also reported vocabulary levels commensurate with nonverbal mental age in children and adolescents. However, a few studies have found lower receptive vocabulary levels in children with DS as compared with those of typically developing children of similar nonverbal mental age (Hick, Botting, & Conti-Ramsden, 2005; Roberts, Price, et al., 2007; Price, Roberts, Vandergrift, & Martin, 2007). Thus, findings as to whether vocabulary comprehension is similar to nonverbal cognitive levels in children with DS differed among studies depending on the children's age, language, and cognitive measure used and whether language and mental age were compared within the same child with DS (within individual) or with typically developing children of the same mental age (between group).

A selective and narrow deficit in comprehension of words for the emotion of fear (e.g., *frightened, scared*), but not for anger (e.g., *mad*), was demonstrated in children with DS who were asked to choose faces that matched the emotion word (Williams, Wishart, Pitcairn, & Willis, 2005; Wishart, Cebula, Willis, & Pitcairn, 2007; Wishart & Pitcairn, 2000). Comprehension of mental state verbs, as well as others' states of mind on theory of mind tasks, also shows additional delay in the later school years (Abbeduto et al., 2001; Abbeduto, Short-Meyerson, Benson, & Dolish, 2004; Yirmiya, Erel, Shaked, & Solomonica-Levi, 1998; Zelazo, Burack, Benedetto, & Frye, 1996).

Receptive Syntax

Findings as to whether children with DS show receptive syntax deficits relative to nonverbal cognitive levels vary by study, partly as a function of the nonverbal tests used to match for mental age and whether hearing loss was examined as a predictor. Comprehension of syntax, as assessed by standardized testing using visual nonverbal cognition and visual short-term memory averages (Thorndike, Hagen, & Sattler, 1986) was commensurate with expectations based on nonverbal mental age in children with DS between the ages of 5 and 12 years (Chapman et al., 1991). Individual performance on syntax comprehension tests ranged in age-equivalent scores from less than 3–4 years in 5- to 8-year-olds and from 3–5 years in 8- to 12-year-olds (Chapman et al., 2002). Longitudinal follow-up of these children across 6 years showed gains for almost all preadolescent children. Most of the 5- to 8-year-old group made a half-year gain, although one child made 2 years of growth, and one child made none. Of the 8- to 12-year-olds in that longitudinal study, three showed almost a year of gain, five showed approximately half a year or less, and one showed no change in the linear trajectories across 6 years (Chapman et al., 2002).

In one recent study (Price, Roberts, Vandergrift, & Martin, 2007), comprehension of grammatical morphology was delayed compared with nonverbal mental age expectations based on the Leiter International Performance Scale–Revised (Roid & Miller, 1997). Comprehension was delayed in a study of children and adolescents with DS that examined the extent of mild hearing impairment (Chapman et al., 1991). Price and colleagues (2007) also compared the comprehension of grammatical morphology and elaborated phrases and sentences of boys with DS and typically developing boys, using a standardized language test. They found that the boys with DS scored lower than the typical group on comprehension of grammatical morphology and elaborated phrases and sentences.

Language Production

Expressive Vocabulary

Expressive vocabulary skills in children with DS appear delayed relative to expectations for mental age (Fidler et al., 2006; Miller, 1995). Children with DS vary widely in the onset of first words. Early studies reported the first spoken words to emerge between 1 and 6 years (Gillham, 1990); a range of 0–85 words at 3 years (Strominger, Winkler, & Cohen 1984); and the first 50 words to emerge between $3^1/_2$ and 6 years (Gillham, 1990). One report indicated that more initial words were spoken than one would expect based on mental age measures (Cardoso-Martins, Mervis, & Mervis, 1985). More recent studies confirm that the growth of spoken vocabulary is slow for most children with DS (Berglund & Eriksson, 2000; Berglund, Eriksson, & Johansson, 2001; Caselli et al., 1998; Mervis & Robinson, 2000). It is possible that speech intelligibility problems may interfere with the identification of words.

The rate of expressive vocabulary learning, including signs, as reported by parents in a longitudinal study of preschool children with DS, was, on average, slower than expected based on mental age, even when signing was taken into account, although it was better than expressive syntax (Miller, 1995). At the same time, individual variability was wide, and 35% of the children with DS studied by Miller had expressive vocabularies consistent with expectations based on mental age. In a large-scale study of word learning in 330 Swedish children with DS ranging in age from 1 to 5 years, parents reported that children with DS used productive words and sentences at 3 years similar to typically developing children of 16 months and at 4 years similar to typically developing children of 20 months (Berglund et al., 2001).

Older children with DS show expressive vocabulary deficits relative to nonverbal cognitive levels. Expressive vocabulary levels on standardized tests and during language samples for children and adolescents with DS were delayed relative to nonverbal cognitive levels and/or comparison groups of younger typically developing boys at similar mental ages (Chapman et al., 1998; Laws & Bishop, 2003; Miller, 1988; Roberts, Price, et al., 2007).

The ability of children and adolescents with DS to label emotions and identify them in stories suggests specific deficits in the labeling of both fear and anger (Kasari, Freeman, & Hughes, 2001). Verbs of emotion and mental state were less frequent in language samples obtained from children and adolescents with DS than expected on the basis of their expressive language level, as indexed by MLU (Hesketh & Chapman, 1998).

Word Learning   Children can learn novel words for new objects and actions in only a few encounters; this process is called *fast mapping* (Chapman, Kay-Raining Bird, & Schwartz, 1990). The child may be able to remember which novel object or action goes with a word, remember the location of the object or action, and even say the word on later testing. The fast-mapping comprehension skill of children with DS is comparable to that of a comparison group matched for nonverbal mental age for a single novel object encountered in a hiding task (Chapman et al., 1990), although increases in the number of items to be fast-mapped reveals less learning (Chapman, 2003). Fast mapping of new vocabulary in production appears similar to groups matched for nonverbal mental age for single words (Chapman et al.,1990) but exhibits some decrement for multiple novel words, as well as for verb vocabulary (Chapman, 2003).

Expressive Syntax

Expressive syntax is delayed relative to mental age expectations in children with DS. In one study, two-word combinations appeared as early as nonverbal cognitive performance would be expected (Miller, 1995), but the emergence of two-word combinations was delayed in many children with DS, with a more prolonged period in which single words co-occur with gestures observed among 4-year-olds (Iverson, Longobardi, & Caselli, 2003). In comparison to typically developing children matched for expressive vocabulary size, preschool children with DS lag slightly on expressive grammar scales, and these delays in grammar are greater than delays in expressive vocabulary for preschoolers with DS (Berglund & Eriksson, 2000; Berglund et al., 2001).

In children with DS, there is considerable evidence for expressive language delays, both as measured by shorter utterances (MLU) compared with younger mental age–matched typically developing children (Chapman et al., 1998; Miller, 1988) and measured by grammatical morpheme production compared with MLU-matched typically developing children (Chapman et al., 1998; Eadie et al., 2002). The children with DS had more frequent omissions of grammatical function words (e.g., articles, prepositions, forms of the verb and auxiliary *be*, verb past tense *-ed*, third person singular *-s*, noun plurals). Children with DS used fewer modal auxiliaries (e.g., *can, may, will*) and lexical verbs (e.g., main verbs other than *have, do,* and *be*) than a comparison group of MLU-matched typically developing children (Hesketh & Chapman, 1998). In another study, grammatical complexity of sentences spoken in conversation by older school-age boys with DS as compared with typically developing boys of similar mental age showed deficits in MLU and overall grammatical complexity, including noun phrases, verb phrases, questions and negations, and sentence structure (Price, Roberts, et al., in press). Although children with DS acquire grammatical morphemes in the same developmental order as typically developing children, morphosyntactic acquisition is delayed relative to expressive sentence length (Berglund et al., 2001).

Pragmatics

Pragmatics is an area of both strengths and weaknesses for children with DS. Toddlers with DS show strengths in social interaction (Dykens et al., 2006) that extend to some but not all communicative interchanges. When compared with children who were typically developing and language age–matched, children with DS show similar rates of commenting but lower rates of requesting (Mundy, Kasari, Sigman, & Ruskin, 1995). This finding may be related to the observation that children with DS prefer face-to-face interaction over object play in nonverbal communication (Mundy, Sigman, Kasari, & Yirmiya, 1988). However, one study of four children found that children with DS use the same range of communicative functions in conversation with their mothers as typically developing children of the same language level (Coggins, Carpenter, & Owings, 1983). Coggins and Stoel-Gammon (1982) found that four children with DS repaired all communication breakdowns when their conversational partner asked for clarification.

Preschoolers with DS stay on topic in interaction with their mothers as often as children matched for mental age and communication level (Tannock, 1988), but they are less likely to introduce new topics. A similar finding was reported by Beeghly, Weiss-Perry, and Cicchetti (1990) in a larger sample of children with DS who used fewer requests with adults but who did not differ in topic maintenance or their use of answers, comments, and protests compared with developmental age–matched children. In comparison to MLU-matched children who were developmentally younger, the children with DS stayed on topic for more turns and offered more appropriate conversational responses to adults.

In a more recent study, Roberts, Martin, and colleagues (2007) compared the conversational interactions of boys with DS talking with a trained examiner with those of typically developing boys of similar cognitive level. The boys with DS were less elaborative when maintaining topics and produced a higher proportion of turns that were only adequate in quality (e.g., simple responses and acknowledgments) when compared with typically developing boys at similar mental levels.

For narratives, mention of salient events, themes, and plot elements in narrative reports of wordless video events and storybooks are at levels commensurate with cognitive level and language comprehension in children and adolescents with DS despite their more limited MLU, sentence complexity, and vocabulary use (Boudreau & Chapman, 2000; Miles & Chapman, 2002). The narratives produced by participants with DS have more utterances than those of typically developing children matched for nonverbal mental age (Chapman et al., 1998). In contrast, the amount recalled in retelling of stories presented verbally without picture support was less for children and adolescents with DS than for mental age–matched children (Kay-Raining Bird, Chapman, & Schwartz, 2004).

Summary

A wide range of individual differences in language skills can be found in children with DS, but the relation of skills to one another in an individual child shows an emerging phenotypic pattern typical of DS. As they grow older, children with DS show increasing lags in expressive language relative to their skills in comprehension and nonverbal cognition. Expressive vocabulary, sentence length, syntactic complexity, and the use of grammatical morphemes are all affected, with the greatest lags seen in syntax and grammatical morpheme use. Pragmatic skills are strengths when they do not depend on syntactic skills and lexical access. Language comprehension is overall less delayed than language production in children with DS. In some language areas such as comprehension of vocabulary, the findings are not clear whether children with DS have nonverbal cognitive levels that are stronger than their language levels. Differences in findings of studies examining whether a particular language domain differs from mental age expectations are due to differences in children's ages when they were tested (i.e., the relation between language and cognition changes as children with DS get older) (Roberts, Price, et al., 2007; Chapman, Seung, Schwartz, & Kay-Raining Bird, 2000), methods of language assessment (e.g., linguistic complexity elicited, standardized test versus conversational sample), method of cognitive assessment (e.g., demand for visual memory), and whether language–nonverbal cognitive comparisons were made within or between samples (i.e., among children with DS versus comparing a DS group with a mental age–matched typical group).

   Future studies of language learning in children with DS should focus on individual differences in acquisition of vocabulary, syntax, and pragmatics. Of particular interest in vocabulary development is verb acquisition, especially for emotional and mental state verbs, and the relation of this learning to children's emotion recognition and the subsequent emergence of complex syntax. For syntax, the effect of providing visual and auditory support for comprehension of and the use of grammatical morphemes is important. Identification of contexts in addition to narratives that encourage the use of complex syntax, and ways to support speed of lexical access in these more complex language tasks (e.g., the wordless picture books studied by Miles, Chapman, & Sindberg, 2006), are important for understanding expressive syntax acquisition. Pragmatic skills should be studied in both conversation and narration, with a particular focus on the ways in which children initiate interactions and make requests for clarification. Comparisons of whether language skills are more delayed relative to mental age, especially for language comprehension measures, requires further study. Longitudinal studies also are needed to examine growth in language skills in children with DS and factors that affect growth.

Possible Mechanisms Underlying Language Learning in Children with Down Syndrome

Multiple factors contribute to the rate of language learning in children in general and in children with DS. To understand the language phenotype of DS and the considerable individual differences in language profiles, it is important to consider potential mechanisms underlying language difficulties in DS. First, hearing loss that occurs in approximately two thirds of children with DS due to conductive or sensorineural hearing losses or both (Roizen, 2002) may affect language development. Conductive hearing loss is typically caused by otitis media or middle ear disease. More than 80% of preschool children with DS require tympanostomy tube placement to manage otitis media, and of those requiring medical treatment, 81% had abnormal hearing prior to treatment (Shott, Joseph, & Heithaus, 2001). Persistent otitis media–associated hearing loss is thought to place children with DS at increased risk for language learning difficulties (American Academy of Family Physicians, American Academy of Otolaryngology-Head and Neck Surgery, and American Academy of Pediatrics Subcommittee on Otitis Media with Effusion [AAFP/AAO-HNS/AAP], 2004; Roberts et al., 2004). Hearing impairment—either conductive or sensorineural—in individuals with DS was related concurrently to difficulties in comprehension of vocabulary and grammatical morphology (Chapman et al., 1991; Miolo, Chapman, & Sindberg, 2005).

Second, it is likely that variation in gene expression associated with trisomy 21, which causes 98% of cases of DS, will ultimately be linked to variations in the phenotype in DS, but the identification of biobehavioral associations has just begun. Third, the presence of an enriched environment for learning and the number of opportunities for language learning encountered also affect the language development of children with DS. For example, maternal responsivity, which has been shown to be related to the language development of typically developing children (Landry, Smith, Swank, & Miller-Loncar, 2000; National Institute of Child Health and Human Development Early Child Care Research Network [NICHD ECCRN], 2000, 2002), has also been shown to be related to language skills in children with DS (Fey et al., 2006; Girolametto, Weitzman, & Clements-Baartman, 1998).

Fourth, nonverbal cognition and working memory deficits may also affect individual differences in language learning in DS. Comprehension of vocabulary is predicted by cognitive level, as indexed by nonverbal visual cognition and visual short-term memory, and chronological age in children with DS (Chapman et al., 1991). Specific deficits in auditory-verbal short-term memory and visual short-term memory were correlated with syntax comprehension, expressive vocabulary, and expressive syntax delays in individuals with DS (Chapman et al., 2002; Hick et al., 2005). Laws and Bishop (2004) identified similarities in the profiles of children with DS and children with specific language impairment in their language skills and underlying difficulties with auditory short-term memory. Difficulties in auditory-verbal short-term memory in children with DS may be attributed to phonological short-term memory storage and the phonological loop connecting listening and speaking (Imada et al., 2006) but are not due to a slower speaking rate in the recall of digits or sentences (Jarrold, Cowan, Hewes, & Riby, 2004; Seung & Chapman, 2000, 2004) or to an unusual lack of intentional rehearsal or hearing impairment (Jarrold & Baddeley, 2001; Jarrold, Baddeley, & Hewes, 2000; Jarrold, Baddeley, & Phillips, 1999). Whether working memory difficulties extend to central executive processes and attention, as well as to language difficulties, in individuals with DS is not clear (Miolo et al., 2005).

Fifth, speech motor function and phonological delay may play a role in explaining the variation in the language skills of children with DS. Difficulties in oral motor structure (e.g., muscular and innervation variances) and function (e.g., reduced speed, limited range of motion) along with apraxia (i.e., difficulty executing the motor programming of speech) and dysarthria (i.e., weakness or incoordination of the articulators) are evident in children with DS (Barnes, Roberts, Mirrett, Sideris, & Misenheimer, 2006; Dodd & Thompson, 2001; Miller & Leddy, 1998). Preschool and school-age boys with DS have poor speech intelligibility and are delayed in their speech development with both similar and different error patterns than younger typically developing children (Roberts, Long, et al., 2005; Shriberg & Widder, 1990; see Chapters 6 and 9). Miller, Miolo, Sedey, Pierce, and Rosin (1989) found that speech motor function and phonetic inventory predicted 80% of the variation in the number of different words produced by children with DS in a spontaneous speech sample 5 months later. They concluded that speech motor function and phonetic inventory were the best speech predictors of vocabulary diversity 18 months later in children with DS. Poor speech intelligibility and phonological delay may contribute to the delayed emergence of expressive vocabulary, as well as to later vocabulary, syntax, and pragmatic development, when intended words and the overall function of communication are harder for adults and others to interpret. This may then limit interactions of adults and others with children, which given the importance of caregiver input to language learning, has implications for language development.

Summary

There are many potential factors (e.g., hearing loss, variation in gene expression, maternal responsivity, cognitive profile, speech motor function, speech delay) that may explain individual differences in language abilities in children with DS. There are few studies examining how these factors affect the language phenotype in DS. Research is needed to identify whether these factors explain individual differences in the language of children with DS and if certain periods in development are more sensitive to these mechanisms.

LANGUAGE OF PRESCHOOL AND SCHOOL-AGE CHILDREN WITH FRAGILE X SYNDROME

Although there is considerable variability, preschool and school-age boys with FXS generally have moderate to severe delays in receptive and expressive language skills, whereas girls with FXS show considerably less language delay (Abbeduto, Brady, & Kover, 2007; Abbeduto & Hagerman, 1997; Rice et al., 2005). There is some indication from longitudinal data that boys with FXS have greater delays in expressive language as compared with receptive language over time (Roberts, Mirrett, & Burchinal, 2001). Both boys and girls with FXS have difficulty with the pragmatic aspects of language (Abbeduto et al., 2007; Abbeduto & Hagerman, 1997; Rice et al., 2005). Also, boys with FXS often have poor speech intelligibility, which may further affect their pragmatic skills and language development in general. (This is discussed in Chapter 9.) Gender differences in the language of boys and girls with FXS appear to reflect their cognitive differences (Abbeduto et al., 2007).

The findings of studies on language comprehension and production in vocabulary, syntax, and pragmatics will be discussed in this chapter. Because of gender differences in language skills in FXS, findings for boys and girls are discussed separately. Although a few studies report combined findings for children, adolescents, and adults (Abbeduto et al., 2001, 2003; Lewis et al., 2006), this chapter includes group studies of primarily preschool and school-age children under 12 years of age. Also, because there are fewer studies of the language of children with FXS as compared with DS, it is stated whether studies are case studies or group studies. In this section, the language findings of studies that compared children with FXS and children with DS are reported. The section concludes with the description of mechanisms that may explain individual differences in the language skills of children with FXS.

Language Comprehension

Receptive Vocabulary

Receptive vocabulary is a relative strength for boys with FXS in some aspects of vocabulary (Madison, George, & Moeschler, 1986; Roberts, Price, et al., 2007). For boys with FXS, one case study (Madison et al., 1986) found comprehension of vocabulary to be commensurate with nonverbal mental age expectations, and one group study (Roberts, Price, et al., 2007) also found that vocabulary comprehension did not differ from younger typically developing children of similar nonverbal mental age. These studies measured vocabulary using the Peabody Picture Vocabulary Test–Revised (Dunn & Dunn, 1981) or the Peabody Picture Vocabulary Test–III (Dunn & Dunn, 1997), a measure that assesses experience-related vocabulary. However, when receptive vocabulary was assessed with the Test for Auditory Comprehension of Language–Third Edition (TACL-3; Carrow-Woolfolk, 1999), a measure of comprehension including more conceptually complex items than items on the Peabody Picture Vocabulary Test–III, boys with FXS scored lower than a control group of typical boys of similar mental age (Price et al., 2007). Thus, when words are conceptually more difficult, boys with FXS appear to have more impaired vocabulary comprehension.

Two studies have examined whether having both FXS and autism spectrum disorder (ASD) further affects receptive vocabulary (Price et al., 2007; Roberts, Price, et al., 2007). Boys who had both FXS and ASD did not differ from boys with FXS without ASD in their comprehension of more concrete and also conceptually difficult vocabulary words (Price et al., 2007; Roberts, Price, et al., 2007). Thus, it appears that autism status does not significantly affect comprehension of vocabulary in boys with FXS.

Two studies (Price et al., 2007; Roberts, Price, et al., 2007) compared lexical comprehension for boys with FXS and boys with DS. Boys with a diagnosis of FXS only (without a diagnosis of ASD) scored higher than boys with DS in both the experience-based and conceptually difficult receptive vocabulary measures. However, boys who had both FXS and ASD did not differ from the DS group on either of these vocabulary measures.

Studies of the receptive vocabulary of girls are markedly absent from the literature. There are two case studies of receptive vocabulary in girls with FXS (Hagerman, Hills, Scharfenaker, & Lewis, 1999; Madison et al., 1986) and two group studies that report combined data for girls and boys (Palmer, Gordon, Coston, & Stevenson, 1988; Prouty et al., 1988). However, it is not possible to make any conclusions about the receptive vocabulary of girls with FXS from the limited data.

Receptive Syntax

There is some indication that receptive syntax is delayed compared with nonverable cognitive level in boys with FXS. Although receptive syntax was found to be commensurate with nonverbal mental age in a report of case studies of boys with FXS (Paul, Cohen, Breg, Watson, & Herman, 1984), one group study found that receptive syntax was lower than mental age expectations of a typically developing group (Price et al., 2007). Price et al. (2007) found that boys with FXS scored lower than younger typically developing boys at similar mental ages on comprehension of grammatical morphology and elaborated utterances as measured by the TACL-3 (Carrow-Woolfolk, 1999).

In one study, receptive syntax was not affected by autism status in boys with FXS. Comprehension of grammatical morphology and elaborated utterances did not differ among boys with FXS with and without ASD (Price et al., 2007). The study also compared comprehension of syntax in boys with FXS and boys with DS (Price et al., 2007). Boys with a diagnosis of FXS without a diagnosis of ASD scored higher than boys with DS in syntax comprehension, although the boys with DS and boys with both FXS and ASD did not differ.

As in studies of receptive vocabulary, it is not possible to draw conclusions about receptive syntax in girls with FXS. There are two group studies that report data for receptive syntax, and data are combined for girls and boys (Palmer et al., 1988; Prouty et al., 1988).

Language Production

Expressive Vocabulary

Expressive vocabulary, like receptive vocabulary, may be a relative strength for boys with FXS. In fact, in some sampling contexts, expressive vocabulary is comparable to mental age expectations for boys with FXS. However, initial case studies of boys with FXS (Madison et al., 1986), group studies of girls and boys with FXS without a comparison sample (Spinelli, Rocha, Giacheti, & Richieri-Costa, 1995), and a group study of children and adults with FXS (Sudhalter, Maranion, & Brooks, 1992) reported expressive vocabulary difficulties relative to chronological age, and in one study, relative to mental age (Sudhalter et al., 1992). Specifically, Sudhalter and colleagues (1992) found that when controlling for overall communication level, boys and adult males with FXS without ASD made more semantic errors on a sentence completion test than did younger typically developing children. More recently, Roberts, Mirrett, Anderson, Burchinal, and Neebe (2002) found that the total number of different words used by preschool and early elementary school–age boys with FXS who did not have characteristics of ASD was delayed but was a relative strength compared with the use of gestures and repair strategies (i.e., there was no typical comparison sample).

More recent studies of the expressive vocabulary of boys with FXS using comparison samples of typically developing boys who were matched for mental age found that the sampling method affected whether expressive vocabulary was delayed relative to mental age expectations. Roberts, Price, et al. (2007) used a standardized expressive vocabulary measure, the Expressive Vocabulary Test (Williams, 1997), and found that boys with FXS without ASD did not differ in their expressive vocabulary from the younger typical boys when compared at similar levels of nonverbal cognitive skills. However, Roberts, Hennon, Dear, Anderson, and Vandergrift, (2007), who used some of the same study participants as Roberts, Price, et al. (2007), reported that boys with FXS who did not meet the criteria for autism on the Autism Diagnostic Observation Schedule–General (Lord, Rutter, DiLavore, & Risi, 2002) produced fewer different words during a language sample than did typically developing boys after controlling for the boys' nonverbal mental level, speech intelligibility, and maternal education. The differences in findings for the two studies may reflect the differences in the cognitive and linguistic demands of the elicitation methods. A language sample as compared with a standardized vocabulary test may demand more processing capacity, greater vocabulary, syntax, and pragmatic knowledge and thus may possibly elicit more anxiety.

The presence of ASD did not generally appear to affect expressive vocabulary in boys with FXS (Roberts, Price, et al., 2007). On a standardized vocabulary test, boys with both FXS and ASD did not differ in their expressive vocabulary as compared with boys with FXS who did not have ASD. However, boys with both FXS and ASD scored lower than the typically developing boys of similar mental age (Roberts, Price, et al., 2007), although boys with FXS who did not have ASD did not differ from the typically developing boys. Therefore, although there was no significant difference in expressive vocabulary between the boys with FXS with and without ASD in this study, a larger sample size may have resulted in significant differences for expressive vocabulary.

In one study, expressive vocabulary of boys with FXS was also compared with that of boys with DS (Roberts, Price, et al., 2007). Boys with FXS with and without ASD did not differ from boys with DS in their overall levels of expressive vocabulary.

Due to the lack of studies, it is not possible to comment on the expressive vocabulary of girls with FXS. Only two reports of case studies in this area have been recognized (Madison et al., 1986; Spinelli et al., 1995).

Expressive Syntax

Boys with FXS appear to have delays in their syntactic skills. Early studies of syntactic skills in boys with FXS had mixed results. Case reports of boys with FXS reported shorter utterance lengths and less complex syntax than expected based on chronological age (Madison et al., 1986; Paul et al., 1984) and mental age (Paul et al., 1984), although a case study (Madison et al., 1986) and two group studies (Sudhalter et al., 1992; Sudhalter, Scarborough, & Cohen, 1991) did not find syntactic delays relative to mental age. However, in another study of a group of preschool and early elementary school–age boys with FXS, delays in use of word combinations relative to children's own chronological age were reported (Roberts et al., 2002).

Three recent studies support findings that the expressive syntax of boys with FXS may not keep pace with expectations based on mental age in early childhood but also suggest that some aspects of syntax may be particular strengths for boys with FXS (Levy, Gottesman, Borochowitz, Frydman, & Sagi, 2006; Price, Roberts, et al., in press; Roberts, Hennon, et al., 2007). Levy and colleagues (2006) found that eight boys with FXS without ASD used fewer complex clauses in a language sample than typically developing boys matched on MLU; however, they had fewer errors on some constructions such as grammatical agreement and past tense. In this study, the use of MLU as a group matching criteria may affect the specific syntactic forms.

In two studies that included some of the same participants, boys with FXS without autism used shorter, less complex utterances than younger typically developing boys in conversational speech after controlling for the boys' nonverbal mental age, speech intelligibility, and mothers' education (Price, Roberts, et al., in press; Roberts, Hennon, et al., 2007). Furthermore, in both studies, the boys with FXS used less complex noun phrases, verb phrases, and sentence structure, but did not use fewer questions and negations than the typically developing boys. Interestingly, the group differences found for syntactic skills in the Roberts, Hennon, et al. (2007) study were not found once vocabulary skills also assessed during conversational speech were used as a predictor of overall syntax scores. Thus, the authors proposed that the boys with FXS have an overall expressive language delay that is not specific to syntax and that the shorter, less complex utterances produced by the boys with FXS were related to vocabulary limitations.

Autism status did not affect syntactic complexity in one study. Boys with FXS classified as having or not having ASD did not differ in utterance length or syntactic complexity overall, or more specifically, in the use of the four syntax complexity forms examined: noun phrases, verb phrases, sentence structures, and questions/negations (Price, Roberts, et al., in press). In comparison to the younger typically developing boys at a similar mental age, the boys with both FXS and ASD scored lower on all four subscales, but boys with FXS who did not have ASD scored lower on only three subscales (e.g., noun phrases, verb phrases, sentence structures) and did not score lower on questions/negations.

It is not possible to make substantial conclusions regarding the expressive syntax of girls with FXS. Except for two case studies (Hagerman et al., 1999; Madison et al., 1986), no studies of syntax in girls with FXS have been reported.

Pragmatics

There is general agreement that conversational discourse skills are impaired in boys with FXS (Abbeduto et al., 2007; Abbeduto & Chapman, 2005; Rice et al., 2005). Earlier case studies (Madison et al., 1986) and group studies that did not include comparison samples (Ferrier, Bashir, Meryash, Johnston, & Wolff, 1991; Fryns, Jacobs, Kleczkowska, & Van den Berghe, 1984; Hanson, Jackson, & Hagerman, 1986; Roberts et al., 2002; Sudhalter et al., 1991; Wolf-Schein et al., 1987) reported difficulties in the conversational skills of children with FXS, including frequent perseveration, atypical turn-taking, poor topic maintenance, and tangential language. Several of these studies reported group data combining both boys and adult males with FXS (Ferrier et al., 1991; Hanson et al., 1986; Madison et al., 1986; Sudhalter et al., 1991; Wolf-Schein et al., 1987). Roberts et al. (2002) did not include a comparison sample but reported delays in the pragmatic aspects of communication for a group of preschool and early elementary school-age boys with FXS, with the use of gestures and reciprocity (i.e., topic maintenance, repair strategies) as relative weaknesses compared with verbal and vocal communication. Interestingly, a relative strength was reported in the use of appropriate gaze shifts in these children, which conflicts with previous reports of gaze avoidance in older males with FXS (Cohen, Vietze, Sudhalter, Jenkins, & Brown, 1989).

More recent studies have also reported greater pragmatic difficulties in boys with FXS than in typically developing children. Levy et al. (2006) found that eight boys with FXS used more perseveration than typically developing children matched on MLU during conversation while looking at a picture book. Roberts, Martin, et al. (2007) compared the discourse skills during conversation of boys with FXS who were not diagnosed with ASD with that of boys who were typically developing and of a similar mental age. After controlling for mental age, boys with FXS without ASD produced more perseveration and less elaborative topic maintenance than the typically developing boys.

Autism status also appears to affect pragmatic skills in boys with FXS. Roberts, Martin, et al. (2007) found that boys with both FXS and ASD produced significantly more noncontingent (i.e., language that is tangential, that is unrelated, or that does not appropriately maintain or change the topic) turns than boys with only FXS and typically developing boys after controlling for mental age. This finding was observed regardless of whether the topic was maintained or changed and whether the turn type was a response or an initiation. Boys with FXS with and without autism did not significantly differ in their use of perseveration; both groups produced more perseveration than typically developing boys. These findings suggest that some aspects of the conversational discourse difficulties attributed to FXS may be functions of the high rate of comorbidity between FXS and ASD and that some difficulties may be characteristic of FXS.

A few studies have compared the pragmatic skills of individuals with FXS to those with ID or autism (Belser & Sudhalter, 2001; Ferrier et al., 1991; Sudhalter & Belser, 2001; Sudhalter, Cohen, Silverman, & Wolf-Schein, 1990; Wolf-Schein et al., 1987). For example, Sudhalter and colleagues (1990) reported that 12 boys and adult males with FXS without autism produced more deviant repetitive language (i.e., perseveration, echolalia, jargon, "affirming by repetition") during conversation than boys and adult males with DS. The FXS group also used less echolalia, more perseverations, better turn-taking ability (i.e., more turns per topic), and less repetitive language than individuals with ASD who did not have FXS. In two follow-up studies, boys and adult males with FXS (autism status unknown) used more repetitive speech as well as more tangential language (i.e., language loosely related to the topic) than individuals with ASD or ID and not FXS (Belser & Sudhalter, 2001; Sudhalter & Belser, 2001). More recently, Roberts, Martin, et al. (2007) found that boys with FXS without ASD produced significantly more perseveration during conversation than 29 boys with DS, after controlling for mental age. Thus, as many in the field have contended, perseveration may be a defining characteristic of FXS.

A few case studies (Hagerman et al., 1999; Spinelli et al., 1995) and a few group studies (Freund, Reiss, & Abrams, 1993; Hagerman et al., 1992; Lesniak-Karpiak, Mazzocco, & Ross, 2003; Mazzocco, Kates, Baumgardner, Freund, & Reiss, 1997) have reported pragmatic or related difficulties in girls with FXS. All of these group studies report combined data for girls, adolescents, and/or adult females with FXS. Females with FXS were reported to have more difficulties initiating and sustaining conversations (Freund, Reiss, & Abrams, 1993; Hagerman et al., 1999; Lesniak-Karpiak et al., 2003; Mazzocco et al., 1997). For example, Lesniak-Karpiak et al. (2003) reported that girls and adolescents with FXS took longer to initiate interactions and produced more hand movements during a videotaped role-play interaction with an unfamiliar adult, and their parents reported more social problems than for unaffected females.

Summary

Although there appears to be a specific language phenotype associated with FXS, there is also considerable variability in the language profile. Boys with FXS have delays in receptive and expressive language, with vocabulary a relative strength in some sampling contexts. Both comprehension and production of syntax do not appear to keep pace with mental age expectations in boys with FXS, and there is general agreement that pragmatic skills are impaired. The presence of ASD in boys with FXS appears to have a specific effect only on particular aspects of language. In contrast to boys with FXS, there are almost no studies of the vocabulary and syntax development of girls with FXS, and there are very few studies of their pragmatic skills. Although there has been an increase of studies on boys with FXS in the past few years, several of the group studies did not separate the children's data from those of adolescent and adult males. Furthermore, there are few longitudinal studies of boys and no longitudinal studies of girls examining language development over time.

Future studies should examine receptive and expressive vocabulary, syntax, and pragmatics longitudinally in the same group of children with FXS to determine what aspects of language are affected and the ways in which language patterns change over time. Studies of vocabulary in children with FXS should examine whether there are delays in vocabulary milestones such as the onset of first words, more conceptually complex vocabulary, specific vocabulary such as emotional and mental state verbs, and the process of how children learn new words or fast mapping. Syntax studies of children with FXS should examine the acquisition of specific morphosyntactic forms and more complex syntax, as well as whether the sampling context (e.g., conversational speech versus narration) affects syntax. Future research on pragmatic skills in children with FXS should study aspects of discourse that could be specific to FXS (e.g., perseveration, excessive question asking, interruptions), difficulties with conversational repair (i.e., how the speaker modifies or asks for a modification when communication is unclear), and narrative skills to retell a story or an experience. The effects of a comorbid diagnosis of FXS and ASD should be examined by comparing boys and girls with FXS who have or do not have ASD. The language profiles of boys and girls with FXS should be compared with each other, as well as with the profiles of children who have other developmental disabilities, specifically children with ASD only and children with other types of ID. Such studies will define the language phenotype in FXS and whether individual differences in language skills relate to FXS specifically or to ID, autism, or gender.

Possible Mechanisms Underlying Language Learning in Fragile X Syndrome

To understand the phenotypic language characteristics of FXS and the considerable variability in profiles among both boys and girls with FXS, it is important to consider potential mechanisms underlying language difficulties in FXS. Although each of these factors is discussed individually, it is likely that many of the factors are interrelated. First, gender is one factor that affects language, although gender likely reflects the degree of ID. The majority of males with FXS have moderate to severe ID (Bennetto & Pennington, 2002). About one quarter of carrier females with FXS have ID; one third have mild ID; and the remaining females are functioning in the average range, although many have learning disabilities (Bennetto & Pennington, 2002; see Chapter 2). Second, the insufficient functioning of the fragile X mental retardation (FMR1) gene and the subsequent failure to produce fragile X mental retardation protein (FMRP) may also explain some variability in language skills. A few studies have reported a relationship between the level of FMRP expressed in blood and cognitive, adaptive, and motor skills and gross measures of language in individuals with FXS (Bailey, Hatton, Skinner, & Mesibov, 2001; Hagerman et al., 1994; Merenstein et al., 1996; Tassone et al., 1999; see also Chapter 2).

Third, hearing loss that occurs when children have otitis media in early childhood may also affect language development in children with FXS. Otitis media is thought to be highly prevalent among young children with FXS (Hagerman, Altshul-Stark, & McBogg, 1987), yet it is unclear if there is an increased incidence of otitis media and hearing loss in individuals with FXS during the first few years of life, when having intact hearing is thought to be critical for later language learning. Furthermore, although persistent otitis media–associated hearing loss is thought to be particularly problematic for children who are at increased risk for language learning difficulties (AAFP/AAO-HNS/AAP, 2004; Roberts et al., 2004), the effect of persistent otitis media in early childhood on later language development in children with FXS has not been examined (see Chapter 6).

Fourth, specific cognitive strengths and weaknesses may also influence language skills in children with FXS. Boys and adult males with FXS have been reported to have specific impairments in executive functioning, attention, working memory, sequential processing, and visuospatial skills (Cornish, Munir, & Cross, 1998, 1999; Cornish, Sudhalter, & Turk, 2004; Dykens, Hodapp, & Leckman, 1987; Freund & Reiss, 1991; Munir, Cornish, & Wilding, 2000), whereas girls with FXS have also been reported to show deficits in executive functioning, attention, and visuospatial skills (Cornish et al., 1998; Kirk, Mazzocco, & Kover, 2005; Mazzocco, Pennington, & Hagerman, 1993; Munir, Cornish, & Wilding, 2000). Reported strengths for males with FXS include simultaneous processing, long-term memory, visual memory, and verbal imitation (Dykens, Hodapp, & Leckman, 1989; Harris-Schmidt, & Fast, 1998; Schoenbrodt & Smith, 1995; Spiridigliozzi et al., 1994). For females, reported strengths are inductive reasoning, verbal processing, and some aspects of memory and spatial ability when task content is meaningful (Bennetto & Pennington, 2002; Freund & Reiss, 1991; Jakala et al., 1997).

Fifth, environmental influences—specifically maternal responsivity—likely affect the language development of children with FXS. Maternal responsivity is well documented as influencing the language development of typically developing children (Landry et al., 2000; NICHD ECCRN, 2000, 2002) and children with developmental disabilities other than FXS (Camarata & Yoder, 2002; Dawson & Galpert, 1990; Landry, Smith, Miller-Loncar, & Swank, 1997; see also Chapter 7).

Several other mechanisms that relate to the psychopathology and autistic characteristics seen in some children with FXS have also been proposed as explaining their specific profile of language difficulties, particularly the pragmatic difficulties. Some of these mechanisms are believed to stem from abnormalities in the frontal lobe of the brain and problems in regulating the autonomic nervous system (Abbeduto et al., 2007; Abbeduto & Hagerman, 1997; Cornish, Turk, et al., 2004; Sudhalter et al., 1990). First, high anxiety/arousal levels may account for the variation in language abilities of individuals with FXS. Males with FXS display symptoms of social anxiety, including gaze aversion and overt signs of discomfort and avoidance, and exhibit elevated levels of arousal, particularly in situations involving social stress (Hessl et al., 2001; Roberts, Boccia, Bailey, Hatton, & Skinner, 2001). Females with FXS also show symptoms of anxiety, including discomfort interacting with peers, social withdrawal, and a need for more time than typically developing peers to initiate interactions (Freund et al., 1993; Lesniak-Karpiak, Mazzocco, & Ross, 2003; Mazzocco, Baumgardner, Freund, & Reiss, 1998). Individuals with FXS appear to be interested in initiating social interactions (Simon & Finucane, 1996; Turk & Cornish, 1998). The social demands of conversation and social interaction, however, may possibly overstimulate children with FXS and lead to a heightened state of arousal, thus triggering atypical language use such as noncontingent language and perseveration.

Second, deficits in sensory processing, integration, and sensorimotor coordination may also affect language skills in males with FXS. Tactile sensitivity, increased sensitivity to sensory stimuli, hyper- and hyposensitivity of the oral musculature, and sensory defensiveness have been reported in males with FXS (Baranek et al., 2002; Miller, Reisman, McIntosh, & Simon, 2001; Rogers, Hepburn, & Wehner, 2003). Increased arousal due to sensory input may make it difficult for a child with FXS to integrate sensory information in the environment and respond appropriately to meet the demands for using language to initiate and maintain conversational interactions.

Third, the presence of autistic characteristics or ASD may also explain the characteristics of the language phenotype in FXS. Approximately 15%–25% of males (with some reports as high as 30%–35%) and 3% of females with FXS have autism (Bailey et al., 1998; Hagerman, 2006; Mazzocco et al., 1997; Turk & Graham, 1997). Autistic behaviors in boys with FXS include poor eye contact, social withdrawal, stereotypic/repetitive behaviors, and hyperactivity (Cohen et al., 1988; Dykens, Hodapp, Ort, & Leckman, 1993; Kerby & Dawson, 1994; Reiss & Freund, 1992). Furthermore, 5.5% of males with autism and 5%–12% of females with autism test positive for FXS (Bailey, Bolton, Butler, & Le Couteur, 1993; Cohen et al., 1989; Dykens & Volkmar, 1997; Hagerman, 2002). Children with FXS with more characteristics of autism score lower in overall language (Bailey, Hatton, et al., 2001; Bailey, Mesibov, et al., 1998; Philofsky, Hepburn, Hayes, Hagerman, & Rogers, 2004; Rogers, Wehner, & Hagerman, 2001) and produce more noncontingent language (Roberts, Martin, et al., 2007) than children with fewer characteristics associated with ASD or no ASD diagnosis.

Finally, some other behavioral characteristics may also account for some of the language difficulties reported in children with FXS. For example, males with FXS have been described as hyperactive, impulsive, and inattentive (Baumgardner, Reiss, Freund, & Abrams, 1995; Dykens et al., 1989; Turk, 1998), and females with FXS have also been described as distractible and hyperactive (Hessl et al., 2001; Lachiewicz & Dawson, 1994).

Summary

Many factors (e.g., a child's gender, hearing loss, cognitive profile, level of FMRP, arousal/anxiety, sensory deficits, autistic and behavioral characteristics, maternal responsivity) have been proposed as explaining the specific language phenotype in FXS, thus accounting for the individual differences in language abilities. There are, however, very few studies actually examining how these factors affect the language phenotype in FXS. Research should determine the role of these factors in explaining individual differences in the language skills of boys and girls with FXS and whether there are certain periods in development when language skills may be more susceptible to these mechanisms.

ASSESSMENT AND INTERVENTION

The wide range of individual differences in language and communication skills of children with DS and children with FXS suggests that assessment should consider the profile of each child's strengths and weaknesses in language skills and provide intervention geared to the needs and abilities of the individual with DS or FXS. Assessment and intervention strategies that seem particularly important based on review of the DS and FXS phenotypes and potential mechanisms explaining those phenotypes are presented. Intervention for children with DS and children with FXS is guided by the same principles that govern enriched language learning in typically developing children and specific interventions that are used with children with specific language learning impairment and other developmental disabilities. These principles include 1) providing a responsive linguistic environment by responding to the child's communicative behaviors, attentional focus, and intended meaning; 2) providing language models at the child's current levels of comprehension; 3) intervening when possible during social interactions in natural contexts that engage the child; 4) expanding and elaborating on children's communication; and 5) offering opportunities for the child to use current forms in new contexts and for new purposes and meanings (e.g., using new vocabulary for requesting rather than commenting; or in narration storytelling rather than conversation) (Chapman, 2000; Fey et al., 2006; Mahoney, Perales, Wiggers, & Herman, 2006). Language intervention programs helping parents to foster these skills are discussed in Chapter 7. See Paul (2007) and McCauley and Fey (2006) for reviews of language assessment and intervention methods.

Manage Otitis Media with Effusion and Hearing Loss

Children with DS or FXS should be routinely screened for otitis media and associated hearing loss (Roberts et al., 2004). Hearing should be tested when otitis media persists for 3 months or longer (AAFP/AAO-HNS/AAP, 2004), following the American Speech-Language-Hearing Association (ASHA) Audiologic Assessment Panel (1996) protocol. When otitis media lasts longer than 4 months, tympanostomy tubes are recommended for at-risk individuals (AAFP/AAO-HNS/AAP, 2004). Language skills should also be monitored, paying particular attention to a child's comprehension and production of grammatical morphemes. When there is hearing loss, low gain hearing aids or other amplification devices such as FM sound field systems in classrooms can be useful (ASHA, 2002; Bennetts & Flynn, 2002). Environmental strategies to optimize language learning and listening for children with otitis media and hearing loss, such as reducing background noise and providing close access to the speaker, have been suggested (AAFP/AAO-HNS/AAP, 2004; Roberts et al., 2004; Roberts & Wallace, 1997). Future studies should examine the impact of low gain hearing aids and other amplification devices such as FM sound field systems on the language skills of children with DS or FXS.

Consider Cognitive Profile in Intervention

The specific strengths and weaknesses in cognitive skills of children with DS and children with FXS can have important implications for language assessment and intervention. For example, for a child with DS, focus can be placed on the relative weaknesses in auditory-verbal working memory and phonological working memory, and the relative strength of visual-spatial short-term memory can be built upon and utilized for learning language. Similarly, the relative strengths in visual memory, verbal imitation, simultaneous processing and long-term memory of meaningful verbal information can be utilized for boys with FXS. For example, a child with FXS may be taught language skills using picture cues and modeling, and memory for vocabulary words can be enhanced by associating the words with a meaningful context. Furthermore, interventions should capitalize on children's strengths in simultaneous rather than sequential processing in which children need to observe and comprehend the whole task rather than the individual steps. In addition, assessment of phonological working memory and short-term memory using nonword repetition and memory-span tasks (ASHA, 2001) may provide important insights into language difficulties and may have implications for intervention. For example, a child with short-term and working memory impairments may benefit from repeated opportunities to hear words and sentences, visual supports to understand meaning and recall information, repeated, brief, and simple instructions, tasks that are broken down into different steps, and encouragement to ask for forgotten information (Alloway & Gathercole, 2006; Gathercole, Alloway, Willis, & Adams, 2006; Miolo et al., 2005). Visually based materials such as storybooks with pictures (see Chapter 10) may be particularly helpful for children with DS or FXS, given their visual memory strengths (Chapman, 2003; Hick et al., 2005).

Consider Speech Skills in Intervention

A child's ability to use speech to communicate and his or her level of speech intelligibility also affects a listener's understanding of the child and a child's communication effectiveness. Language competence may be underestimated when speech intelligibility is poor or when a child needs or relies on an augmentative or alternative communication system. Knowledge of the contexts in which the communication of a child with DS or FXS is more effective or particularly difficult due to speech difficulties has important implications for defining and focusing language intervention strategies. See Chapters 6 and 9 for a discussion of strategies to improve speech skills in individuals with DS or FXS.

Consider the Role of Anxiety/Hyperarousal and Sensory Deficits in Fragile X Syndrome

For children with FXS, sensory deficits and levels of anxiety/hyperarousal should be considered in language assessment and intervention. Interventions targeting sensory deficits may possibly decrease sensory defensiveness, help children to manage their sensory environment, and optimize arousal levels for learning (Hessl, Rivera, & Reiss, 2004; Rogers, 1998b; Scharfenaker, O'Connor, Stackhouse, Braden, & Gray, 2002). A number of techniques have been suggested for use in speech and language intervention, including cotreatment of occupational and speech-language therapy, sensory integration therapy, and calming techniques (e.g., deep pressure, bouncing on an exercise ball, reducing visual and auditory distractions) (Scharfenaker et al., 2002). High levels of anxiety/hyperarousal should also be considered in language assessment, intervention, and behavior management strategies for children with FXS. For example, being too close to a child, demanding eye contact, or requiring the child to look at the clinician's face may provoke anxiety in children with FXS. Hyperarousal or sensory defensiveness may be decreased in some children with FXS when a less directive, more incidental approach to teaching or therapy is used. Other children with FXS who are anxious and who seek predictability and routine, however, may benefit from a more structured approach. Although approaches to managing anxiety/hyperarousal and sensory integration issues are conceptually compelling, seem promising, and have considerable support based on clinical reports, systematic intervention studies demonstrating their efficacy are lacking (Dawson & Watling, 2000; Schaaf & Miller, 2005) and are needed.

Consider Approaches for Children with Autism

Given that 15%–25% of individuals with FXS (Bailey et al., 1998; Dykens & Volkmar, 1997; Hagerman, 2002) and at least 5%–7% of individuals with DS (Ghaziuddin, Tsai, & Ghaziuddin, 1992; Kent, Evans, Paul, & Sharp, 1999) meet the diagnostic criteria for autism, and other children with FXS or DS have characteristics of autism without meeting the diagnostic criteria for autism, intervention strategies used for children with ASD should be considered when working with a child with DS or FXS. Language interventions for children with ASD include developmental approaches (e.g., the SCERTS® Model; Prizant, Wetherby, Rubin, & Laurent, 2003; Prizant, Wetherby, Rubin, Laurent, & Rydell, 2005), naturalistic behavioral models (e.g., Pivotal Response Training; Koegel et al., 1989), and models that are more consistent with traditional applied behavior analysis (e.g., early intensive behavioral intervention) (Smith, 1999, 2001). It has been suggested that more structured behavioral approaches might be more effective in teaching vocabulary and syntax, whereas more naturalistic approaches (e.g., incidental teaching) might be more useful in teaching the pragmatic aspects of language and generalization to new contexts (Carr & Durand, 1985; Jones, Carr, & Feeley, 2006). Although there is substantial literature on the effectiveness of behavioral approaches in increasing children's language skills, there is less published outcome data on developmental models. However, behavioral and developmental approaches may be used for different children in different situations, depending on the needs of the child, the child's abilities, and the nature of the language skills being taught. For example, Yoder and colleagues (1995) reported that children at lower language levels responded better to milieu teaching than to a responsive approach intervention, whereas children at higher language levels responded better to a responsive interaction approach. See reviews by Goldstein (2002), Koegel (2000), Landa (2007), Paul (2003), and Rogers (1998a, 2000) for overviews of language and communication interventions for children with autism. Future research is needed to determine whether the behavioral and developmentally based language interventions recommended for children with ASD are effective for children who have FXS or DS.

Assess Language in a Variety of Contexts

Children with DS or FXS should have their language assessed with a variety of elicitation methods, and the effect of language sampling and environmental context should be considered when determining the profile of strengths and weaknesses in vocabulary, syntax, and pragmatics. Given that sampling context has been shown to affect language performance for both children with DS and children with FXS, it is important to assess language in a variety of contexts (e.g., in standardized tests, in conversation, in narration) and to consider which aspects of language are being measured. Conversational speech can elicit different language complexity than standardized measures (Chapman et al., 1998; Glenn & Cunningham, 2005; Price et al., in press; Roberts, Hennon, et al., 2007; Roberts, Price, et al., 2007), narratives can elicit more complex language than conversational speech samples (Miles et al., 2006), and different standardized tests (e.g., tests of vocabulary) can elicit different language complexity (Miolo et al., 2005; Price et al., 2007; Roberts, Price, et al., 2007). It is also important to determine if certain language functions, environmental contexts, and conversational partners affect language in children with DS and children with FXS. Since children with DS are reported to have more difficulty with some pragmatic aspects of language (e.g., requesting, introducing new topics, elaboration) (Beeghly et al., 1990; Mundy et al., 1995; Roberts, Martin, et al., 2007), assessing these specific aspects of language and comparing them with other language functions and topic use is particularly important for children with DS. Because of the potential influence of arousal, anxiety, and sensory issues, particularly on the pragmatic aspects of language in children with FXS (Abbeduto et al., 2007; Abbeduto & Chapman, 2005; Cornish, Turk, et al., 2004; Sudhalter et al., 1990), assessment during contexts with differing social demands (e.g., interacting in large groups, one to one, and/or with a familiar and unfamiliar person) should be conducted and compared for children with FXS. Asking teachers and caregivers about children's language skills (e.g., contexts where topic maintenance, elaboration, or perseveration occur more or less frequently) can be very helpful.

Target Developmentally Appropriate
Vocabulary, Syntax, and Pragmatic Skills

The phenotypic characterization of the communication skills of children with DS and boys with FXS as previously described would suggest that language intervention should focus on expressive language skills, with successive, developmentally sequenced goals of early vocabulary development using augmentative/alternative communication systems (if helpful), simple sentence acquisition in conversational contexts, and complex sentence acquisition in narrative contexts. Many children with DS need to focus particularly on the appropriate use of grammatical morphology, and many boys and girls with FXS need to concentrate on pragmatic aspects of language. Interventions that consider the effect of speech intelligibility (see Chapters 6 and 9) and that incorporate the need for augmentative or alternative communication methods in language intervention (see Chapter 7) are essential for both populations. Because receptive language and cognitive skills may exceed expressive language skills in both children with DS and children with FXS (Dykens et al., 2006; Roberts, Hennon, et al., 2007), language input should be targeted at a child's receptive language level.

Vocabulary

The targeting of developmentally appropriate vocabulary in children with intellectual disabilities requires that both their current level of conceptual understanding, and their current interests, activities, and social experience be taken into account. As children with ds and fxs grow older, they can be expected to acquire a larger comprehension vocabulary that reflects a wider variety of and more age-appropriate concerns (miolo et al., 2005). At the same time, special attention should be given to creating opportunities to learn to understand and use more complex vocabulary (e.g., mental constructs relating to time, space, number, logical relations; emotional and mental state verbs and adjectives). In addition, repeated opportunities to hear and produce new words in meaningful contexts may facilitate acquisition; practice in a variety of contexts that makes the words familiar may also speed comprehension (chapman, sindberg, bridge, gigstead, & hesketh, 2006). Vocabulary work can be linked to reading as part of the building of word-recognition skills. Literacy activities such as shared book reading and using books with diverse vocabulary and age-appropriate themes could serve as important contexts for ongoing language intervention (see chapter 10).

Syntax

Syntax intervention should target specific syntactic forms (e.g., grammatical morphemes such as third person singular *-s* and past tense *-ed*). Whether intervention should target forms that mark only grammatical finiteness of sentences (see Rice, Wexler, & Cleave, 1995, and Rice & Wexler, 1996, for a discussion of finiteness) such as the third person singular (e.g., *she runs*) and past tense (e.g., *he jumped*) and not other forms such as plurals (e.g., *books*) needs further study. Conversational recasts, for example, may be used to develop complex syntax production, an area of concern for many children with DS. In a conversational recast, the adult expands a child's utterance with semantic or grammatical information so that, for instance, when the child says "doggie bark," the adult responds, "The doggie is barking." See Camarata and Nelson (2006) for a description of the recast approach and research supporting its effectiveness. Books and exercises that provide examples of complex sentence structures in repetitive ways could help children build schema for such structures and their associated grammatical morphemes (e.g., conjunctions, prepositions) or verbs (e.g., verbs of perception, emotion, cognition). Other approaches to develop syntactic skills are described in Paul (1992, 2007) and McCauley and Fey (2006).

Pragmatics

Because perseveration and noncontingent language (e.g., language that is tangential, unrelated, or does not appropriately maintain or change the topic) can present specific challenges for some children with FXS, and initiations and elaboration of topics can present particular challenges for some children with DS, interventions focusing on these pragmatic aspects of language are described next. Suggested activities to improve pragmatic aspects of language for children with FXS (Harris-Schmidt & Fast, 2004; Scharfenaker et al., 2002) and children with DS (Fey et al., 2006; Kumin, 2003; Kumin, Goodman, & Councill, 1996; see also Chapter 8) have been described in the literature.

Decrease Perseveration and Noncontingent Language   Frequent perseveration in conversation can interfere with a child's communication effectiveness and can be frustrating for a conversational partner. Identifying the possible underlying causes of perseveration for a particular child in a particular situation should inform intervention. Perseveration may serve a variety of functions for a child with FXS, such as to gain information, reassurance, or attention; to control the interaction; to avoid a stressful situation; or to initiate or maintain an interaction. The most widely cited explanation for perseveration in FXS is hyperarousal and anxiety (Belser & Sudhalter, 1995; Cornish, Sudhalter, et al., 2004; Sudhalter et al., 1990). Other possible reasons for perseveration are deficits in receptive language, expressive language, and cognition; social skills deficits; frequent attention seeking; and a lack of interest/motivation in social interactions. Scharfenaker and colleagues (2002) suggested several strategies to reduce perseveration in children with FXS, such as providing increased time for processing, reducing the complexity of utterances directed at the child, monitoring anxiety level, and utilizing verbal redirection. Other interventions used to reduce perseveration in children with ASD include the use of scripted prompts and conversations to teach the child more effective ways to initiate or maintain a conversation, modeling appropriate (nonperseverative) language, reinforcement of nonperseverative responses, use of visual and verbal cues that clue the child to change his perseverative language, and teaching functionally equivalent alternative responses to replace the perseverative responses (e.g., teaching the child to say "I need a break" instead of perseverating on "What time is it?") (Carr & Durand, 1985; Frea & Hughes, 1997; Koegel & Frea, 1993; Kostinas, Scandlen, & Luiselli, 2001; Mace & Lalli, 1991; Reese, Richman, Zarcone, & Zarcone, 2003; Rehfeldt & Chambers, 2003; Ross, 2002). Schopler, Mesibov, and Hearsey (1995) have suggested strategies that may reduce anxiety-based perseverative behavior in children with ASD (e.g., establishing predictable routines, helping transition by visually displaying what is going to happen, practicing alternative coping behaviors such as relaxation). Another strategy shown to be effective in increasing appropriate social interactions in children with ASD was incorporating a child's perseverative topic into interactions (e.g., one child who perseverated on maps was taught a tag game played on a giant map) (Baker, Koegel, & Koegel, 1998).

Use of noncontingent language also can greatly interfere with communication effectiveness. Increasing a child's use of contingent language and enhancing his or her ability to maintain a topic of a conversation may greatly affect communication effectiveness. Some of the same causes of perseverative language may be affecting the child's use of noncontingent language, and some of the strategies suggested to decrease perseveration may also decrease noncontingent language. Strategies such as peer-mediated interventions to teach initiations and responsiveness (i.e., answering questions) to typically developing peers of children with ASD (see Strain & Kohler, 1998, for a review) have considerable empirical support. Video modeling of targeted language skills (e.g., videotape presentations of target skills and skills later practiced with an adult) have also been used with children with ASD (Charlop & Milstein, 1989). Other strategies to increase topic maintenance, which is similar to contingent language, have been suggested for children with language disorders, such as using games with familiar routines or those that require contingent responding (e.g., collaborating with a group to make a story), balancing conversations to encourage more give and take, and letting the child select the topic and elaborating on the topic (Brinton & Fujiki, 1989; Brinton, Robinson, & Fujiki 2004). Strategies recommended for children with FXS for facilitating pragmatic skills such as reducing tangential language were providing a greater response time, using visual cues, and using parallel talk in which the adult verbalizes what the child is doing or thinking (Scharfenaker et al., 2002).

Increase Initiations and Elaborations   A lack of verbal initiations and elaborations of a topic can also affect communication effectiveness. The reasons for using few initiations and elaborations will vary as with perseveration and noncontingent language, thus informing intervention strategies. Children may infrequently initiate conversational interactions due to such things as shyness or social anxiety, expressive or receptive language deficits, and/or a lack of social motivation or interest. Children may not elaborate on a conversational topic due to cognitive deficits, receptive and expressive language deficits, and/or social anxiety, among other possibilities. A number of strategies have been suggested to increase initiations in children with developmental delays, including milieu language teaching (e.g., Yoder & Warren, 1999; see Chapter 7), and in children with ASD, including visual supports and scripts (e.g., Krantz, MacDuff, & McClannahan, 1993; Krantz & McClannahan, 1993); video modeling (e.g., Bidwell & Rehfeldt, 2004); peer mediation (e.g., Morrison, Kamps, Garcia, Parker, & Dunlap, 2001; Strain & Odom, 1986); Pivotal Response Training (Koegel, Camarata, & Koegel, 1998; Koegel, Carter, & Koegel, 2003); and peer-mediated, teacher-directed interventions (e.g., Odom & Strain, 1986). See also Brinton and Fujiki (1989), Fey (1986), and McCauley and Fey (2006) for specific steps to increase verbal initiations in children.

Techniques to increase contingent language, as previously described, may also result in increases in children's use of elaboration of topics. Specific techniques to increase elaboration of conversational topics have been suggested by Bliss (2002) and Scharfenaker and colleagues (2002). One approach toward increasing elaboration in conversation was suggested by Bliss (2002). The child gives directions or plans an event (e.g., describes how to make a sandwich). The clinician then directs the child to give further information (e.g., "Tell me more"). Other strategies to increase children's elaborative language are to support child-initiated topics with specific questions (e.g., open ended as opposed to yes/no) and comments; pausing to allow a child sufficient time to respond; and focusing on activities, topics, and materials of interest to the child.

Promote Generalization of Language Targets

Since difficulty generalizing may be characteristic of many children with DS or FXS, generalization of targeted language skills should be specifically incorporated into intervention plans. Naturalistic language methods such as milieu language teaching (e.g., arranging the environment to encourage commenting) have considerable research support and promote generalization of language skills (ASHA, 2005; McCauley & Fey, 2006; Paul, 2007) and are also described in Chapters 3 and 7. Providing multiple exemplars of target skills and using specific teaching strategies such as models, prompts, and conversational recasts may also increase generalization. Materials from the child's home or classroom (e.g., storybooks, an older child's textbooks) can also be integrated into intervention. Generalization is more likely when language is worked on in a variety of settings in the child's natural environment (e.g., classroom, home, community) and with a variety of communication partners (e.g., teachers, parents, siblings, classmates). In some service delivery models, it is easier to focus on functional communication in everyday contexts. Given the cognitive deficits characteristic of children with DS or FXS, it is important to facilitate generalization of target skills by providing opportunities to practice multiple exemplars of the target form and/or function, as well as to use communication in multiple contexts.

Summary

The assessment and intervention strategies that were previously suggested are based on the review of the phenotypes of DS and FXS, the potential mechanisms explaining those phenotypes, language learning in typically developing children, and interventions designed for children with DS, FXS, ASD, language impairments, and other developmental disabilities. Although there are case reports and clinical recommendations for language intervention for both children with DS and children with FXS, evidence-based interventions designed to increase the language skills of children with DS or children with FXS are markedly lacking. There is a critical need for well-controlled studies that examine the effectiveness of intervention to foster vocabulary, syntax, and pragmatic skills in children with DS and children with FXS. Studies must determine which interventions result in the most gains in language development and generalization of new skills.

PARENT INVOLVEMENT

Parents and other caregivers play an important role in the language development of their children with DS or FXS. There are several parent intervention programs that educate parents in ways to understand their children's attempts to communicate, tailor their communication to their children's needs, and provide a responsive and enriching communication environment (see Chapter 7). For example, It Takes Two to Talk—The Hanen Program for Parents (Girolametto & Weitzman, 2006) is a developmental approach that includes child-focused strategies (e.g., follow the child's lead), interaction-promoting strategies (e.g., ask questions that continue the conversation, wait for your child to take a turn), language modeling strategies (e.g., label, expand, comment), and using language that is responsive to the child's communicative attempts.

There are several specific strategies parents of children with DS or FXS can use with their children. First, parents may be interviewed regarding specific topics, contexts, or conversational partners around which communication is more effective and/or more problematic. For example, a child with DS or FXS may display more complex, contingent, and elaborative language; more initiations; and/or less perseveration when talking about a topic of interest, speaking in shorter utterances, talking with a familiar person, or during a frequent routine such as mealtime.

Second, parents can interpret the speech of children with DS or FXS when it is less intelligible to unfamiliar listeners and can help their children develop skills to clarify and repair unclear communication. Third, parents can provide a responsive linguistic environment for their children with DS or FXS during their daily interactions, using strategies to facilitate language development (e.g., talking often to their children, modeling speech patterns, repeating and expanding on what their child says) (Girolametto & Weitzman, 2006; Pepper & Weitzman, 2004; Snow, Burns, & Griffin, 1998). Abbeduto et al. (2007) noted that interventions that focus on increasing caregiver responsivity have not been examined in children with FXS, and because some children with FXS have challenging behavior, responsive interaction strategies may be hard to use and thus require some modifications.

Fourth, parents of children with DS or FXS can also support the use of augmentative and alternative communication systems in their home environment with signing or alternative communication as a way to support unclear communication (see Chapter 11). Research is needed to determine which parent interventions are most effective in facilitating the language development of children with DS or FXS.

RESEARCH DIRECTIONS

Although both children with DS and children with FXS experience language delays, there is a specific language phenotype that is characteristic of each syndrome. Many children with DS have particular deficits in expressive syntax, whereas children with FXS have particular deficits in pragmatics skills. The mechanisms that underlie language skills and difficulties appear to differ in the two populations. There are several additional directions for future research on the language skills of children with DS or FXS. First, research is needed to further define the vocabulary, syntax, and pragmatics characteristics specific to both DS and FXS. DS and FXS have most often been the comparison sample for each other. Language characteristics for both of these groups of individuals should be compared with those of other groups of children with ID to understand whether the language profile reflects only differences between the two populations or whether these characteristics are specific to the language phenotype in DS and FXS.

Second, studies should also examine children's rate of growth in language skills using longitudinal designs. This will help determine at what age period changes in language skills occur, if there is continued growth in language, or whether there is a plateau at a specific age. Such findings will have important implications for the timing of language intervention and professionals' ability to define specific language domains on which intervention should focus. It is possible that a specific domain of language may be more vulnerable to language deficits at a certain age period. For example, in the school-age years, the demands of the academic curriculum may place greater demands on language comprehension and production.

Third, studies of girls with FXS are markedly lacking. Future research should examine the vocabulary, syntax, and pragmatic skills of girls with FXS to understand the role of gender in FXS.

Fourth, studies are needed to understand the mechanisms that underlie language development in DS and FXS. For example, the relationship between genetic variations and individual differences in language learning is an area of future research in children with DS and children with FXS. Also, the effects of the fragile X premutation on language (see Abbeduto et al., 2007, for a review) must be studied. For children with DS, it is important to determine the role of factors such as phonological working memory, hearing loss due to otitis media, and the presence of ASD on language skills. For children with FXS, it is important to examine the effects of working memory, anxiety/arousal, sensory processing issues, and the presence of ASD or autism-like symptoms on language skills. Identification of these mechanisms has important implications for understanding which children are at greatest risk for language difficulties and where to focus intervention strategies.

Fifth, medical interventions may have important implications for language for both of these populations. For example, donepezil cholinergic therapy has been shown to affect language performance in adults with DS and in one small trial of seven children with DS, in which expressive language skills increased significantly on standardized testing after 16 weeks of treatment (Heller et al., 2004). Finally, well-controlled intervention studies are needed to examine the efficacy of intervention that is specific to children with DS and children with FXS. Intervention studies must examine which methods cause the most gains in vocabulary, syntax, and pragmatics and then generalize to other contexts.

REFERENCES

Abbeduto, L., Brady, N., & Kover, S. (2007). Language development and fragile X syndrome: Profiles, syndrome specificity, and within-syndrome differences. *Mental Retardation and Developmental Disabilities Research Reviews, 13,* 36–46.

Abbeduto L., & Chapman, R.S. (2005). Language development in Down syndrome and fragile X syndrome: Current research and implications for theory and practice. In P. Fletcher & J.F. Miller (Eds.), *Developmental theory and language disorders.* Amsterdam: John Benjamins Publishing.

Abbeduto, L., & Hagerman, R.J. (1997). Language and communication in fragile X syndrome. *Mental Retardation and Developmental Disabilities Research Reviews, 3,* 313–322.

Abbeduto, L., Murphy, M.M., Cawthon, S.W., Richmond, E., Weissman, M.D., Karadottir, S., et al. (2003). Receptive language skills of adolescents and young adults with Down or fragile X syndrome. *American Journal of Mental Retardation, 108*(3), 149–160.

Abbeduto, L., Pavetto, M., Kesin, E., Weissman, M., Karadottir, S., O'Brient, A., et al. (2001). The linguistic and cognitive profile of Down syndrome: Evidence from a comparison with fragile X syndrome. *Down Syndrome Research and Practice, 7,* 9–16.

Abbeduto, L., Short-Meyerson, K., Benson, G., & Dolish, J. (2004). Relationship between theory of mind and language ability in children and adolescents with intellectual disability. *Journal of Intellectual Disability Research, 48,* 150–159.

Alloway, T.P., & Gathercole, S.E. (Eds.). (2006). *Working memory and neurodevelopmental conditions*. Hove, England: Psychology Press.

American Academy of Family Physicians, American Academy of Otolaryngology-Head and Neck Surgery, and American Academy of Pediatrics Subcommittee on Otitis Media with Effusion. (2004). Otitis media with effusion: Clinical practice guideline. *Pediatrics, 113,* 1412–1429.

American Speech-Language-Hearing Association. (2001). *Roles and responsibilities of speech language pathologists with respect to reading and writing in children and adolescents* [Guidelines]. Available from http://www.asha.org/policy

American Speech-Language-Hearing Association. (2002*). Guidelines for fitting and monitoring FM systems* [Guidelines]. Available from http://www.asha.org/policy

American Speech-Language-Hearing Association. (2005). *Roles and responsibilities of speech language pathologists serving persons with mental retardation/developmental disabilities* [Guidelines]. Available from http://www.asha.org/policy

American Speech-Language-Hearing Association Audiologic Assessment Panel. (1996). *Guidelines for audiologic screening.* Rockville, MD: Author.

Bailey, A.J., Bolton, P., Butler, L., & Le Couteur, A. (1993). Prevalence of the fragile X anomaly amongst autistic twins and singletons. *Journal of Child Psychology and Psychiatry, 34*(5), 673–688.

Bailey, D.B., Hatton, D.D., Skinner, M., & Mesibov, G. (2001). Autistic behavior, FMR1 protein, and developmental trajectories in young males with fragile X syndrome. *Journal of Autism and Developmental Disorders, 31*(2), 165–174.

Bailey, D.B., Mesibov, G.B., Hatton, D.D., Clark, R.D., Roberts, J.E., & Mayhew, L. (1998). Autistic behavior in young boys with fragile X syndrome. *Journal of Autism and Developmental Disorders, 28*(6), 499–508.

Baker, M.J., Koegel, R.L., & Koegel, L.K. (1998). Increasing the social behavior of young children with autism using their obsessive behaviors. *Journal of the Association for Persons with Severe Handicaps, 23*(4), 300–308.

Baranek, G.T., Chin, Y.H., Hess, L.M.G., Yankee, J.G., Hatton, D.D., & Hooper, S.R. (2002). Sensory processing correlates of occupational performance in children with fragile X syndrome: Preliminary findings. *American Journal of Occupational Therapy, 56*(5), 538–546.

Barnes, E.F., Roberts, J., Mirrett, P., Sideris, J., & Misenheimer, J. (2006). A comparison of oral structure and oral motor function in young males with fragile X syndrome and Down syndrome. *Journal of Speech, Language, and Hearing Research, 49,* 903–917.

Baumgardner, T.L., Reiss, A.L., Freund, L.S., & Abrams, M.T. (1995). Specification of the neurobehavioral phenotype in males with fragile X syndrome. *Pediatrics, 95,* 744–752.

Beeghly, M., Weiss-Perry, B., & Cicchetti, D. (1990). Beyond sensorimotor functioning: Early communicative and play development of children with Down syndrome. In D. Cicchetti & M. Beeghly (Eds.), *Children with Down syndrome: A developmental perspective.* New York: Cambridge University Press.

Belser, R.C., & Sudhalter, V. (1995). Arousal difficulties in males with fragile X syndrome: A preliminary report. *Developmental Brain Dysfunction, 8*(4), 270–279.

Belser, R.C., & Sudhalter, V. (2001). Conversational characteristics of children with fragile X syndrome: Repetitive speech. *American Journal on Mental Retardation, 106*(1), 28–38.

Bennetto, L., & Pennington, B.F. (2002). The neuropsychology of fragile X syndrome. In R.J. Hagerman & A.C. Cronister (Eds.), *Fragile X syndrome: Diagnosis, treatment, and research* (2nd ed., pp. 210–248). Baltimore: The Johns Hopkins University Press.

Bennetts, L.K., & Flynn, M.C. (2002). Improving the classroom listening skills of children with Down syndrome by using sound-field amplification. *Down Syndrome Research and Practice, 8,* 19–24.

Berglund, E., & Eriksson, M. (2000). Communicative development in Swedish children 16–28 months old: The Swedish Early Communicative Development Inventory—words and sentences. *Scandinavian Journal of Psychology, 41*(2), 133–144.

Berglund, E., Eriksson, M., & Johansson, I. (2001). Parental reports of spoken language skills in children with Down syndrome. *Journal of Speech, Language, and Hearing Research, 44,* 179–191.

Bidwell, M., & Rehfeldt, R.A. (2004). Using video modeling to teach a domestic skill with an embedded social skill to adults with severe mental retardation. *Behavioral Interventions, 19*(4), 263–274.

Bliss, L.S. (2002). *Discourse impairments: Assessment and intervention applications.* Boston: Allyn & Bacon.

Boudreau, D.M., & Chapman, R.S. (2000). The relationship between event representation and linguistic skill in narratives of children and adolescents with Down syndrome. *Journal of Speech, Language, and Hearing Research, 43,* 1146–1159.

Brinton, B., & Fujiki, M. (1989). *Conversational management with language-impaired children: Pragmatic assessment and intervention.* Gaithersburg, MD: Aspen Publishers.

Brinton, B., Robinson, L.A., & Fujiki, M. (2004). Description of a program for social language intervention: "If you can have a conversation, you can have a relationship." *Language, Speech, and Hearing Services in Schools, 35*(3), 283–290.

Camarata, S.M., & Nelson, K.E. (2006). In R.J. McCauley & M.E. Fey (Eds.), *Conversational recast intervention with preschool and older children.* Baltimore: Paul H. Brookes Publishing Co.

Camarata, S., & Yoder, P. (2002). Language transactions during development and intervention: Theoretical implications for developmental neuroscience. *International Journal of Developmental Neuroscience, Special Issue: NICHD Mental Retardation Research Centers, 20*(3–5), 459–465.

Cardoso-Martins, C., Mervis, C.B., & Mervis, C.A. (1985). Early vocabulary acquisition by children with Down syndrome. *American Journal of Mental Deficiency, 90*(2), 177–184.

Carr, E.G., & Durand, V.M. (1985). Reducing behavior problems through functional communication training. *Journal of Applied Behavioral Analysis, 18*(2), 111–126.

Carrow-Woolfolk, C. (1999). *Test for Auditory Comprehension of Language–Third Edition.* Austin, TX: PRO-ED.

Caselli, M.C., Vicari, S., Longobardi, E., Lami, L., Pizzoli, C., & Stella, G. (1998). Gestures and words in early development of children with Down syndrome. *Journal of Speech, Language, and Hearing Research, 41*(5), 1125–1135.

Chapman, R.S. (2000). Children's language learning: An interactionist perspective. *Journal of Child Psychology and Psychiatry, 41,* 33–54.

Chapman, R.S. (2003). Language and communication in individuals with DS. In L. Abbeduto (Ed.), *International review of research in mental retardation: Language and communication* (pp. 1–34). San Diego: Academic Press.

Chapman, R.S., & Hesketh, L.J. (2000). Behavioral phenotype of individuals with Down syndrome. *Mental Retardation and Developmental Disabilities Research Reviews, 6*(2), 84–95.

Chapman, R.S., Hesketh, L.J., & Kistler, D.J. (2002). Predicting longitudinal change in language production and comprehension in individuals with Down syndrome: Hierarchical linear modeling. *Journal of Speech, Language, and Hearing Research, 45,* 902–915.

Chapman, R.S., Kay-Raining Bird, E., & Schwartz, S.E. (1990). Fast mapping of words in event contexts by children with Down syndrome. *Journal of Speech and Hearing Disorders, 55,* 761–770.

Chapman, R.S., Schwartz, S.E., & Kay-Raining Bird, E. (1991). Language skills of children and adolescents with Down syndrome: I. Comprehension. *Journal of Speech and Hearing Research, 34*(5), 1106–1120.

Chapman, R.S., Seung, H., Schwartz, S.E., & Kay-Raining Bird, E. (1998). Language skills of children and adolescents with Down syndrome: II. Production deficits. *Journal of Speech, Language, and Hearing Research, 41*(4), 861–873.

Chapman, R.S., Seung, H.K., Schwartz, S.E., & Kay-Raining Bird, E. (2000). Predicting language production in children and adolescents with Down syndrome: The role of comprehension. *Journal of Speech, Language, and Hearing Research, 43,* 340–350.

Chapman, R.S., Sindberg, H., Bridge, C., Gigstead, K., & Hesketh, L.J. (2006). Effect of memory support and elicited production on fast mapping of new words by adolescents with Down syndrome. *Journal of Speech, Language, & Hearing Research, 49,* 3–15.

Charlop, M.H., & Milstein, J.P. (1989). Teaching autistic children conversational speech using video modeling. *Journal of Applied Behavior Analysis, 22,* 275–285.

Coggins, T.E., Carpenter, R.L., & Owings, N.O. (1983). Examining early intentional communication in Down syndrome and nonretarded children. *British Journal of Disorders of Communication, 18*(2), 98–106.

Coggins, T.E., & Stoel-Gammon, C. (1982). Clarification strategies used by four Down syndrome children for maintaining normal conversational interaction. *Education Training Mental Retardation, 16,* 65–67.

Cohen, I.L., Fisch, G.S., Sudhalter, V., Wolf-Schein, E.G., Hanson, D., Hagerman, R., et al. (1988). Social gaze, social avoidance, and repetitive behavior in fragile X males: A controlled study. *American Journal on Mental Retardation, 92*(5), 436–446.

Cohen, I.L., Vietze, P.M., Sudhalter, V., Jenkins, E.C., & Brown, W.T. (1989). Parent–child dyadic gaze patterns in fragile X males and in non-fragile X males with autistic disorder. *Journal of Child Psychology and Psychiatry, 30*(6), 845–856.

Cornish, K.M., Munir, F., & Cross, G. (1998). The nature of the spatial deficit in young females with fragile-X syndrome: A neuropsychological and molecular perspective. *Neuropsychologia, 36*(11), 1239–1246.

Cornish, K.M., Munir, F., & Cross, G. (1999). Spatial cognition in males with fragile-X syndrome: Evidence for a neuropsychological phenotype. *Cortex, 35,* 263–271.

Cornish, K., Sudhalter, V., & Turk, J. (2004). Attention and language in fragile X. *Mental Retardation and Developmental Disabilities Research Reviews, 10*(1), 11–16.

Cornish, K.M., Turk, J., Wilding, J., Sudhalter, V., Munir, F., Kooy, F., et al. (2004). Deconstructing the attention deficit in fragile X syndrome: A developmental neuropsychological approach. *Journal of Child Psychology and Psychiatry, 45*(6), 1042–1053.

Dawson, G., & Galpert, L. (1990). Others' use of imitative play for facilitating social responsiveness and toy play in young autistic children. *Development and Psychopathology, 2*(2), 151–162.

Dawson, G., & Watling, R. (2000). Interventions to facilitate auditory, visual, and motor integration in autism: A review of the evidence. *Journal of Autism and Developmental Disorders, Special Issue: Treatments for People with Autism and Other Pervasive Developmental Disorders: Research Perspectives, 30*(5), 415–421.

Dodd, B., & Thompson, L. (2001). Speech disorder in children with Down syndrome. *Journal of Intellectual Disabilities Research, 45,* 308–316.

Dunn, L.M., & Dunn, L.M. (1981). *Peabody Picture Vocabulary Test–Revised.* Circle Pines, MN: American Guidance Service.

Dunn, L.M., & Dunn, L.M. (1997). *Peabody Picture Vocabulary Test–Third Edition.* Circle Pines, MN: American Guidance Service.

Dykens, E.M., Hodapp, R.M., & Evans, D.W. (2006). Profiles and development of adaptive behavior in children with Down syndrome. *Down Syndrome Research and Practice, 9,* 45–50.

Dykens, E.M., Hodapp, R.M., & Leckman, J.F. (1987). Strengths and weaknesses in the intellectual functioning of males with fragile X syndrome. *American Journal of Mental Deficiency, 92*(2), 234–236.

Dykens, E.M., Hodapp, R.M., & Leckman, J.F. (1989). Adaptive and maladaptive functioning of institutionalized and noninstitutionalized fragile X males. *Journal of the American Academy of Child and Adolescent Psychiatry, 28*(3), 427–430.

Dykens, E.M., Hodapp, R.M., Ort, S.I., & Leckman, J.F. (1993). Trajectory of adaptive behavior in males with fragile X syndrome. *Journal of Autism and Developmental Disorders, 23*(1), 135–145.

Dykens, E.M., & Volkmar, F. (1997). Medical conditions associated with autism. In D. Cohen & F. Volkmar (Eds.), *Autism and pervasive developmental disorders* (2nd ed.). New York: John Wiley & Sons.

Eadie, P.A., Fey, M.E., Douglas, J.M., & Parsons, C.L. (2002). Profiles of grammatical morphology and sentence imitation in children with specific language impairment and Down syndrome. *Journal of Speech, Language, and Hearing Research, 45,* 720–732.

Fenson, L., Dale, P.S., Reznick, J.S., Thal, D., Bates, E., Hartung, J.P., et al. (1992). *MacArthur-Bates Communicative Development Inventories (CDIs).* Baltimore: Paul H. Brookes Publishing Co.

Ferrier, L.J., Bashir, A.S., Meryash, D.L., Johnston, J., & Wolff, P. (1991). Conversational skills of individuals with fragile-X syndrome: A comparison with autism and Down syndrome. *Developmental Medicine and Child Neurology, 33,* 776–778.

Fey, M.E. (1986). *Language intervention with young children.* San Diego: College-Hill Press.

Fey, M.E., Warren, S.F., Brady, N., Finestack, L.H., Bredin-Oja, S.L., Fairchild, M., et al. (2006). Early effects of responsivity education/prelinguistic milieu teaching for children with developmental delays and their parents. *Journal of Speech, Language, and Hearing Research, 49,* 526–547.

Fidler, D.J. (2005). The emerging Down syndrome behavioral phenotype in early childhood: Implications for practice. *Infants and Young Children, 18,* 86–103.

Fidler, D.J., Hepburn, S., & Rogers, S. (2006). Early learning and adaptive behavior in toddlers with Down syndrome: Evidence for an emerging behavioral phenotype. *Down Syndrome Research and Practice, 9,* 37–44.

Fowler, C.A. (1988). Differential shortening of repeated content words produced in various communicative contexts. *Language and Speech, 31*(4), 307–319.

Frea, W.D., & Hughes, C. (1997). Functional analysis and treatment of social-communicative behavior of adolescents with developmental disabilities. *Journal of Applied Behavior Analysis, 30*(4), 701–704.

Freund, L.S., & Reiss, A.L. (1991). Rating problem behaviors in outpatients with mental retardation: Use of the aberrant behavior checklist. *Research in Developmental Disabilities, 12*(4), 435–451.

Freund, L.S., Reiss, A.L., & Abrams, M.T. (1993). Psychiatric disorders associated with fragile X in the young female. *Pediatrics, 91*(2), 321–329.

Fryns, J.P., Jacobs, J., Kleczkowska, A., & Van den Berghe, H. (1984). The psychological profile of the fragile X syndrome. *Clinical Genetics, 25,* 131–134.

Gathercole, S.E., Alloway, T.P., Willis, C., & Adams, A. (2006). Working memory in children with reading disabilities. *Journal of Experimental Child Psychology, 93*(3), 265–281.

Ghaziuddin, M., Tsai, L.Y., & Ghaziuddin, N. (1992). Autism in Down syndrome: Presentation and diagnosis. *Journal of Intellectual Disability Research, 36*(5), 449–456.

Gillham, B. (1990). First words in normal and Down syndrome children: A comparison of content and wordform categories. *Child Language Teaching and Therapy, 6,* 25–32.

Girolametto, L., & Weitzman, E. (2006). It takes two to talk—The Hanen program for parents: Early intervention through caregiver training. In S.F. Warren & M.E. Fey (Series Eds.) & R.J. McCauley & M.E. Fey (Vol. Eds.), *Communication and language intervention series: Treatment of language disorders in children* (pp. 77–103). Baltimore: Paul H. Brookes Publishing Co.

Girolametto, L., Weitzman, E., & Clements-Baartman, J. (1998). Vocabulary intervention for children with Down syndrome: Parent training using focused stimulation. *Infant-Toddler Intervention, 8*(2), 109–125.

Gleason, J.B. (2005). *The development of language* (6th ed.). Boston: Allyn & Bacon.

Glenn, S., & Cunningham, C. (2005). Performance of young people with Down syndrome on the Leiter-R and British picture vocabulary scales. *Journal of Intellectual Disability Research, 49*(4), 239–244.

Goldstein, H. (2002). Communication intervention for children with autism: A review of treatment efficacy. *Journal of Autism and Developmental Disorders, 32,* 373–396.

Hagerman, R.J. (2002). The physical and behavioral phenotype. In R.J. Hagerman & P.J. Hagerman (Eds.), *Fragile X syndrome: Diagnosis, treatment, and research* (pp. 3–109). Baltimore: The Johns Hopkins University Press.

Hagerman, R.J. (2006). Lessons from fragile X regarding neurobiology, autism, and neurodegeneration. *Journal of Developmental & Behavioral Pediatrics, 27,* 63–74.

Hagerman, R.J., Altshul-Stark, D., & McBogg, P. (1987). Recurrent otitis media in boys with the fragile X syndrome. *American Journal of Diseases of Children, 141,* 184–187.

Hagerman, R.J., Hills, J., Scharfenaker, S., & Lewis, H. (1999). Fragile X syndrome and selective mutism. *American Journal of Medical Genetics, 83,* 313–317.

Hagerman, R.J., Hull, C.E., Safanda, J.F., Carpenter, I., Staley, L.W., O'Connor, R., et al. (1994). High functioning fragile X males: Demonstration of an unmethylated, fully expanded FMR-1 mutation associated with protein expression. *American Journal of Medical Genetics, 51,* 298–308.

Hagerman, R.J., Jackson, C., Amiri, K., Silverman, A.C., O'Connor, R., & Sobesky, W. (1992). Girls with fragile X syndrome: Physical and neurocognitive status and outcome. *Pediatrics, 89,* 395–400.

Hanson, D.M., Jackson, A.W., & Hagerman, R.J. (1986). Speech disturbances (cluttering) in mildly impaired males with the Martin-Bell/fragile X syndrome. *American Journal of Medical Genetics, 23,* 195–206.

Harris-Schmidt, G., & Fast, D. (1998). Fragile X syndrome: Genetics, characteristics, and educational implications. In A.F. Rotatori, J.O. Schwenn, & S. Burkhardt (Eds.), *Advances in special education: Issues, practices, and concerns in special education* (Vol. 2, pp. 187–222). Greenwich, CT: Elsevier Science/JAI Press.

Harris-Schmidt, G., & Fast, D. (2004). *The Source for fragile X syndrome.* East Moline, IL: LinguiSystems.

Heller, J.H., Spiridigliozzi, G.A., Doraiswarmy, P.M., Sullivan, J.A., Crissman, B.G., & Kishnani, P.S. (2004). Donepezil effects on language in children with Down syndrome: Results of the first 22-week pilot clinical trial. *American Journal of Medical Genetics, 130,* 325–326.

Hesketh, L.J., & Chapman, R.S. (1998). Verb use by individuals with Down syndrome. *American Journal on Mental Retardation, 103,* 288–304.

Hessl, D., Dyer-Friedman, J., Glaser, B., Wisbek, J., Barajas, R.G., Taylor, A., et al. (2001). The influence of environmental and genetic factors on behavior problems and autistic symptoms in boys and girls with fragile X syndrome. *Pediatrics, 108*(5), 88–104.

Hessl, D., Rivera, S.M., & Reiss, A.L. (2004). The neuroanatomy and neuroendocrinology of fragile X syndrome. *Mental Retardation and Developmental Disabilities Research Reviews, 10,* 17–24.

Hick, R.F., Botting, N., & Conti-Ramsden, G. (2005). Short-term memory and vocabulary development in children with Down syndrome and children with specific language impairment. *Developmental Medicine and Child Neurology, 47,* 532–538.

Imada, T., Zhang, Y., Cheour, M., Taulu, S., Ahonen, A., & Kuhl, P.K. (2006). Infant speech perception activates Broca's area: A developmental magnetoencephalography study. *Neuroreport, 17,* 957–962.

Iverson, J.M., Longobardi, E., & Caselli, M.C. (2003). Relationship between gestures and words in children with Down's syndrome and typically developing children in the early stages of communicative development. *International Journal of Language and Communication Disorders, 38,* 179–197.

Jakala, P., Hanninen, T., Ryynanen, M., Laakso, M., Partanen, K., Mannermaa, A., et al. (1997). Fragile-X: Neuropsychological test performance, CGG triplet repeat lengths, and hippocampal volumes. *Journal of Clinical Investigation, 100,* 331–338.

Jarrold, C., & Baddeley, A.D. (2001). Short-term memory in Down syndrome: Applying the working memory model. *Down Syndrome Research and Practice, 7,* 17–23.

Jarrold, C., Baddeley, A.D., & Hewes, A.K. (2000). Verbal short-term memory deficits in Down syndrome: A consequence of problems in rehearsal. *Journal of Child Psychology and Psychiatry, 41,* 233–244.

Jarrold, C., Baddeley, A.D., & Phillips, C. (1999). Down syndrome and the phonological loop: The evidence for and importance of a specific verbal short-term memory deficit. *Down Syndrome Research and Practice, 6,* 61–75.

Jarrold, C., Cowan, N., Hewes, A.K., & Riby, D.M. (2004). Speech timing and verbal short-term memory: Evidence for contrasting deficits in Down syndrome and Williams syndrome. *Journal of Memory and Language, 51,* 365–380.

Jones, E.A., Carr, E.G., & Feeley, K.M. (2006). Multiple effects of joint attention intervention for children with autism. *Behavior Modification, 30,* 782–834.

Kasari, C., Freeman, S.F., & Hughes, M.A. (2001). Emotion recognition by children with Down syndrome. *American Journal on Mental Retardation, 106,* 59–72.

Kay-Raining Bird, E., Chapman, R.S., & Schwartz, S.E. (2004). Fast mapping of words and story recall by individuals with Down syndrome. *Journal of Speech, Language, and Hearing Research, 47,* 1286–1300.

Kent, L., Evans, J., Paul, M., & Sharp, M. (1999). Comorbidity of autistic spectrum disorders in children with Down syndrome. *Developmental Medicine and Child Neurology, 41*(3), 153–158.

Kerby, D.S., & Dawson, B.L. (1994). Autistic features, personality, and adaptive behavior in males with the fragile X syndrome and no autism. *American Journal on Mental Retardation, 98*(4), 455–462.

Kirk, J.W., Mazzocco, M.M., & Kover, S.T. (2005). Assessing executive dysfunction in girls with fragile X or Turner syndrome using the contingency naming test (CNT). *Developmental Neuropsychology, 28*(3), 755–777.

Koegel, L. (2000). Intervention to facilitate communication in autism. *Journal of Autism and Developmental Disorders, 30,* 383–391.

Koegel, L.K., Carter, C.M., & Koegel, R.L. (2003). Teaching children with autism self-initiations as a pivotal response. *Topics in Language Disorders, 32,* 134–145.

Koegel, R.L., Camarata, S., & Koegel, L.K. (1998). Increasing speech intelligibility in children with autism. *Journal of Autism and Developmental Disorders, 28*(3), 241–251.

Koegel, R.L., & Frea, W.D. (1993). Treatment of social behavior in autism through the modification of pivotal social skills. *Journal of Applied Behavior Analysis, 26,* 369–377.

Koegel, R.L., Koegel, L.K., & Carter, C.M. (1999). Pivotal teaching interactions for children with autism. *School Psychology Review, 28*(4), 576–594.

Koegel, R.L., O'Dell, M.C., & Koegel, L.K. (1987). A natural language teaching paradigm for nonverbal autistic children. *Journal of Autism and Developmental Disorders, 17*(2), 187–200.

Koegel, R.L, Schreibman, L., Good, A., Cerniglia, L., Murphy, C., & Koegel, L.K. (1989). *How to teach pivotal behaviors to children with autism: A training manual.* Santa Barbara: University of California.

Kostinas, G., Scandlen, A., & Luiselli, J.K. (2001). Effects of DRL and DRL combined with response cost on perseverative verbal behavior of an adult with mental retardation and obsessive compulsive disorder. *Behavioral Interventions, 16*(1), 27–37.

Krantz, P.J., MacDuff, M.T., & McClannahan, L.E. (1993). Programming participation in family activities for children with autism: Parents' use of photographic activity schedules. *Journal of Applied Behavior Analysis, 26*(1), 137–138.

Krantz, P.J., & McClannahan, L.E. (1993). Teaching children with autism to initiate to peers: Effects of a script-fading procedure. *Journal of Applied Behavior Analysis, 26*(1), 121–132.

Kumin, L. (2003). *Early communication skills for children with Down syndrome: A guide for parents and professionals.* Bethesda, MD: Woodbine House.

Kumin, L., Goodman, M., & Councill, C. (1996). Comprehensive speech and language intervention for school-aged children with Down syndrome. *Down Syndrome Quarterly, 1*(1), 1–8.

Lachiewicz, A.M., & Dawson, D.V. (1994). Behavior problems of young girls with fragile X syndrome: Factor scores on the Conners' Parent's Questionnaire. *American Journal of Medical Genetics, 51*(4), 364–369.

Landa, R. (2007). Early communication development and intervention for children with autism. *Mental Retardation and Developmental Disabilities Research Reviews, 13*(1), 16–25.

Landry, S.H., Smith, K.E., Miller-Loncar, C.L., & Swank, P.R. (1997). Predicting cognitive-language and social growth curves from early maternal behaviors in children at varying degrees of biological risk. *Developmental Psychology, 33*(6), 1040–1053.

Landry, S.H., Smith, K.E., Swank, P.R., & Miller-Loncar, C.L. (2000). Early maternal and child influences on children's later independent cognitive and social functioning. *Child Development, 71,* 358–375.

Laws, G., & Bishop, D.V. (2003). A comparison of language abilities in adolescents with Down syndrome and children with specific language impairment. *Journal of Speech, Language, and Hearing Research, 46,* 1324–1339.

Laws, G., & Bishop, D.V. (2004). Verbal deficits in Down's syndrome and specific language impairment: A comparison. *International Journal of Language and Communication Disorders, 39,* 423–451.

Lesniak-Karpiak, K., Mazzocco, M.M., & Ross, J.L. (2003). Behavioral assessment of social anxiety in females with Turner or fragile X syndrome. *Journal of Autism and Developmental Disorders, 33*(1), 55–67.

Levy, Y., Gottesman, R., Borochowitz, Z., Frydman, M., & Sagi, M. (2006). Language in boys with fragile X syndrome: Erratum. *Journal of Child Language, 33*(2), 437.

Lewis, P., Abbeduto, L., Murphy, M., Richmond, E., Giles, N., Bruno, L., & Schroeder, S. (2006). Cognitive, language and social-cognitive skills of individuals with fragile X syndrome with and without autism. *Journal of Intellectual Disability Research, 50*(7), 532–545.

Lord, C., Rutter, M., DiLavore, P.C., & Risi, S. (2002). *Autism Diagnostic Observation Schedule.* Los Angeles: Western Psychological Services.

Madison, L.S., George, C., & Moeschler, J.B. (1986). Cognitive functioning in the fragile X syndrome: A study of intellectual, memory, and communication skills. *Journal of Mental Deficiency Research, 30*(2), 129–148.

Mahoney, G., Perales, F., Wiggers, B., & Herman, B. (2006). Responsive teaching: Early intervention for children with Down syndrome and other disabilities. *Down Syndrome Research and Practice, 11,* 18–28.

Mazzocco, M.M., Baumgardner, T., Freund, L., & Reiss, A. (1998). Social functioning among girls with fragile X or Turner syndrome and their sisters. *Journal of Autism and Developmental Disorders, 28*(6), 509–517.

Mazzocco, M.M., Kates, W.R., Baumgardner, T.L., Freund, L.S., & Reiss, A.L. (1997). Autistic behaviors among girls with fragile X syndrome. *Journal of Autism and Developmental Disorders, 27*(4), 415–435.

Mazzocco, M.M., Pennington, B.F., & Hagerman, R.J. (1993). The neurocognitive phenotype of female carriers of fragile X: Additional evidence for specificity. *Journal of Developmental and Behavioral Pediatrics, 14*(5), 328–335.

McCauley, R.J., & Fey, M.E. (Vol. Eds.) & S.F. Warren & M.E. Fey (Series Eds.) (2006). *Communication and language intervention series: Treatment of language disorders in children.* Baltimore: Paul H. Brookes Publishing Co.

Merenstein, S.A., Sobesky, W.E., Taylor, A.K., Riddle, J.E., Tran, H.X., & Hagerman, R.J. (1996). Molecular-clinical correlations in males with an expanded FMR1 mutation. *American Journal of Medical Genetics, 64,* 388–394.

Mervis, C.B., & Robinson, B.F. (2000). Expressive vocabulary ability of toddlers with Williams syndrome or Down syndrome: A comparison. *Developmental Neuropsychology, 17*(1), 111–126.

Miles, S., & Chapman, R.S. (2002). Narrative content as described by individuals with Down syndrome and typically developing children. *Journal of Speech, Language, and Hearing Research, 45,* 175–189.

Miles, S., Chapman, R., & Sindberg, H. (2006). Sampling context affects MLU in the language of adolescents with Down syndrome. *Journal of Speech, Language, and Hearing Research, 49,* 325–337.

Miller, J.F. (1988). The developmental asynchrony of language development in children with Down syndrome. In L. Nadel (Ed.), *The psychobiology of Down syndrome* (pp. 167–198). Cambridge: MIT Press.

Miller, J.F. (1995). Individual differences in vocabulary acquisition in children with Down syndrome. *Progress in Clinical Biology Research, 393,* 93–103.

Miller, J.F., & Leddy, M. (1998). Down syndrome: The impact of speech production on language development. In S.F. Warren & J. Reichle (Series Eds.) & R. Paul (Vol. Ed.), *Exploring the speech-language connection* (pp. 163–177). Baltimore: Paul H. Brookes Publishing Co.

Miller, J.F., Miolo, G., Sedey, A., Pierce, K., & Rosin, M. (1989). *Predicting lexical growth in children with Down syndrome.* Poster presented at the annual meeting of the American Speech-Language-Hearing Association, St. Louis, MO.

Miller, L.J., Reisman, J., McIntosh, D.N., & Simon, J. (2001). The ecological model of sensory modulation: Performance of children with fragile X syndrome, autism, ADHD, and SMD. In S. Roley, R. Schaaf, & E. Blanche (Eds.), *Sensory integration and developmental disabilities.* San Antonio: Therapy Skill Builders.

Miolo, G., Chapman, R.S., & Sindberg, H.A. (2005). Sentence comprehension in adolescents with Down syndrome and typically developing children: Role of sentence voice, visual context, and auditory-verbal short-term memory. *Journal of Speech, Language, and Hearing Research, 48,* 172–188.

Morrison, L., Kamps, D., Garcia, J., Parker, D., & Dunlap, G. (2001). Peer mediation and monitoring strategies to improve initiation and social skills for students with autism. *Journal of Positive Behavior Interventions, 3*(4), 237.

Mundy, P., Kasari, C., Sigman, M., & Ruskin, E. (1995). Nonverbal communication and early language acquisition in children with Down syndrome and in normally developing children. *Journal of Speech and Hearing Research, 38,* 157–167.

Mundy, P., Sigman, M., Kasari, C., & Yirmiya, N. (1988). Nonverbal communication skills in Down syndrome children. *Child Development, 59*(1), 235–249.

Munir, F., Cornish, K.M., & Wilding, J. (2000). Nature of the working memory deficit in fragile X syndrome. *Brain and Cognition, 44*(3), 387–401.

National Institute of Child Health and Human Development Early Child Care Research Network. (2000). The relation of child care to cognitive and language development. *Child Development, 71*(4), 960–980.

National Institute of Child Health and Human Development Early Child Care Research Network. (2002). Early child care and children's development prior to school entry: Results from the NICHD study of early child care. *American Educational Research Journal, 39,* 133–164.

Odom, S.L., & Strain, P.S. (1986). A comparison of peer initiation and teacher-antecedent interventions for promoting reciprocal social interactions of autistic preschoolers. *Journal of Applied Behavior Analysis, 19,* 59–71.

Palmer, K.K., Gordon, J.S., Coston, G.N., & Stevenson, R.E. (1988). Fragile X syndrome IV. Speech and language characteristics. *Proceedings of Greenwood Genetic Center, 7,* 93–97.

Paul, R. (1992). *Pragmatic activities for language intervention: Semantics, syntax, and emerging literacy.* Austin, TX: PRO-ED.

Paul, R. (2003). Promoting social communication in high functioning individuals with autistic spectrum disorders. *Child and Adolescent Psychiatric Clinics of North America, 12,* 87–106.

Paul, R. (2007). *Language disorders from infancy through adolescence* (3rd ed.). Philadelphia: Mosby Elsevier.

Paul, R., Cohen, D.J., Breg, W.R., Watson, M., & Herman, S. (1984). Fragile X syndrome: Its relations to speech and language disorders. *Journal of Speech and Hearing Disorders, 49,* 326–336.

Pepper, J., & Weitzman, E. (2004). *It takes two to talk: A practical guide for parents of children with language delays* (2nd ed.). Toronto: The Hanen Centre.

Philofsky, A., Hepburn, S.L., Hayes, A., Hagerman, R., & Rogers, S. (2004). Linguistic and cognitive functioning and autism symptoms in young children with fragile X syndrome. *American Journal on Mental Retardation, 109*(3), 208–218.

Price, J.R., Roberts, J.E., Hennon, E.A., Berni, M.C., Anderson, K.L., & Sideris, J. (in press). Syntactic complexity during conversation of boys with fragile X syndrome and Down syndrome. *Journal of Speech, Language, and Hearing Research.*

Price, J.R., Roberts, J.E., Vandergrift, N., & Martin, G. (2007). Language comprehension in boys with fragile X syndrome and boys with Down syndrome. *Journal of Intellectual Disability Research, 51*(4), 318–326.

Prizant, B.M., Wetherby, A.M. Rubin, E., & Laurent, A.C. (2003). The SCERTS Model: A transactional, family-centered approach to enhancing communication and socioemotional abilities of children with Autism Spectrum Disorder. *Infants and Young Children, 16,* 296–316.

Prizant, B.M., Wetherby, A.M., Rubin, E., Laurent, A.C., & Rydell, P.J. (2005). *The SCERTS® Model: A comprehensive educational approach for children with autism spectrum disorders* (Vols. I and II). Baltimore: Paul H. Brookes Publishing Co.

Prouty, L.A., Rogers, R.C., Stevenson, R.E., Dean, J.H., Palmer, K.K., Simensen, R.J., et al. (1988). Fragile X syndrome: Growth, development, and intellectual function. *American Journal of Medical Genetics, 30,* 123–142.

Rehfeldt, R.A., & Chambers, M.R. (2003). Functional analysis and treatment of verbal perseverations displayed by an adult with autism. *Journal of Applied Behavior Analysis, 36,* 259–261.

Reiss, A.L., & Freund, L. (1992). Behavioral phenotype of fragile X syndrome: DSM-III-R autistic behavior in male children. *American Journal of Medical Genetics, 43,* 35–46.

Rice, M.L., Warren, S.F., & Betz, S.K. (2005). Language symptoms of developmental language disorders: An overview of autism, Down syndrome, fragile X, specific language impairment, and Williams syndrome. *Applied Psycholinguistics, 26,* 7–27.

Rice, M.L., & Wexler, K. (1996). Toward tense as a clinical marker of specific language impairment in English-speaking children. *Journal of Speech and Hearing Research, 39,* 1239–1257.

Rice, M.L., Wexler, K., & Cleave, P.L. (1995). Specific language impairment as a period of extended optional infinitive. *Journal of Speech and Hearing Research, 38,* 850–863.

Roberts, J.E., Boccia, M.L., Bailey, D.B., Hatton, D.D., & Skinner, M. (2001). Cardiovascular indices of physiological arousal in boys with fragile X syndrome. *Developmental Psychobiology, 39*(2), 107–123.

Roberts, J.E., Hennon, E.A., Anderson, K., Roush, J., Gravel, J., Skinner, M., et al. (2005). Auditory brainstem responses in young males with fragile X syndrome. *Journal of Speech, Language, and Hearing Research, 48,* 494–500.

Roberts, J.E., Hennon, E.A., Dear, E., Anderson, K., & Vandergrift, N.A. (2007). Expressive language during conversational speech in boys with fragile X syndrome. *American Journal on Mental Retardation, 112,* 1–15.

Roberts, J.E., Hunter, L., Gravel, J., Rosenfeld, R., Berman, S., Haggard, M., et al. (2004). Otitis media, hearing loss, and language learning: Controversies and current research. *Journal of Developmental and Behavioral Pediatrics, 25*(2), 1–13.

Roberts, J., Long, S.H., Malkin, C., Barnes, E., Skinner, M., Hennon, E.A., et al. (2005). A comparison of phonological skills of boys with fragile X syndrome and Down syndrome. *Journal of Speech, Language, and Hearing Research, 48,* 980–985.

Roberts, J., Martin, G.E., Moskowitz, L., Harris, A.A., Foreman, J., & Nelson, L. (2007). Discourse skills of boys with fragile X syndrome in comparison to boys with Down syndrome. *Journal of Speech, Language, and Hearing Research, 50,* 475–492.

Roberts, J.E., Mirrett, P., Anderson, K., Burchinal, M., & Neebe, E. (2002). Early communication, symbolic behavior, and social profiles of young males with fragile X syndrome. *American Journal of Speech Language Pathology, 11,* 295–304.

Roberts, J.E., Mirrett, P., & Burchinal, M. (2001). Receptive and expressive communication development of young males with fragile X syndrome. *American Journal on Mental Retardation, 106*(3), 216–230.

Roberts, J., Price, J., Nelson, L., Burchinal, M., Hennon, E., Barnes, E., et al. (2007). Receptive vocabulary, expressive vocabulary, and speech production of boys with fragile X syndrome in comparison to boys with Down syndrome. *American Journal on Mental Retardation, 112,* 177–193.

Roberts, J.E., & Wallace, I.F. (1997). Language and otitis media. In J.E. Roberts, I.F. Wallace, & F.W. Henderson (Eds.), *Otitis media in young children* (1st ed., pp. 133–161). Baltimore: Paul H. Brookes Publishing Co.

Rogers, S.J. (1998a). Empirically supported comprehensive treatments for young children with autism. *Journal of Clinical Child Psychology, 27,* 168–179.

Rogers, S.J. (1998b). Neuropsychology of autism in young children and its implications for early intervention. *Mental Retardation and Developmental Disabilities Research Reviews, 4,* 104–112.

Rogers, S.J. (2000). Interventions that facilitate socialization in children with autism. *Journal of Autism and Developmental Disorders, 30,* 399–409.

Rogers, S.J., Hepburn, S., & Wehner, E. (2003). Parent reports of sensory symptoms in toddlers with autism and those with other developmental disorders. *Journal of Autism and Developmental Disorders, 33,* 631–642.

Rogers, S.J., Wehner, E.A., & Hagerman, R. (2001). The behavioral phenotype in fragile X: Symptoms of autism in very young children with fragile X syndrome, idiopathic autism, and other developmental disorders, *Developmental and Behavioral Pediatrics, 22*(6), 409–417.

Roid, G.H., & Miller, L.J. (1997). *Leiter International Performance Scale–Revised.* Wood Dale, IL: Stoelting.

Roizen, N.J. (2002). Down syndrome. In M.L. Batshaw (Ed.), *Children with disabilities* (5th ed., pp. 307–320). Baltimore: Paul H. Brookes Publishing Co.

Ross, D.E. (2002). Replacing faulty conversational exchanges for children with autism by establishing a functionally equivalent alternative response. *Education and Training in Mental Retardation and Developmental Disabilities, 37,* 343–362.

Schaaf, R.C., & Miller, L.J. (2005). Occupational therapy using a sensory integrative approach for children with developmental disabilities. *Mental Retardation and Developmental Disabilities Research Reviews, 11*(2), 143–148.

Scharfenaker, S.R., O'Connor, R., Stackhouse, M., Braden, L., & Gray, K. (2002). An integrated approach to intervention. In R.J. Hagerman & P.J. Hagerman (Eds.), *Fragile X syndrome diagnosis, treatment, and research* (3rd ed., pp. 363–427). Baltimore: The Johns Hopkins University Press.

Schoenbrodt, L., & Smith, R.A. (1995). *Communication disorders and interventions in low incidence pediatric populations.* San Diego: Singular Publishing Group.

Schopler, E., Mesibov, G.B., & Hearsey, K. (1995). In E. Schopler & G.B. Mesibov (Eds.), *Structured teaching in the TEACCH system.* New York: Kluwer Academic/Plenum.

Seung, H-K., & Chapman, R.S. (2000). Digit span in individuals with Down syndrome and typically developing children: Temporal aspects. *Journal of Speech, Language, and Hearing Research, 43,* 609–620.

Seung, H.K., & Chapman, R.. (2004). Sentence memory of individuals with Down's syndrome and typically developing children. *Journal of Intellectual Disabilities Research, 48,* 160–171.

Shott, S.R., Joseph, A., & Heithaus, D. (2001). Hearing loss in children with Down syndrome. *International Journal of Pediatric Otorhinolaryngology, 61,* 199–205.

Shriberg, L.D., & Widder, C.J. (1990). Speech and prosody characteristics of adults with mental retardation. *Journal of Speech and Hearing Research, 33,* 627–653.

Simon, E.W., & Finucane, B.M. (1996). Facial emotion identification in males with fragile X syndrome. *American Journal of Medical Genetics, 16*(1), 77–80.

Smith, T. (1999). Outcome of early intervention for children with autism. *Clinical Psychology: Research and Practice, 6,* 33–49.

Smith, T. (2001). Discrete trial training in the treatment of autism. *Focus on Autism and Other Developmental Disabilities, 16,* 86–106.

Snow, C.E., Burns, M.S., & Griffin, P. (1998). *Preventing reading difficulties in young children.* Washington, DC: National Academies Press.

Spinelli, M., Rocha, A., Giacheti, C., & Richieri-Costa, A. (1995). Word-finding difficulties, verbal paraphasias, and verbal dyspraxia in ten individuals with fragile X syndrome. *American Journal of Medical Genetics, 60,* 39–43.

Spiridigliozzi, G.A., Lachiewicz, A.M., MacMurdo, C.S., Vizoso, A.D., O'Donnell, C.M., McConkie-Rosell, A., et al. (1994). *Educating boys with fragile X syndrome: A guide for parents and professionals.*

Strain, P.S., & Kohler, F.W. (1998). Peer-mediated social intervention for young children with autism. *Seminars in Speech and Language, 19,* 391–405.

Strain, P.S., & Odom, S.L. (1986). Peer social initiations: Effective intervention for social skills development of exceptional children. *Exceptional Children, 52*(6), 43–51.

Strominger, A.Z., Winkler, M.R., & Cohen, L.T. (1984). Speech and language evaluation. In S.M. Pueschel (Ed.), *The young child with Down syndrome* (pp. 253–261). New York: Human Sciences Press.

Sudhalter, V., & Belser, R.C. (2001). Conversational characteristics of children with fragile X syndrome: Tangential language. *American Journal on Mental Retardation, 106*(5), 389–400.

Sudhalter, V., Cohen, I., Silverman, W., & Wolf-Schein, E. (1990). Conversational analyses of males with fragile X, Down syndrome, and autism: Comparison of the emergence of deviant language. *American Journal on Mental Retardation, 94,* 431–441.

Sudhalter, V., Maranion, M., & Brooks, P. (1992). Expressive semantic deficit in the productive language of males with fragile X syndrome. *American Journal of Medical Genetics, 43,* 65–71.

Sudhalter, V., Scarborough, H.S., & Cohen, I.L. (1991). Syntactic delay and pragmatic deviance in the language of fragile X males. *American Journal of Medical Genetics, 38,* 493–497.

Tannock, R. (1988). Mother directiveness in their interactions with their children with and without Down syndrome. *American Journal of Mental Retardation, 93,* 154–165.

Tassone, F., Hagerman, R.J., Iklé, D.N., Dyer, P.N., Lampe, M., Willemsen, R., et al. (1999). FMRP expression as a potential prognostic indicator in fragile X syndrome. *American Journal of Medical Genetics, 84,* 250–261.

Thorndike, R.L., Hagen, E.P., & Sattler, J.M. (1986). *The Stanford-Binet intelligence scale* (4th ed). Chicago: Riverside.

Turk, J. (1998). Fragile X syndrome and attentional deficits. *Journal of Applied Research in Intellectual Disabilities, 11*(3), 175–191.

Turk, J., & Cornish, K. (1998). Face recognition and emotion perception in boys with fragile-X syndrome. *Journal of Intellectual Disability Research, 42*(6), 490–499.

Turk, J., & Graham, P. (1997). Fragile X syndrome, autism, and autistic features. *Autism, 1*(2), 175–197.

Vicari, S., Caselli, M.C., & Tonucci, F. (2000). Asynchrony of lexical and morphosyntactic development in children with Down syndrome. *Neuropsychologia, 38*, 634–644.

Williams, K.R., Wishart, J.G., Pitcairn, T.K., & Willis, D.S. (2005). Emotion recognition by children with Down syndrome: Investigation of specific impairments and error patterns. *American Journal on Mental Retardation, 110*, 378–392.

Williams, K.T. (1997). *Expressive vocabulary test.* Circle Pines, MN: American Guidance Service.

Wishart, J.G., Cebula, K.R., Willis, D.S., & Pitcairn, T.K. (2007). Understanding of facial expressions of emotion by children with intellectual disabilities of differing aetiology. *Journal of Intellectual Disability Research, 51*, 551–563.

Wishart, J.G., & Pitcairn, T.K. (2000). Recognition of identity and expression in faces by children with Down syndrome. *American Journal on Mental Retardation, 105*, 466–479.

Wolf-Schein, E.G., Sudhalter, V., Cohen, I., Fisch, G.S., Hanson, D., Pfadt, A.G., et al. (1987). Speech-language and the fragile X syndrome: Initial findings. *American Speech-Language-Hearing Association, 29*, 35–38.

Yirmiya, N., Erel, O., Shaked, M., & Solomonica-Levi, D. (1998). Meta-analyses comparing theory of mind abilities of individuals with autism, individuals with mental retardation and normally developing individuals. *Psychological Bulletin, 124*, 283–307.

Yoder, P.J., Kaiser, A., & Alpert, C. (1991). An exploratory study of the interaction between language teaching methods and child characteristics. *Journal of Speech and Hearing Research, 34*, 155–167.

Yoder P.J., Kaiser A., Goldstein H., Alpert, C., Mousetis, L., Kaczmarek, L., et al. (1995). An exploratory comparison of milieu teaching and responsive interaction in classroom applications. *Journal of Early Intervention, 19*, 218–242.

Yoder, P., & Warren, S.F. (1999). Maternal responsivity mediates the relationship between prelinguistic intentional communication and later language. *Journal of Early Intervention, 22*, 126–136.

Zelazo, P.D., Burack, J.A., Benedetto, E., & Frye, D. (1996). Theory of mind and rule use in individuals with Down syndrome: A test of the uniqueness and specificity claims. *Journal of Child Psychology and Psychiatry, 37*, 479–484.

CHAPTER 5

Language Profiles of Adolescents and Young Adults with Down Syndrome and Fragile X Syndrome

ANDREA MCDUFFIE, ROBIN S. CHAPMAN, AND LEONARD ABBEDUTO

D own syndrome (DS) and fragile X syndrome (FXS) are the two most common genetic causes of intellectual disability (Dykens, Hodapp, & Finucane, 2000). This chapter compares and contrasts the language profiles of adolescents and young adults with DS and FXS. Such a comparison is useful for at least two reasons. First, because these syndromes affect a large proportion of the individuals encountered by speech-language pathologists, special educators, and other professionals who provide services to individuals with intellectual disability, information about similarities and differences between language profiles can be used to plan assessment and treatment. Second, a substantial body of literature exists on the language profile specific to adolescents and young adults with DS, and this literature can guide us in continuing to determine the language characteristics of individuals with FXS, which have been less well studied.

It is already clear from the existing literature that some features of the FXS behavioral phenotype distinguish it from DS in ways that are likely to have important consequences for language development across the life span (Murphy & Abbeduto, 2003). This chapter reviews the literature addressing receptive and expressive language development in adolescents and young adults with DS and is followed by a corresponding review for adolescents and young adults with FXS. It also explores how language development in FXS is affected by gender or a comorbid diagnosis of FXS and autism. Each review provides suggestions for supporting language development through assessment, intervention, and parent involvement and concludes by proposing research that will continue to advance our understanding of language development in adolescents and young adults with DS and FXS.

Preparation of this chapter was supported by National Institutes of Health (NIH) Grants R01 HD24356 and T32 HD007489 awarded to L. Abbeduto; by NIH Grant RO1 HD23353 awarded to R. Chapman, with additional support from the National Down Syndrome Society; and by NIH Grant P30 HD03352 awarded to the Waisman Center.

LANGUAGE IN ADOLESCENTS AND YOUNG ADULTS WITH DOWN SYNDROME

Adolescents and young adults with DS show a specific phenotypic language profile with problems in receptive language, expressive language, speech, and theory
of mind—over and above delays in visual nonverbal cognition (Abbeduto &
Chapman, 2005; Abbeduto et al., 2001; Fowler, Gelman, & Gleitman, 1994; Laws
& Bishop, 2003; Rice, Warren, & Betz, 2005; Roberts et al., 2005; Roberts, Price,
et al., 2007). Intelligibility is a problem frequently reported as an area of concern
for adolescents with DS (Buckley & Sacks, 1987; Kumin, 1994; Roberts et al.,
2005), although intelligibility typically does improve with age (Chapman, Seung,
Schwartz, & Kay-Raining Bird, 1998). Problems in language for adolescents with
DS are associated with specific, additional problems in auditory short-term verbal
memory (Kay-Raining Bird & Chapman, 1994; Laws, 2004; Laws & Gunn, 2004;
Miolo, Chapman, & Sindberg, 2005) and, to a lesser degree, visual short-term
memory (Chapman, Hesketh, & Kistler, 2002). Hearing impairment, a problem
for many individuals with DS, is particularly related to problems of grammatical
morpheme comprehension (Miolo et al., 2005), slower response times in production of "fast mapped" novel words (Chapman, Sindberg, Bridge, Gigstead, &
Hesketh, 2006), and problems in spoken intelligibility (Chapman et al., 1998).
Strengths in vocabulary are associated with nonverbal mental age and maternal
education (Price, Roberts, Vandergrift, & Martin, 2007). The following sections
review the current research on language comprehension and production in adolescents with DS (for reviews of earlier work, see Chapman, 1995, 2003; Chapman & Hesketh, 2000; Miller, 1987).

Language Comprehension

In adolescents and young adults with DS, language comprehension skills show a
complex trajectory as a function of chronological age, nonverbal mental age,
visual and auditory working memory, linguistic domain, and hearing status.
Younger children with DS show comprehension skills commensurate with measures of visual nonverbal cognition (Chapman et al., 2000; Price et al., 2007). In
adolescence, however, vocabulary skills have sometimes been reported to exceed
nonverbal cognition (Chapman et al., 1998, 2000; Chapman, Schwartz, & Kay-
Raining Bird, 1991; Rosin, Swift, Bless, & Vetter, 1988), although this profile also
characterizes adolescents and young adults with intellectual disability of unknown
or mixed etiology (Chapman, 2006; Facon, Facon-Bollengier, & Grubar, 2002;
Facon, Grubar, & Gardez, 1998). In contrast, syntax comprehension in DS begins
to lag nonverbal cognition and vocabulary comprehension in adolescence (Miolo
et al., 2005; Vicari, Caselli, & Tonucci, 2000), showing actual losses over time in a
longitudinal study of individuals in late adolescence and young adulthood (17
years onward; Chapman et al., 2002).

Vocabulary Comprehension

Studies reporting vocabulary comprehension to be a strength for adolescents and
young adults with DS have most often relied on the Peabody Picture Vocabulary
Test (PPVT; Dunn & Dunn, 1981, 1997). With vocabulary based on both pictura-

bility and frequency criteria, the PPVT appears to tap the increased life experience of teenagers with cognitive impairment, compared with younger typically developing children of similar nonverbal cognitive skills. Thus, the PPVT is a fair test of comprehension vocabulary size but not of conceptual difficulty. Use of a comparison group of typically developing children matched for mental age based on the PPVT, as was the practice in older studies of adolescents with DS, puts the group with DS at a serious disadvantage in other skill areas, whether the match is viewed as one of mental age (a mistake) or vocabulary comprehension. That is, vocabulary and conceptual ability are commensurate for typically developing individuals but discrepant for individuals with DS, resulting in a cognitive advantage on experimental tasks for the comparison group.

In contrast, vocabulary tests based on words chosen on the basis of conceptual difficulty, rather than frequency of use, show a different picture of lexical comprehension in both adolescents with DS and adolescents with cognitive impairment of unknown origin; this picture is more consistent with their performance in syntax comprehension (Chapman, 2006; Miolo et al., 2005). For example, much of the vocabulary on subtest I of the Test for Auditory Comprehension of Language–3 (TACL-3; Carrow-Woolfolk, 1999) becomes harder in conceptual content (e.g. "half," "some," "few," "equal"). On this test, adolescents with DS do not show the same exceptional strengths in vocabulary compared with their typically developing peers, relative to nonverbal visual cognition or syntax comprehension. Rather, lexical comprehension for these items is generally consistent with nonverbal cognitive skills and similar to comparison groups of typically developing children matched for syntax comprehension (Abbeduto et al., 2003; Miolo et al., 2005) or adolescents with cognitive impairment of unknown origin (Chapman, in press).

Variation in performance by 10- to 12-year-old boys with DS is predicted by both nonverbal mental age and mother's education (Price et al., 2007). Thus, adolescents and young adults with DS have a larger comprehension vocabulary, but not necessary a conceptually more advanced vocabulary, than typically developing children matched for cognition or syntax comprehension. An exception to this pattern is found for understanding words that convey emotion, particularly those related to fear; 8- to 18-year-old individuals with DS showed poorer ability to recognize these emotions (Williams, Wishart, Pitcairn, & Willis, 2005).

Fast Mapping of Vocabulary in Comprehension

Learning the conventional meaning of a word requires the learner to form an arbitrary link between a label that is heard and an object or action (referent) that is observed incidentally in the word-learning context. The rapid associative process by which label and referent are paired following one or very few exposures was termed *fast mapping* in a classic study by Carey and Bartlett (1978). Theoretically, the initial fast-mapping process is followed by a more protracted period of *slow mapping* during which the partial representation of each new word is elaborated, both linguistically and conceptually, and fully incorporated into the individual's expanding lexicon.

Many subsequent studies have employed the construct of fast mapping as a theoretical explanation for how typically developing children acquire new vocabulary words (Akhtar & Tomasello, 1996; Baldwin, 1991, 1993a, 1993b; Tomasello

& Barton, 1994; Woodward, Markman, & Fitzsimmons, 1994). The general design for these types of studies has been to provide exposure to a label–referent pairing, followed by assessing whether a novel word has been learned. The incidental learning of novel nouns and verbs by individuals with DS has been studied in a variety of hiding tasks reviewed by Chapman (2003). Adolescents with DS, ages 12–20 years, have been found to learn a single novel noun encountered once in a hiding game about as often as a group matched on nonverbal mental age and to remember its location equally well when tested after an hour delay (Chapman, Kay-Raining Bird, & Schwartz, 1990). These findings mean that adolescents with DS, despite their learning impairments, are remembering novel objects and their actions on them (hiding in a particular location) and are drawing conclusions about speaker referential intent without the assistance of referential pointing about as well as would be expected for their levels of (nonverbal) cognitive functioning. Performance on fast-mapping tasks reflects the strength in vocabulary learning that, over years of opportunity, could result in greatly increased comprehension vocabulary on PPVT-type measures, compared with nonverbal mental age expectations.

Other studies have attempted to manipulate the phonological complexity and utterance position of novel words in ways that might tax hearing and auditory–verbal short-term memory (Chapman, 2003), thereby revealing individual differences in comprehension skill. Chapman, Miller, Sindberg, and Seung (1996) tested participants with DS, 9–24 years of age, with six fast-mapping tasks requiring participants to hide a series of three objects (one familiar, one novel and named, one novel and unnamed) on a trial, varying the order of mention and the number of syllables (one versus three) in the novel word. In this more taxing task, participants with DS performed significantly more poorly than a group of typically developing children matched for nonverbal mental age.

Effects of Memory Support and Elicited Production on Fast Mapping
Chapman and colleagues (2006) were interested in the impact of memory support on fast mapping. These investigators tested the possibility that repeated mentions of a novel word (five versus one) would improve fast-mapping comprehension of nouns for adolescents with DS compared with a group of preschool-age typically developing children matched for syntax comprehension. The authors also examined whether asking the participant to say the word twice would improve fast mapping. Memory support facilitated comprehension and increased speed of responding for the individuals in the DS group, which performed similarly to the comparison group overall. Standard comprehension measures predicted individual differences in fast-mapped comprehension for both groups—vocabulary in the DS group, syntax in the comparison group.

Fast Mapping of Vocabulary in Story Contexts   Learning new vocabulary from a story context, particularly stories unaccompanied by pictures, can be expected to require more listener resources than fast mapping in event contexts. A fast-mapping task involving two novel nouns, presented three times each within a brief story, was conducted with participants with DS ages 13–20 years who were matched on nonverbal mental age to a preschool-age comparison group (Kay-Raining Bird, Chapman, & Schwartz, 2004). Participants were asked to listen to and retell stories, then to define novel words and say what they

remembered about them. Strikingly, fast-mapped comprehension measured by word definition was poor for both groups. In addition, text units associated with the novel words were less likely to be recalled than text units not containing novel words, suggesting a trade-off effect in fast mapping versus sentence processing.

Syntax Comprehension

In contrast to vocabulary comprehension and expressive syntax, syntax comprehension in adolescents and young adults with DS shows a relative plateau (at a level lower than nonverbal mental age predictions) followed, at about ages 17–27 years, by actual declines in performance on standardized tests of comprehension (Chapman et al., 2002). In a 6-year longitudinal study of language development in children, adolescents, and young adults with DS, three variables—age at study start, visual short-term memory, and auditory–verbal short-term memory—predicted age-equivalent scores for the Test for Auditory Comprehension of Language–Revised (TACL-R; Carrow-Woolfolk, 1985) at the study start, whereas chronological age predicted the changing slope of linear growth in syntax comprehension (Chapman et al., 2002).

An experimental test of comprehension of information-dense active and passive sentences requiring participants to act out the meaning of the sentence with manipulatives revealed similar performance by adolescents with DS and typically developing children matched for syntax comprehension (Miolo et al., 2005). Auditory–verbal short-term memory (but not visual short-term memory) predicted syntax comprehension skills in both groups on most measures. Of the domains of syntax comprehension tested, grammatical morphology showed the greatest impairment (Chapman, 1997; Chapman, Schwartz, & Kay-Raining Bird, 1991; Miolo et al., 2005). Hearing impairment predicted grammatical morpheme comprehension but not elaborated sentence comprehension (Miolo et al., 2005).

Language Production

In contrast to the findings for language comprehension, studies have revealed clear evidence of a specific deficit in expressive language for individuals with DS, relative to their own comprehension performance or to mental age–matched controls (Chapman, Seung, Schwartz, & Kay-Raining-Bird, 2000). This deficit extends across the domains of both vocabulary and syntax. Variations in comprehension predict a substantial portion of the variance in expressive language performance. In the following sections, a closer look at the domains of language production for individuals with DS is provided.

Vocabulary Production

In studies of lexical use in narrative language samples, the number of different words produced by adolescents with DS is often fewer than typically developing peers matched for mental age (Chapman et al., 1998; for boys 10–12 years old, Roberts, Martin, et al., 2007). Relative to mean length of utterance, individuals with DS use fewer lexical verbs, particularly mental state verbs (Hesketh & Chapman, 1998). Nonetheless, vocabulary use is less affected than grammatical morphology.

Fast Mapping of Vocabulary in Production

In adolescents with DS, the production of newly fast-mapped words has been shown to be more challenging than comprehension of the same words (Chapman, 2003; Chapman et al., 1990), especially when novel vocabulary was introduced in the context of a story (Kay-Raining Bird et al., 2004). When memory support and requests for elicited production were introduced, elicited production improved fast mapping for all participants. Moreover, memory support aided both groups when elicited production was not required (Chapman et al., 2006). Chapman and colleagues (2006) also found that auditory verbal short-term memory measures predicted individual variation in typically developing preschoolers' fast-mapped production of words, but hearing status and grammatical morpheme comprehension predicted production for individuals with DS.

Syntax Production

Studies of the narrative language of adolescents with DS reveal both the limitations and the strengths of their expressive language skills. In language samples based on personal narratives, recalled television programs and favorite stories, and pictures of complex events, mean length of utterance has been found to be longer than in conversation and does not show the plateauing in sentence length reported for conversational samples in adolescents (Fowler et al., 1994). Rather, a longitudinal study of narrative performance found that mean length of utterance increased across 6 years for individuals with DS ages 12–20 years at the outset (Chapman et al., 2002). For stories told from wordless picture books, in particular, sentence length and complexity for individuals with DS were found to be comparable to that of typically developing children matched for syntax comprehension (Miles, Chapman, & Sindberg, 2006; Thordardottir, Chapman, & Wagner, 2002; but see Abbeduto et al., 2001, for an exception), although grammatical morphology lagged behind (Eadie, Fey, Douglas, & Parsons, 2002).

The variation in expressive narrative language among children and adolescents with DS, relative to a nonverbal mental age–matched typically developing comparison group, was modeled in hierarchical regression analyses by Chapman and colleagues (2000) using group, chronological age, cognition, socioeconomic status, and hearing status as predictors in one model and adding comprehension performance as a predictor in an alternate model. For participants with DS, results revealed that the model including comprehension as a variable accounted for significantly more variance in expressive language performance, explaining 68% of the variance in number of different words, 80% in mean length of utterance, and 32% in intelligibility. Similar percentages or variance were observed for the typically developing comparison group.

The Pragmatics of Language Use

Conversational skills in boys with DS who are 10–12 years old reveal strengths in the ability to maintain topic, in contrast to boys with FXS. Noncontingent language and perseveration, which are problems for males with FXS, are not particular weaknesses for boys with DS compared with a typically developing group matched for nonverbal mental age (Roberts, Martin, et al., 2007). The discourse-level content of stories told by adolescents with DS has been investigated in a series of studies by Chapman and colleagues.

When stories were presented auditorily, and individuals had to rely on online comprehension and short-term memory to recall the story, both adolescents with DS and mental age–matched, typically developing peers recalled few story propositions (Seung & Chapman, 2003). When stories were presented visually in a short film, adolescents with DS recalled as many events as mental age–matched typically developing peers, although adolescents with DS constructed their narratives out of more, but shorter, utterances (Boudreau & Chapman, 2000).

When telling stories from wordless picture books, adolescents with DS incorporated as many story elements into their narratives as did typically developing children matched for syntax comprehension and incorporated significantly more elements than did typically developing children matched for mean length of utterance (Miles & Chapman, 2002). Once again, the facilitative effects of picture support were observed, in tandem with strengths in vocabulary, on the narrative performance of individuals with DS, as well as how conceptual understanding is expressed despite limitations in mean length of utterance.

Miles, Sindberg, Bridge, and Chapman (2002) examined the effects of adult scaffolding on narrative content in microgenetic studies in which adolescents with DS were asked to practice telling stories from wordless picture books over six sessions separated by approximately 1 week each. The story in the *low* scaffolding condition was supported by the story pictures, the adult's encouragement of spontaneous story expression, nonspecific prompts to "tell more," and repetition of the participant's spontaneous story content with the addition of missing grammatical morphemes. The *high* scaffolding condition, accompanying a second story, included all the elements of the low scaffolding condition and added specific *wh-* questions ("who," "what," "where," "what's happening," and "when") for missing content. Mention of the setting information (boy protagonist, the place where the story began, and the time of day or night) was analyzed in the two conditions for 15 participants. Almost all participants mentioned the protagonist on all tellings, few mentioned the time of day on any telling, and the scaffolding questions significantly increased the mentions of spatial information, which was otherwise infrequent. It appears that direct questions can increase the inclusion of missing content in subsequent retellings by adolescents with DS, provided that those questions are within the storyteller's comprehension repertoire.

In a follow-up study, Miles and Chapman (2005) analyzed the full content of the stories told across 6 days under the two scaffolding conditions. In general, plot line/theme expression and mean length of utterance increased over time for both the DS and the typically developing groups. Narrative content was greater in the high scaffold condition for the groups as well. The high scaffold condition was more effective in increasing only the measure of semantic diversity over time. No significant differences were found between groups in conceptual understanding of the stories; however, the syntax-comprehension comparison group's greater growth in syntactic complexity, semantic diversity, and automaticity demonstrated more rapid simultaneous change in multiple domains, and more integration of change into narrative performance, than the group with individuals with DS.

And finally, Miles, Chapman, and Sindberg (2004) used the microgenetic method to study storytelling strategies over the six retellings; that is, ways participants solved the problems of construing the task, interacting with the examiner, and narrating the storybooks. In contrast to other narrative studies by Chapman and colleagues, almost all of the participants, even at the lowest developmental levels, approached the task as one of telling related events. The adolescents with DS, however, were more likely to use a multiple-utterance strategy and were also more likely to use the developmentally advanced strategy of including character voice than syntax comprehension–matched comparison typically developing children. Multiple-utterance strategies were also more likely in the condition in which high scaffolding was provided. Thus, participants with DS may be compensating for limitations in expressive language by producing multiple utterances to convey their more advanced conceptual understanding of narrative.

Implications for Assessment, Intervention, and Parent Involvement

Understanding the phenotypical language characteristics of individuals with DS results in important clinical implications for the ways in which language and cognition are measured, for the ways interventions are designed and implemented, and for the ways in which parents can be involved in facilitating positive language outcomes for their children.

Assessment

The studies reviewed in this chapter underscore the failure of frequency-based vocabulary comprehension tests, such as the various versions of the PPVT, to accurately reflect the status of conceptual or syntactic levels of comprehension or of nonverbal problem-solving skills in adolescents with cognitive impairment. The PPVT, however, is useful for assessing some facets of vocabulary comprehension. The findings in the studies reviewed also underscore the importance of considering how a language sample was obtained when evaluating its evidence for expressive language level. Samples based on conversation and free play are not sufficient to evaluate the emergence of complex sentence structures and the control of extended discourse structures (e.g., stories) in adolescence. A further detail, of particular importance for evaluating language samples from individuals with DS, is whether visual support for the sample was provided.

Intervention

Of chief importance for intervention is the evidence that language learning is ongoing in adolescence for individuals with DS. Individuals with DS demonstrate large gains in vocabulary comprehension size and have expected gains in concept comprehension; continued development in expressive language, including complex sentence structure, lexicon, and story content; and fast mapping new vocabulary in contexts offering minimal memory support and requiring attention to speaker intent. This evidence suggests the possibility of progress in language learning during adolescence and leads to the strong recommendation for *ongoing access to language intervention and literacy instruction for individuals with DS during education in adolescence.*

The observed pattern of correlations of language skills of individuals with DS with (at most) mild hearing impairment suggests that *aiding hearing in the learning environment* may have a substantial impact on three areas: intelligibility of speech, comprehension of grammatical morphology, and fast mapping of new vocabulary in production. Encouraging continuing use of aids and monitoring the listening demands of communicative settings will also be important.

The studies reviewed in this chapter also make clear that *visual support* is helpful for individuals with DS in both comprehension and production tasks. The findings imply that picture support for telling stories—in addition to adult encouragement, confirmation, and questioning—will lead to increased narrative skills, both immediately and with practice, and that visual referents and demonstrations facilitate comprehension. These studies also demonstrate how little information is retained from (even brief) stories that are simply presented aloud. More thought to providing photos, videos, demonstrations, enactments, and, in general, visual support to the content to be conveyed may greatly improve effective communication for individuals with DS.

Parent Involvement

Parent involvement in the lives of their children with DS requires, of course, attention to their health, well-being, independent living skills, and social and vocational life. In each domain, there are new communication demands to master and new patterns of communicative interaction to learn. Awareness that each of these learning domains will include opportunities—and demands—for language learning and use, in addition to the parent's support and practice of that learning, will always be helpful. What is important to recognize is that, for adolescents and young adults with DS, language is still being learned, so multiple avenues for teaching new content (and learning its language) should be made available.

Directions for Future Research

The observation that syntax comprehension skills of individuals with DS, in contrast to expressive language skills, are plateauing in adolescence and actually declining in young adulthood—with variability predicted by chronological age, auditory–verbal short-term memory, and visual short-term memory—raises two serious possibilities requiring further research. One possibility, connected to chronological age as a predictor, is that lack of access to language and literacy instruction in adolescence (as individuals are shifted into vocational programming) and even greater lack of stimulation in language input in adult living situations contribute to the losses in comprehension. A second possibility is that comprehension test items are sensitive indicators of age-related losses associated with DS, if, for example, overexpression of APP (beta-amyloid precursor) or another gene on chromosome 21 is causing cumulative neuronal losses evident by the third decade of life. If such a mechanism is at work, individual variability in comprehension loss should reflect the variability of gene expression, and longitudinal studies of young adults in their 20s and 30s should reveal ongoing loss of syntax comprehension skill on standardized testing. A recent pilot study of a cholinergic drug, donepezil, as a treatment for cognitive loss related to Alzheimer's disease, has shown efficacy specifically for language impairments

(Heller et al., 2003; Heller et al., 2004). In a brief, open-label clinical trial for adults with DS, expressive language improved across the entire group and comprehension skills improved for those with the highest language skills (Heller et al., 2003). An additional pilot study with children with DS also showed language benefits (Heller et al., 2004) that should be explored in future research.

LANGUAGE IN ADOLESCENTS AND YOUNG ADULTS WITH FRAGILE X SYNDROME

Numerous cognitive skills thought to be important for language are delayed or impaired in FXS (Belser & Sudhalter, 1995; Cohen, 1995; Cornish et al., 2004; Mirrett et al., 2003; Munir et al., 2000; Murphy & Abbeduto, 2003). In the following sections, the language characteristics of individuals with FXS is presented and the syndrome specific associations between cognitive and performance in the domains of language comprehension and production are considered.

Language Comprehension

On average, males with FXS show substantial delays relative to chronological age in all facets of language comprehension (Abbeduto & Hagerman, 1997). The few studies of males with FXS that have focused on either the relation between language comprehension and cognition or on the relation between different domains of receptive language (Madison, George, & Moeschler, 1986; Paul et al., 1987), however, have yielded findings that are contradictory or difficult to interpret. In part, these ambiguous findings are due to the use of small and restricted samples with wide ranges of ages and ability levels (e.g., a single family in the Madison and colleagues study and 12 institutionalized adults in the Paul and colleagues study). Interpretation of empirical results is also complicated by the failure of many studies to include a typically developing comparison group. Such a comparison is necessary when each domain of language is measured with a different standardized test (Mervis & Robinson, 1999, 2005). Individuals on whom different tests are normed can differ in potentially important and unknown ways, including in average ability level. This makes it impossible to know what scores would be achieved on the different tests by an "average" child. As a result, it is not clear what magnitude of difference between scores on two different language tests is needed to conclude that there is a reliable difference in achievement across different domains for individuals with FXS (Murphy & Abbeduto, 2003).

Few studies have provided an in-depth examination of receptive language abilities in females with FXS, but existing data indicate a relative strength in verbal ability, at least when measured by global measures of language competence that collapse across receptive and expressive modalities (Freund & Reiss, 1991; Hagerman, 1996). That is, females with FXS display higher verbal than nonverbal performance on standardized tests of intelligence, a finding that reflects a relative strength within the individual but not relative to age-matched peers (Mazzocco, 2000). Only three studies of females with FXS have specifically addressed receptive language development (Abbeduto et al., 2003; Madison et al., 1986; Simon, Keenan, Pennington, Taylor, & Hagerman, 2001). Problems with generalizing from the receptive language results of the Madison and colleagues study have already been mentioned. Simon and colleagues (2001) examined discourse comprehension in high-functioning females with FXS. The authors found that females with the full mutation had difficulty selecting appropriate humorous endings for written stories, suggesting problems in creating cohesive representations of events. This finding is noteworthy given that the participants in the Simon and colleagues study were functioning in the normal range of cognitive ability. It is reasonable to expect more serious comprehension problems if language skills are examined in females with FXS who also have cognitive impairments.

Many limitations in previous studies examining receptive language in adolescents and young adults with FXS have been addressed in recent research. Abbeduto and colleagues (2003) administered the TACL-R to adolescents and young adults with FXS. Both male and female participants with FXS were included in this study in order to reveal the nature and extent of gender differences within the syndrome. Participants with FXS were matched with participants with DS based on chronological age and nonverbal mental age and were matched with a group of typically developing 3- to 6-year-olds based on nonverbal mental age. There was not a significant difference in overall TACL-R age-equivalent scores between participants with FXS and mental age–matched typically developing children. Total age-equivalent scores of participants with FXS, however, were significantly higher than participants with DS. In addition, females with FXS achieved higher total language scores than males, but this gender difference was not significant after controlling for differences in nonverbal mental age.

Vocabulary Comprehension

Limitations in cognition and social functioning in males with FXS suggest that vocabulary learning will be a special challenge, given the dependence of lexical learning on social interaction and on understanding a speaker's referential intentions (Baldwin, 1995). In fact, existing data indicate that males with FXS achieve well below chronological age expectations on measures of receptive vocabulary (Madison et al., 1986; Paul et al., 1987; Sudhalter, Maranion, & Brooks, 1992). The data, however, are inconsistent as to whether lexical learning keeps pace with, exceeds, or lags behind achievements in nonverbal cognition as well as other domains of language. In addition, given that word learning extends past the childhood years, adolescents and young adults with FXS may continue to progress in acquiring new words and may compensate, to some degree, for early delays in the domain of vocabulary knowledge.

The Abbeduto and colleagues (2003) study reviewed previously presented four findings relevant to vocabulary comprehension in adolescents and young adults with FXS. First, participants with FXS did not differ in vocabulary age-equivalent scores from either of the two mental age–matched comparison groups (adolescents and young adults with DS and typically developing 3- to 6-year-olds). Second, participants with FXS and typically developing comparison children attained TACL-R vocabulary age-equivalent scores commensurate with scores obtained on the two TACL-R subtests measuring syntactical skills. Third, all participants achieved vocabulary age-equivalent scores that were commensurate with their nonverbal mental ages. Finally, within the group of FXS participants, males achieved lower vocabulary scores than did females. These data suggest that adolescents and young adults with FXS demonstrate synchrony between lexical understanding and nonverbal cognition and between lexical understanding and understanding of syntax and morphology. This profile contrasts with the profile observed for DS, which is characterized by receptive vocabulary that is in advance of receptive syntax and is as developed as, or in advance of, nonverbal cognition.

An important limitation on our understanding of receptive vocabulary (and other domains of language) in FXS is that the emphasis has been on characterizing the absolute level of competence achieved rather than the processes by which language is learned. Thus, in contrast to Chapman and colleagues' numerous fast-mapping studies with adolescents and young adults with DS, there are no comparable data for individuals with FXS, and virtually nothing is known about the processes of new word learning for individuals with FXS. In addition, the ways in which learning new vocabulary (both in comprehension and in production) is affected by the cognitive phenotype of individuals with FXS is not well understood.

Syntax Comprehension

As a group, males with FXS consistently perform below chronological age–level expectations on measures of syntax comprehension (Abbeduto & Hagerman, 1997), which, however, appears to keep pace with nonverbal cognition (Abbeduto et al., 2003; Paul et al., 1987). As discussed previously, Abbeduto and colleagues (2003) found that participants with FXS did not differ from nonverbal mental age–matched typically developing children on either of the two syntactically focused TACL-R subtests, but the participants with FXS did outperform the nonverbal mental age–matched DS group on these same subtests. In contrast to individuals with DS, therefore, adolescents and young adults with FXS demonstrate neither an asynchrony in individual domains of language comprehension nor an asynchrony between language comprehension and nonverbal cognition.

Language Production

When language production is considered, individuals with FXS do not demonstrate the specific expressive language deficit, relative to comprehension, that is considered characteristic of individuals with DS. As is discussed in the following paragraphs, individuals with FXS also present profiles of synchronous performance across the domains of vocabulary and syntax. However, the use of language in social contexts with ongoing demands in both the roles of speaker and listener proves to be an area of special challenge, at least for males with FXS.

Vocabulary Production

Males with FXS achieve well below chronological age level expectations on measures of expressive vocabulary (Madison et al., 1986; Paul et al., 1987; Sudhalter et al., 1992). Studies using summary measures that collapse across vocabulary and other domains of language have reported that males with FXS have more difficulty with expressive than receptive language skills (Roberts, Mirrett, & Burchinal, 2001). Little understanding exists, however, as to whether receptive and expressive vocabularies are delayed to a similar extent in males with FXS. Indeed, Madison and colleagues (1986) and Sudhalter, Maranion, and Brooks (1992) have reported higher scores on expressive measures of vocabulary compared with receptive measures, whereas Paul and colleagues (1987) found no differences. These results, however, are problematic to interpret given differences in measures and participants across studies, as well as relatively small sample sizes.

Syntax Production

Few studies have provided data on expressive syntax for individuals with FXS. Madison and colleagues (1986) examined conversations of males with FXS and found that the mean length of utterance was at or above expectations relative to nonverbal mental age. In contrast, Paul and colleagues (1987) found no differences on several measures of expressive syntax in conversational language between adult males with FXS who had been institutionalized and age- and IQ score–matched individuals with other etiologies of intellectual disability. Similarly, Ferrier, Bashir, Meryash, Johnston, and Wolff (1991) found that males with FXS did not differ from cognitively matched individuals with DS or younger typically developing children on syntactic measures derived from conversation.

Using the Oral Expression subtest of the Oral and Written Language Scales (OWLS; Carrow-Woolfolk, 1995), Abbeduto and colleagues (2001) found that adolescents and young adults with FXS did not differ in age-equivalent scores from typically developing 3- to 6-year-olds matched on nonverbal mental age. Like the typically developing group, participants with FXS did not show a discrepancy between receptive language performance (as measured by the TACL-R) and expressive language performance (as measured by the OWLS). As expected, participants with FXS demonstrated significantly better expressive language performance than did cognitively matched individuals with DS.

In studies of language production in FXS, measures of expressive syntax (e.g., mean length of utterance) are typically derived from conversational language samples (Murphy & Abbeduto, 2003). Yet, as demonstrated for individuals with DS (Chapman et al., 1998), there is abundant evidence that sampling context can have a substantial impact on the nature of the language produced by individuals with intellectual disability (Abbeduto, Benson, Short, & Dolish, 1995), as well as by typically developing children (Dollaghan, Campbell, & Tomlin, 1990). Thus, reliance on conversation is likely to provide an incomplete picture of the productive syntax of adolescents and young adults with FXS. In fact, Abbeduto and colleagues (2001) found differences in mean length of utterance between individuals with DS and FXS in a story-telling (i.e., narrative) context, but not in a conversational context, with the narrative data showing a significant advantage on mean length of utterance for individuals with FXS. In addition, comparison with a nonverbal mental age–matched typically developing group indicated that in narration, the mean length of utterance of adolescents and young adults with FXS was commensurate with their nonverbal mental ages.

The Pragmatics of Language Use

The ways in which an individual with FXS uses language within the context of social interaction likely will influence the way conversational partners will respond to him or her. The inability to engage in reciprocal interaction also may limit the amount of linguistic input an individual with FXS receives. Thus, failure to acquire pragmatic skills may reflect a slowing of development in the lexical and syntactic domains or may reflect constraints imposed from maladaptive behaviors such as social anxiety, hyperarousal, and inattention (Belser & Sudhalter, 1995, 2001; Cornish, Sudhalter, & Turk, 2004; Ferrier et al., 1991; Murphy & Abbeduto, 2003; Sudhalter, Cohen, Silverman, & Wolf-Schein, 1990). It is likely that initial behavioral challenges for individuals with FXS will affect language development over time.

Some insight into the pragmatic language abilities of males with FXS has been provided through informant reports of adaptive behavior that include communication items, such as the Communication Domain of the Vineland Adaptive Behavior Scales (Sparrow, Balla, & Cicchetti, 1984). Dykens, Leckman, Paul, and Watson (1988) found that the Vineland scores of males with FXS were closer to mental age than to chronological age expectations. In addition, scores on the Communication Domain began to fall behind scores on the Daily Living Domain during adolescence. This suggests that pragmatics is not only an area of relative weakness in FXS but also one that becomes an increasing challenge with age (Dykens, Hodapp, & Leckman, 1994; Dykens, Hodapp, Ort, & Finucane, 1989; Dykens, Ort, Cohen, & Finucane, 1996).

Referential talk is critical to successful communication because listeners must use the speaker's intended referent as the foundation for constructing meaning within the conversational context (Graesser, Millis, & Zwaan, 1997). Abbeduto and colleagues (2006) used a barrier task in which the participant assumed the role of speaker. Participants were adolescents and young adults with FXS, matched for nonverbal mental age and chronological age with adolescents and young adults with DS and for nonverbal mental age with typically developing 3- to 6-year-olds. Both males and females with FXS were included. Participants with FXS or DS were less likely than typically developing children to provide a unique description for individual shapes; instead, participants with FXS or DS extended the same description to multiple shapes. In addition, participants with FXS were less likely than both comparison groups to provide a consistent descriptor for a shape each time it appeared.

In a second study using a barrier task, Abbeduto and colleagues (2007) examined noncomprehension signaling with participants taking the role of listeners following simple directions from the examiner. Failure to signal and repair noncomprehension early in a conversation may greatly reduce the length and number of conversational turns. The participants were again nonverbal mental age–matched groups of adolescents and young adults with FXS or DS and typically developing children. Participants with FXS or DS signaled noncomprehension less often than typically developing children. Across all groups, noncomprehension signaling was more likely when the speaker referred to an item that was not present. Importantly, when the speaker's directions were informative, all participant groups were able to successfully complete the task. Thus, it appears that adolescents and young adults with FXS are poor at monitoring and resolving problems in comprehension, even when they understand task requirements and have the ability to process the types of linguistic forms uttered.

Researchers have suggested that perseverative language is a unique and distinguishing characteristic of males with FXS (Abbeduto & Hagerman, 1997; Bennetto & Pennington, 1996). In particular, males with FXS display especially high rates of self-repetition as well as off-topic or tangential utterances (Belser & Sudhalter, 2001; Ferrier et al., 1991; Sudhalter & Belser, 2001). Cornish and colleagues (2004) suggested that one consequence of the hyperarousal and social anxiety characteristic of individuals with FXS is the impulsive tendency to talk about favorite and very narrow topics, regardless of the actual demands of conversation. Both tangential and repetitive language may be impulsively reintroduced because this well-rehearsed verbal language can be used to maintain a conversation and avoid the need to exchange new information. Depending on the willingness of a listener to tolerate challenges to conversation, it is likely that the use of repetitive and tangential language may contribute to difficulties in sustaining conversational interactions for individuals with FXS. Interestingly, the occurrence of perseveration is context dependent, being more likely in relatively unstructured contexts, such as conversation, than in relatively more structured contexts, such as story telling. Thus, as seen for DS, scaffolding in the form of pictures and highly circumscribed task demands leads to improved performance in adolescents and young adults with FXS.

Males with FXS also characteristically demonstrate eye gaze aversion in contexts of social interaction (Cohen, Vietze, Sudhalter, Jenkins, & Brown, 1989; Reiss, & Freund, 1992; Wolff, Gardner, Paccla, & Lappen, 1989). The underlying causes and adaptive functions of gaze aversion have yet to be determined, and it is possible that gaze aversion represents a response to either cognitive processing load or social demands (Belser & Sudhalter, 2001; Doherty-Sneddon & Phelps, 2005). Regardless of the cause and function, this phenotypic pattern of behavior is likely to add to pragmatic challenges faced by males with FXS.

Gender Differences in Language in Fragile X Syndrome

Despite differences in the severity of affectedness, the profile of relative cognitive strengths and weaknesses and risk for psychopathology associated with FXS is not thought to vary according to gender (Dykens et al., 2000). In the following section, research examining gender differences in language comprehension and production for individuals with FXS will be presented.

Language Comprehension

Direct comparisons of males and females with FXS within the same study have been surprisingly rare in the literature. It has been suggested that, despite differences in severity of affectedness, the language profile associated with FXS does not vary based on gender. With respect to language comprehension, this conclusion is supported by the Abbeduto and colleagues (2003) study reviewed previously. In this study, female participants with FXS had higher scores than the males, although the magnitude of the gender difference was constant across TACL-R subtests. In addition to flat profiles of language comprehension, both males and females achieved language scores commensurate with nonverbal cognition. These results are consistent with a pattern of quantitative, not qualitative, differences in receptive language between males and females with FXS.

Language Production

Pavetto and Abbeduto (2002) compared the expressive language produced by males and females with FXS in both conversation and narration on talkativeness, fluency, lexical diversity, and syntactic complexity. Although no gender differences were observed for fluency or lexical diversity, two aspects of production were influenced by gender: Males were more talkative than females, and females produced utterances of greater syntactic complexity. Both males and females demonstrated longer mean lengths of utterance in narration, and the magnitude of the gender difference in syntactic complexity was greater for narration than for conversation.

As noted previously, perseverative language is considered a defining feature of the language produced by males with FXS (Abbeduto & Hagerman, 1997; Bennetto & Pennington, 1996). Murphy and Abbeduto (2007) examined the relationship between repetitive language and sampling context in both male and female adolescents with FXS. Language samples were coded for utterance level, topic, and conversational device repetitions. Males produced more conversational device repetitions than females, and this difference was not explained by controlling for nonverbal cognition or expressive language ability. Regardless of gender, more topic repetitions and marginally more utterance level repetitions occurred in conversation than in narration. Observed gender difference in repetition use suggests that although speakers of both genders are influenced by context, males with FXS may rely more heavily on rote phrases in expressive language. The less structured context of conversation leads to increases in this type of maladaptive verbal behavior for individuals of both genders.

Language Profiles of Individuals with Comorbid Fragile X Syndrome and Autism

An association between FXS and autism is well documented (Bailey, Hatton, Skinner, & Mesibov, 2001), with conservative estimates placing the prevalence of FXS and autism at 25%. Recent studies using standardized diagnostic criteria inclusive of pervasive developmental disorder-not otherwise specified (PDD-NOS), however, have documented prevalence rates of autism as high as 47% in young children with FXS (Demark, Feldman, & Holden, 2003; Kaufmann et al., 2004; Philofsky, Hepburn, Hayes, Hagerman, & Rogers, 2004). The term *PDD-NOS* is used as the diagnostic classification for children who do not meet the more stringent criteria for autistic disorder due to late age of onset, atypical symptoms, or symptoms that are evident at subthreshold levels. Individuals with PDD-NOS, while not receiving a diagnosis of autistic disorder, are considered to be on the autism spectrum. Thus, PDD-NOS is a more inclusive diagnostic classification than is autistic disorder. It is not yet clear whether the characteristics of autism are distributed on a continuum in the population of individuals with FXS or whether the comorbid diagnosis of autism spectrum disorder (ASD) in FXS represents a qualitatively distinct subtype of the FXS phenotype. Most recent studies of autism in FXS have involved samples of preschool-age children (Bailey, Hatton, Mesibov, Ament, & Skinner, 2000; Bailey, Hatton, Tassone, et al., 2001; Bailey et al., 1998; Philofsky et al., 2004; Rogers, Wehner, & Hagerman, 2001). Thus, it is also not clear whether the diagnosis or symptoms of autism change over time in FXS, or whether autism symptom severity is associated with levels of language or nonverbal cognition at any point in development.

Lewis and colleagues (2006) have published a study examining language profiles of adolescents and young adults with comorbid FXS and autism. As expected, adolescents with comorbid FXS and autism ($n = 10$) scored significantly lower than adolescents with FXS only ($n = 44$) on a measure of nonverbal cognition; all 10 participants with both FXS and autism achieved the lowest possible standard score, in contrast to 48% of participants with FXS only. When participants with both FXS and autism were matched with participants with FXS only ($n = 21$) who also achieved the lowest standard score on the Stanford-Binet Intelligence Scale (Thorndike, Hagen, & Sattler, 1986), there were no significant between-group differences in expressive language as measured with the OWLS (Carrow-Woolfolk, 1995). The group with comorbid FXS and autism, however, performed more poorly on all three subtests of the TACL-R than did matched participants with FXS only. This study replicates the greater impairment in cognitive ability observed in younger children with comorbid FXS and autism (Rogers et al., 2001). In addition, the findings suggest that although adolescents and young adults with FXS only typically display a flat profile of language and nonverbal cognitive skills, those with comorbid FXS and autism may display an asynchronous profile, with receptive language more impaired than either expressive language or nonverbal cognition.

Implications for Assessment, Intervention, and Parent Involvement

The profile of cognitive and psychological features characteristic of FXS has been shown to influence language learning outcomes for individuals with this syndrome. The research findings reviewed earlier have important practical implications for assessment, intervention, and parent involvement. These topics are discussed in the following sections.

Assessment

It is clear that assessment measures for individuals with FXS must address individual domains of language because broad measures, yielding summary scores across language domains, are not useful for characterizing within-syndrome language profiles. As has been described in this chapter, comparisons with individuals with different and well-defined forms of intellectual disability can be useful for understanding which language characteristics are unique to a syndrome and which are the results of general cognitive challenges. Although the use of standardized tests of language ability provides a starting point, more detailed information is required for intervention planning. Language performance varies based on the context in which an aspect of language is measured. Thus, it is important to assess language skills in both conversational and narrative contexts to obtain a more complete description of strengths and weaknesses. In addition, tasks that are more taxing may be successful in revealing potential areas for intervention. The barrier tasks developed by Abbeduto, Murphy, Richmond, and colleagues (2006), in which the individual takes the role of speaker or listener, provide a template for the types of activities that would be helpful for assessing language and planning intervention activities.

Intervention

Understanding the associations between receptive and expressive language and nonverbal cognition, as well as between the lexical and syntactic domains, is critical for developing interventions for individuals with FXS that can target areas of greatest challenge or exploit areas of relative strength when teaching new language skills (Hodapp & Dykens, 2001; Hodapp & Fidler, 1999). Studies using the TACL-R reveal that vocabulary and syntax comprehension are equally affected in adolescents and young adults with FXS and that language comprehension is commensurate with measures of nonverbal cognition. This finding suggests that both areas should be addressed in the course of language intervention for individuals with FXS.

Results across studies also suggest that the behavioral characteristics of the broader phenotype of FXS (e.g., social anxiety, gaze aversion, inability to direct and sustain attention) may influence the acquisition and use of language skills by interfering with an individual's ability to achieve successful interpersonal communication. It is important for clinicians to take phenotypic characteristics into consideration when selecting goals and developing language intervention activities. Indeed, it may be beneficial to target a particular language skill while simultaneously intervening on the behavioral characteristics that affect use of the skill in naturalistic contexts. Intervention activities for individuals with FXS would be valuable if they addressed skills that, once acquired, might serve to maintain successful conversational interactions. The use of a narrative context has been shown to elicit longer utterances for individuals with FXS. Thus, in addition to its use in assessment, narrative tasks can be used in intervention, as new vocabulary and syntactic targets can be introduced and practiced during reciprocal storytelling.

Parent Involvement

Considerable evidence demonstrates that the development of language in both typically developing children and children with developmental disabilities is influenced by the environment, especially interactions with parents and other adult caregivers (Abbeduto, Brady, & Kover, 2007). Thus, high rates of parental interaction and linguistic input are associated with increased rates of linguistic and cognitive development (Hart & Risley, 1995; Hauser-Cram, Warfield, Shonkoff, & Drauss, 2001). In addition, high rates of responding to child initiations combined with low rates of directiveness on the part of mothers is also associated with better language outcomes for children over a range of ability levels (Girolametto, Verbey, & Tannock, 1994; Mahoney, 1988).

There have been no direct comparisons across DS and FXS on those dimensions of adult–child interaction related to language outcomes. Nevertheless, it is likely that relatively higher rates of challenging behaviors will make interaction more difficult for children with FXS (Abbeduto et al., 2007). Moreover, the lower levels of psychological well-being seen in mothers of youth with FXS compared with mothers of youth with DS (Abbeduto et al., 2004) suggest that the former may be less able to engage in frequent and responsive interactions with their children. In other words, parent and child may both contribute to interactions that are less facilitative of language development in the case of FXS than in DS. Testing this hypothesis is important because it implies that interventions designed to reduce challenging child behavior or treating mental health challenges in parents may indirectly facilitate language learning in these children.

Directions for Future Research

One important methodological strategy that should be used in language research for individuals with FXS is to employ measures of individual domains of language rather than broad summary-level measures of language skills. Use of measures sensitive to well-defined aspects of language performance is of primary importance to identify and intervene on those areas of language that present problems for individuals with FXS. In addition, the continued approach of conducting comparisons across syndromes will allow assessment of the specificity of language challenges for these individuals.

Few studies to date have examined trajectories of language development in individuals with FXS through the collection of longitudinal data. This is important because it is not known if changes occur across development in either the relative levels of performance in different domains of language or between levels of performance in language and nonverbal cognition. In addition, as perseveration appears to be a defining characteristic of language in FXS, it is important to examine the developmental trajectories of perseverative and repetitive language to determine when and why it emerges.

Previous studies of language development in individuals with FXS have emphasized measuring levels of achievement rather than processes of language acquisition. Studies of the processes by which language is acquired, as addressed in the fast-mapping studies of Chapman and colleagues, may better inform the development of successful intervention approaches. Studies of language comprehension and use within the context of reciprocal interactions, such as the barrier tasks developed by Abbeduto and colleagues (2006), may reveal challenges to communication that will not be obvious in response to standardized language tests. The question of whether there are qualitative differences in the language profiles of males and females with FXS will need to be addressed in studies that include participants of both genders. These participants must be administered the same measures under the same experimental conditions. In this way, it will be possible to partial out the effects of gender on language development in FXS.

The use of gold-standard instruments for the diagnosis of ASD, such as the Autism Diagnostic Interview–Revised (ADI-R; Lord, Rutter, & LeCouteur, 1994) and the Autism Diagnostic Observation Schedule (ADOS; Lord, Rutter, LeCouteur, DiLavore, & Risi, 1999), will provide researchers with increased precision in characterizing the language profiles of individuals with comorbid FXS and autism. In addition, studies distinguishing between participants with FXS who have diagnoses on the autism spectrum and including comparison groups of participants with FXS only and autism only will be necessary for advancing our understanding of the language differences between FXS and autism.

CONCLUSION

Comparing and contrasting the behavioral and language characteristics of DS and FXS helps us to understand how genes and the environment interact to shape behavior. Individuals with DS have delays in receptive and expressive syntax relative to nonverbal cognition, with strengths in comprehending and using vocabulary and challenges in speech intelligibility. Alternatively, individuals with FXS have language skills commensurate with nonverbal cognition, but they have high rates of social anxiety, inattentiveness, and behavioral challenges. Examination of language learning and use in a variety of contexts by individuals with identifiable genetic syndromes will allow continued progress in understanding the indirect effects of genes on development.

REFERENCES

Abbeduto, L., Benson, G., Short, K., & Dolish, J. (1995). Effects of sampling context on the expressive language of children and adolescents with mental retardation. *Mental Retardation, 33,* 279–288.

Abbeduto, L., Brady, N., & Kover, S. (2007). Language development and fragile X syndrome: Profiles, syndrome-specificity, and within-syndrome differences. *Mental Retardation and Developmental Disabilities Research Reviews, 13,* 36–46.

Abbeduto, L., & Chapman, R. (2005). Language and communication skills in children with DS and fragile X. In P. Fletcher & J. Miller (Eds.), *Trends in language acquisition research: Developmental theory and language disorders* (Vol. 4, pp. 53–72). Amsterdam, Netherlands: John Benjamins.

Abbeduto, L., & Hagerman, R. (1997). Language and communication in fragile X syndrome. *Mental Retardation and Developmental Disabilities Research Reviews, 3,* 313–322.

Abbeduto, L., Murphy, M., Cawthon, S., Richmond, E., Weissman, M., Karadottir, S., et al. (2003). Receptive language skills of adolescents and young adults with mental retardation: A comparison of DS and fragile X syndrome. *American Journal on Mental Retardation, 108,* 149–160.

Abbeduto, L., Murphy, M.M., Richmond, E.K., Amman, A., Beth, P., Weissman, M.D., et al. (2006). Collaboration in referential communication: Comparison of youth with Down syndrome or fragile X syndrome. *American Journal on Mental Retardation, 3,* 170–183.

Abbeduto, L., Pavetto, M., Kesin, E., Weissman, M., Karadottir, S., O'Brien, A., et al. (2001). The linguistic and cognitive profile of DS: Evidence from a comparison with fragile X syndrome. *Down Syndrome Research and Practice, 7,* 9–16.

Abbeduto, L., Seltzer, M. M., Shattuck, P., Krauss, M., Orsmond, G., & Murphy, M. (2004). Psychological well-being and coping in mothers of youths with autism, Down syndrome, or fragile X syndrome. *American Journal on Mental Retardation, 109*(3), 237–254.

Akhtar, N., & Tomasello, M. (1996). Twenty-four-month-old children learn words for absent objects and actions. *British Journal of Developmental Psychology, 14,* 79–93.

Bailey, D.B., Hatton, D.D., Mesibov, G., Ament, N., & Skinner, M. (2000). Early development, temperament, and functional impairment in autism and fragile X syndrome. *Journal of Autism and Developmental Disorders, 30*(1), 49–59.

Bailey, D.B., Hatton, D.D., Skinner, M., & Mesibov, G. (2001). Autistic behavior, FMR1 protein, and developmental trajectories in young males with fragile X syndrome. *Journal of Autism and Developmental Disorders, 31,* 165–174.

Bailey, D.B., Hatton, D.D., Tassone, F., Skinner, M., & Taylor, A.K. (2001). Variability in FMRP and early development in males with fragile X syndrome. *American Journal on Mental Retardation, 106,* 16–27.

Bailey, D.B., Mesibov, G.B., Hatton, D.D., Clark, R.D., Roberts, J.E., & Mayhew, L. (1998). Autistic behavior in young boys with fragile X syndrome. *Journal of Autism and Developmental Disorders, 28,* 499–508.

Baldwin, D. (1991). Infants' contribution to the achievement of joint reference. *Child Development, 62,* 875–890.

Baldwin, D. (1993a). Early referential understanding: Young children's ability to recognize referential acts for what they are. *Developmental Psychology, 29,* 1–12.

Baldwin, D. (1993b). Infant's ability to consult the speaker for clues to word reference. *Journal of Child Language, 2,* 395–418.

Baldwin, D. (1995). Understanding the link between joint attention and language. In C. Moore & P. Dunham (Eds.), *Joint attention: Its origins and role in development* (pp. 131–158). Mahwah, NJ: Lawrence Erlbaum Associates.

Belser, R.C., & Sudhalter, V. (1995). Arousal difficulties in males with fragile X syndrome: A preliminary report. *Developmental Brain Dysfunction, 8,* 270–279.

Belser, R.C., & Sudhalter, V. (2001). Conversational characteristics of children with fragile X syndrome: Repetitive speech. *American Journal on Mental Retardation, 106,* 28–38.

Bennetto, L., & Pennington, B. (1996). The neuropsychology of fragile X syndrome. In R.J. Hagerman & A. Cronister (Eds.), *Fragile X syndrome: Diagnosis, treatment, and research* (2nd ed., pp. 210–243). Baltimore: The Johns Hopkins University Press.

Boudreau, D., & Chapman, R. (2000). The relationship between event representation and linguistic skill in narratives of children and adolescents with DS. *Journal of Speech, Language, and Hearing Research, 43,* 1146–1159.

Buckley, S., & Sacks, B. (1987). *The adolescent with Down's syndrome: Life for the teenager and for the family.* Portsmouth, England: University of Portsmouth.

Carey, S., & Bartlett, E. (1978). Acquiring a single new word. *Papers and Reports on Child Language Development, 15,* 17–29.

Carrow-Woolfolk, E. (1985). *Test for Auditory Comprehension of Language* (Rev. ed.) Allen, TX: DLM Teaching Resources.

Carrow-Woolfolk, E. (1995). *Oral and Written Language Scales.* Circle Pines, MN: American Guidance Services.

Carrow-Woolfolk, E. (1999). *Test for Auditory Comprehension of Language* (3rd ed.). Circle Pines, MN: American Guidance Services.

Chapman, R. (1995). Language development in children with Down syndrome. In P. Fletcher & B. MacWhinney (Eds.), *Handbook of child language* (pp. 651–663). Oxford, England: Blackwell Publishing.

Chapman, R.S. (1997). Language development in children and adolescents with Down syndrome. *Mental Retardation and Developmental Disabilities Research Reviews, 3*(4), 307–312.

Chapman, R. (2003). Language and communication in individuals with DS. In L. Abbeduto (Ed.), *International Review of Research in Mental Retardation: Language and Communication* (Vol. 27, pp. 1–34). New York: Academic Press.

Chapman, R. (2006). Language learning in DS: The speech and language profile compared to adolescents with cognitive impairment of unknown origin. *Down Syndrome Research and Practice, 10,* 61–66.

Chapman, R.S., & Hesketh, L. (2000). Behavioral phenotype of individuals with DS. *Mental Retardation and Developmental Disability Research Reviews, 6,* 84–95.

Chapman, R.S., & Hesketh, L. (2001). Language, cognition, and short-term memory in individuals with DS. *Down Syndrome Research and Practice, 7,* 1–7.

Chapman, R.S., Hesketh, L., & Kistler, D. (2002). Predicting longitudinal change in language production and comprehension in individuals with DS: Hierarchical linear modeling. *Journal of Speech, Language, and Hearing Research, 45,* 902–915.

Chapman, R.S., Kay-Raining Bird, E., & Schwartz, S.E. (1990). Fast mapping of words in event contexts by children with Down syndrome. *Journal of Speech and Hearing Disorders, 55*(4), 761–770.

Chapman, R.S., Miller, J., Sindberg, H., Seung, H.-K. (1996). *Fast mapping of novel words by children and adolescents with Down syndrome: Relation to auditory memory.* Poster session presented at the Gatlinburg Research Conference on Mental Retardation, Gatlinburg, TN.

Chapman, R.S., Schwartz, S., & Kay-Raining Bird, E. (1991). Language skills of children and adolescents with DS: I. Comprehension. *Journal of Speech and Hearing Research, 34,* 1106–1120.

Chapman, R.S., Seung, H.-K., Schwartz, S.E., & Kay-Raining Bird, E. (1998). Language skills of children and adolescents with Down syndrome: II. Production deficits. *Journal of Speech, Language, and Hearing Research, 41*(4), 861–873.

Chapman, R.S., Seung, H.-K., Schwartz, S., & Kay-Raining Bird, E. (2000). Predicting language development in children and adolescents with DS: The role of comprehension. *Journal of Speech, Language, and Hearing Research, 43,* 340–350.

Chapman, R.S., Sindberg, H., Bridge, C., Gigstead, K., & Hesketh, L.J. (2006). Effect of memory support and elicited production on fast mapping of new words by adolescents with DS. *Journal of Speech, Language, and Hearing Research, 49,* 3–15.

Cohen, I.L., Vietze, P.M., Sudhalter, V., Jenkins, E.C., & Brown, W.T. (1989). Parent–child dyadic gaze patterns in fragile X males and in non-fragile X males with autistic disorder. *Journal of Child Psychology and Psychiatry and Allied Disciplines, 30,* 845–856.

Cornish, K., Sudhalter, V., & Turk, J. (2004). Attention and language in fragile X. *Mental Retardation and Developmental Disabilities Research Reviews, 10*, 11–16.

Demark, J.L., Feldman, M.A., & Holden, J.J.A. (2003). Behavioral relationship between autism and fragile X syndrome. *American Journal on Mental Retardation, 108*(5), 314–326.

Doherty-Sneddon, G., & Phelps, F. (2005). Gaze aversion: A response to cognitive or social difficulty? *Memory and Cognition, 33*, 727–733.

Dollaghan, C., Campbell, T., & Tomlin, B. (1990). Video narration as a language sampling context. *Journal of Speech and Hearing Disorders, 55*, 582–590.

Dunn, L., & Dunn, L. (1981). *Peabody Picture Vocabulary Test* (Rev. ed.). Circle Pines, MN: American Guidance Service.

Dunn, L., & Dunn, L. (1997). *Peabody Picture Vocabulary Test* (3rd ed.). Circle Pines, MN: American Guidance Service.

Dykens, E.M., Hodapp, R.M., & Finucane, B.M. (2000). *Genetics and mental retardation syndromes: A new look at behavior and interventions.* Baltimore: Paul H. Brookes Publishing Co.

Dykens, E., Hodapp, R., & Leckman, J. (1994). *Behavior and development in fragile X syndrome.* Thousand Oaks, CA: Sage Publications.

Dykens, E.M., Hodapp, R.M., Ort, S., & Finucane, B. (1989). The trajectory of cognitive development in males with fragile X syndrome. *Journal of the American Academy of Child and Adolescent Psychiatry, 28*(3), 422–426.

Dykens, E., Leckman, J., Paul, R., & Watson, M. (1988). Cognitive, behavioral, and adaptive functioning in fragile X and non-fragile X retarded men. *Journal of Autism and Developmental Disorders, 18*(1), 41–52.

Dykens, E., Ort, S., Cohen, I., & Finucane, B. (1996). Trajectories and profiles of adaptive behavior in males with fragile X syndrome: Multicenter studies. *Journal of Autism and Developmental Disorders, 26*(3), 287–301.

Eadie, P., Fey, M., Douglas, J., & Parsons, C. (2002). Profiles of grammatical morphology and sentence imitation in children with specific language impairment and DS. *Journal of Speech, Language, and Hearing Research, 45*, 720–732.

Facon, B., Facon-Bollengier, T., & Grubar, J. (2002). Chronological age, receptive vocabulary, and syntax comprehension in children and adolescents with mental retardation. *American Journal on Mental Retardation, 107*, 91–98.

Facon, B., Grubar, J., & Gardez, C. (1998). Chronological age and receptive vocabulary of persons with DS. *Psychological Reports, 82*, 723–726.

Ferrier, L., Bashir, A., Meryash, D., Johnston, J., & Wolff, P. (1991). Conversational skill of individuals with fragile X syndrome: A comparison with autism and Down syndrome. *Developmental Medicine and Child Neurology, 33*, 776–788.

Fowler, A., Gelman, R., & Gleitman, L. (1994). The course of language learning in children with Down syndrome. In H. Tager-Flusberg (Ed.), *Constraints on language acquisition studies of atypical children* (pp. 91–140). Mahwah, NJ: Lawrence Erlbaum Associates.

Freund, L., & Reiss, A. (1991). Cognitive profiles associated with the fra(X) syndrome in males and females. *American Journal of Medical Genetics, 38*, 542–547.

Girolametto, L., Verbey, M., & Tannock, R. (1994). Improving joint engagement in parent-child interaction: An intervention study. *Journal of Early Intervention, 18*(2), 155–167.

Graesser, A., Millis, K., & Zwaan, R. (1997). Discourse comprehension. In J. Spence, J. Darley, & D. Foss (Eds.), *Annual Review of Psychology* (pp. 163–189). Palo Alto, CA: The Annual Reviews.

Hagerman, R.J. (1996). Physical and behavioral phenotype. In R.J. Hagerman & A. Cronister (Eds.), *Fragile X syndrome: Diagnosis, treatment, and research* (2nd ed., pp. 3–87). Baltimore: The Johns Hopkins University Press.

Hart, B., & Risley, T.R. (1995). *Meaningful differences in the everyday experience of young American children.* Baltimore: Paul H. Brookes Publishing Co.

Hauser-Cram, P., Warfield, M., Shonkoff, J.P., & Drauss, M. (2001). Children with disabilities: A longitudinal study of child development and parental well-being. *Monographs of the Society for Research in Child Development, 66*(3), 1–131.

Heller, J., Spiridigliozzi, G., Doraiswamy, P., Sullivan, J., Crissman, B., & Kishnani, P. (2004). Donepezil effects on language in children with Down syndrome: Results of the first 22-week pilot clinical trial. *American Journal of Medical Genetics, 130*, 325–326.

Heller, J., Spiridigliozzi, G., Sullivan, J., Doraiswamy, P., Krishnan, R., & Kishnani, P. (2003). Donepezil for the treatment of language deficits in adults with Down syndrome: A preliminary 24-week open trial. *American Journal of Medical Genetics, 116,* 111–116.

Hesketh, L., & Chapman, R. (1998). Verb use by individuals with DS. *American Journal on Mental Retardation, 103,* 288–304.

Hodapp, R.M., & Dykens, E.M. (2001). Strengthening behavioral research on genetic mental retardation syndromes. *American Journal on Mental Retardation, 106*(1), 4–15.

Hodapp, R.M., & Fidler, D.J. (1999). Special education and genetics: Connections for the 21st century. *Journal of Special Education, 33*(3), 130–137.

Kaufmann, W.E., Cortell, R., Kau, A.S., Bukelis, I., Tierney, E., Gray, R.M., et al. (2004). Autism Spectrum Disorder in fragile X syndrome: Communication, social interaction, and specific behaviors. *American Journal of Medical Genetics, 129,* 225–234.

Kay-Raining Bird, E., & Chapman, R.S. (1994). Sequential recall in individuals with Down syndrome. *Journal of Speech and Hearing Research, 37*(6), 1369–1380.

Kay-Raining Bird, E., Chapman, R.S., & Schwartz, S. (2004). Fast mapping of words and story recall by children with Down syndrome. *Journal of Speech, Language, and Hearing Research, 47,* 1286–1300.

Kumin, L. (1994). Intelligibility of speech in children with Down syndrome in natural settings: Parents' perspective. *Perception & Motor Skills, 78,* 307–314.

Laws, G. (2004). Contributions of phonological memory, language comprehension and hearing to the expressive language of adolescents and young adults with Down syndrome. *Journal of Child Psychology and Psychiatry, 45*(6), 1085–1095.

Laws, G., & Bishop, D. (2003). A comparison of language abilities in adolescents with DS and children with specific language impairment. *Journal of Speech, Language, and Hearing Research, 46,* 1324–1339.

Laws, G., & Gunn, D. (2004). Phonological memory as a predictor of language comprehension in Down syndrome: A five-year follow-up study. *Journal of Child Psychology and Psychiatry, 45,* 326–337.

Lewis, P., Abbeduto, L., Murphy, M., Richmond, E., Giles, N., & Bruno, L., et al. (2006). Cognitive, language and social-cognitive skills of individuals with fragile X syndrome with and without autism. *Journal of Intellectual Disability Research, 50*(7), 532–545.

Lord, C., Rutter, M., & LeCouteur, A. (1994). Autism Diagnostic Interview-Revised: a revised version of a diagnostic interview for caregivers of individuals with possible pervasive developmental disorders. *Journal of Autism and Developmental Disorders, 24,* 659–685.

Lord, C., Rutter, M., LeCouteur, A., DiLavore, P., & Risi, S. (1999). *Autism Diagnostic Observation Schedule.* Los Angeles: Western Psychological Services.

Madison, L., George, C., & Moeschler, J. (1986). Cognitive functioning in the fragile X syndrome: A study of intellectual, memory, and communication skills. *Journal of Mental Deficiency Research, 30,* 129–148.

Mahoney, G. (1988). Maternal communication style with mentally retarded children. *American Journal on Mental Retardation, 92,* 352–359.

Mazzocco, M.M. (2000). Advances in research on the fragile X syndrome. *Mental Retardation and Developmental Disabilities Research Reviews, 6*(2), 96–106.

Mervis, C., & Robinson, B. (1999). Methodological issues in cross-syndrome comparisons: Matching procedures, sensitivity (Se) and specificity (Sp). *Monographs of the Society for Research in Child Development, 64,* 115–130.

Mervis, C., & Robinson, B. (2005). Designing measures for profiling and genotype/phenotype studies of individuals with genetic syndromes or developmental language disorders. *Applied Psycholinguistics, 26,* 41–64.

Miles, S., & Chapman, R. (2002). Narrative content as described by individuals with Down syndrome and typically-developing children. *Journal of Speech, Language, and Hearing Research, 45,* 175–189.

Miles, S., & Chapman, R. (2005, June). *The relationship between adult scaffolding and narrative expression by adolescents with Down syndrome.* Poster session presented at the Symposium on Research in Child Language Disorders, Madison, WI.

Miles, S., Chapman, R.S., & Sindberg, H. (2004, June). *A microgenetic study of storytelling by adolescents with DS and typically-developing children matched for syntax comprehension.* Poster session presented at the Symposium for Research in Child Language Disorders, Madison, WI.

Miles, S., Chapman, R.S., & Sindberg, H. (2006). Sampling context affects MLU in the language of adolescents with Down syndrome. *Journal of Speech, Language, and Hearing Research, 49*, 325–337.

Miles, S., Sindberg, H., Bridge, C., & Chapman, R. (2002, July). *Scaffolded expression of setting information in narratives by adolescents and young adults with Down syndrome.* Poster session presented at the Joint Symposium for Research in Child Language Disorders and International Association for the Study of Child Language, Madison, WI.

Miller, J. (1987). Language and communication characteristics of children with Down syndrome. In S. Pueschel, S., Tingey, J. Rynders, A. Crocker, & D. Crutcher (Eds.), *New perspectives on Down syndrome* (pp. 233–263). Baltimore: Paul H. Brookes Publishing Co.

Miolo, G., Chapman, R.S., & Sindberg, H. (2005). Sentence comprehension in adolescents with Down syndrome and typically-developing children: Role of sentence voice, visual context, and auditory-verbal short-term memory. *Journal of Speech, Language, and Hearing Research, 48*, 172–188.

Munir, F., Cornish, K.M., & Wilding, J. (2000). Nature of the working memory deficit in fragile-X syndrome. *Brain and Cognition, 44*, 387–401.

Murphy, M., & Abbeduto, L. (2003). Language and communication in fragile X syndrome. In L. Abbeduto (Ed.), *International review of research in mental retardation* (Vol. 26, pp. 83–119). New York: Academic Press.

Murphy, M.M., & Abbeduto, L. (in press). Gender differences in repetitive language in fragile X syndrome. *Journal of Intellectual Disability Research, 51*, 329–407.

Paul, R., Dykens, E., Leckman, F., Watson, M., Breg, W.R., & Cohen, D. (1987). A comparison of language characteristics of mentally retarded adults with fragile X syndrome and those with nonspecific mental retardation and autism. *Journal of Autism and Developmental Disorders, 17*, 457–468.

Pavetto, M., & Abbeduto, L. (2002). *Characteristics of expressive language among males and females with fragile X syndrome.* Poster session presented at the annual meeting of the Academy of Mental Retardation, Orlando, FL.

Philofsky, A., Hepburn, S.L., Hayes, A., Hagerman, R., & Rogers, S.J. (2004). Linguistic and cognitive functioning and autism symptoms in young children with fragile X syndrome. *American Journal on Mental Retardation, 109*(3), 208–218.

Price, J., Roberts, J., Vandergrift, N., & Martin, G. (2007). Language comprehension in boys with fragile X syndrome and boys with Down syndrome. *Journal of Intellectual Disability Research, 51*, 318–326.

Reiss, A., & Freund, L. (1992). Behavioral phenotype of fragile X syndrome: *DSM-III-R* autistic behavior in male children. *American Journal of Medical Genetics, 43*, 35–46.

Rice, M., Warren, S.F., & Betz, S. (2005). Language symptoms of developmental language disorders: An overview of autism, Down syndrome, fragile X, specific language impairment, and Williams syndrome. *Applied Psycholinguistics, 26*, 7–27.

Roberts, J., Long, S., Malkin, C., Barnes, E., Skinner, M., Hennon, E., et al. (2005). A comparison of phonological skills of young males with fragile X syndrome and Down syndrome. *Journal of Speech, Language, and Hearing Research, 48*, 980–995.

Roberts, J., Martin, G.E., Moskowitz, L., Harris, A.A., Foreman, J., & Nelson, L. (2007). Discourse skills of boys with fragile X syndrome in comparison to boys with Down syndrome. *Journal of Speech, Language, and Hearing Research, 50*, 1–18.

Roberts, J.E., Mirrett, P., & Burchinal, M. (2001). Receptive and expressive communication development of young males with fragile X syndrome. *American Journal on Mental Retardation, 106*(3), 216–230.

Roberts, J., Price, J., Nelson, L., Burchinal, M., Hennon, E., Barnes, E., et al. (2007). Receptive vocabulary, expressive vocabulary, and speech production of boys with fragile X syndrome in comparison to boys with Down syndrome. *American Journal on Mental Retardation, 112*, 177–193.

Rogers, S., Wehner, E., & Hagerman, R. (2001). The behavioral phenotype in fragile X: Symptoms of autism in very young children with fragile X syndrome, idiopathic autism, and other developmental disorders. *Journal of Developmental and Behavioral Pediatrics, 22*, 409–418.

Rosin, M., Swift, E., Bless, D., & Vetter, D. (1988). Communication profiles of adolescents with Down syndrome. *Journal of Childhood Communication Disorders, 12*, 49–64.

Seung, H.-K., & Chapman, R. (2003). The effect of story presentation rates on story retelling by individuals with DS. *Applied Psycholinguistics, 24*, 601–618.

Simon, J.A., Keenan, J.M., Pennington, B.F., Taylor, A.K., & Hagerman, R.J. (2001). Discourse processing in women with fragile X syndrome: Evidence for a deficit establishing coherence. *Cognitive Neuropsychology, 18*(1), 1–18.

Sparrow, S., Balla, D., & Cicchetti, D. (1984). *Vineland Adaptive Behavior Scales.* Circle Pines, MN: American Guidance Service.

Sudhalter, V., & Belser, R.C. (2001). Conversational characteristics of children with fragile X syndrome: Tangential language. *American Journal on Mental Retardation, 106*(5), 389–400.

Sudhalter, V., Cohen, I., Silverman, W., & Wolf-Schein, E. (1990). Conversational analysis of males with fragile X, Down syndrome, and autism: Comparison of the emergence of deviant language. *American Journal on Mental Retardation, 94*, 431–441.

Sudhalter, V., Maranion, M., & Brooks, P. (1992). Expressive semantic deficit in the productive language of males with fragile X syndrome. *American Journal of Medical Genetics, 43*, 65–71.

Thordardottir, E., Chapman, R.S., & Wagner, L. (2002). Complex sentence production by adolescents with Down syndrome. *Applied Psycholinguistics, 24*, 163–183.

Thorndike, R., Hagen, E., & Sattler, J. (1986). *Stanford-Binet Intelligence Scale* (4th ed.). Chicago: The Riverside Publishing Company.

Tomasello, M., & Barton, M.E. (1994). Learning words in nonostensive contexts. *Developmental Psychology, 30*(5), 639–650.

Vicari, S., Caselli, M.C., & Tonucci, F. (2000). Asynchrony of lexical and morphosyntactic development in children with Down syndrome. *Neuropsychologia, 38*, 634–644.

Williams, K., Wishart, J., Pitcairn, T., & Willis, D. (2005). Emotion recognition by children with Down syndrome: Investigation of specific impairments and error patterns. *American Journal on Mental Retardation, 110*, 378–392.

Wolff, P., Gardner, J., Paccla, J., & Lappen, J. (1989). The greeting behavior of fragile X males. *American Journal on Mental Retardation, 93*, 406–411.

Woodward, A., Markman, E., & Fitzsimmons, C. (1994). Rapid word learning in 13–18 month-olds. *Developmental Psychology, 30*, 553–566.

CHAPTER 6

Phonological Characteristics of Children with Down Syndrome or Fragile X Syndrome

JOANNE E. ROBERTS, CAROL STOEL-GAMMON, AND ELIZABETH F. BARNES

Many individuals with Down syndrome (DS) have speech difficulties and can be hard to understand. In particular, individuals with DS can have problems with the intelligibility of their spoken language throughout their lifespan. Speech difficulties are also common among males with fragile X syndrome (FXS) but less common among females with FXS (Hanson, Jackson, & Hagerman, 1986; Madison, George, & Moeschler, 1986; Newell, Sanborn, & Hagerman, 1983; Roberts et al., 2005). Boys and adult males with FXS are commonly reported to be difficult to understand in connected speech, although there is a spectrum of speech involvement (Madison et al., 1986; Paul et al., 1987; Spinelli, de Oliveira Rocha, Giacheti, & Richieri-Costa, 1995). Reduced speech intelligibility may be a defining feature of the communication phenotype of individuals with DS and males with FXS. Examining the nature of speech disorders in individuals with DS and FXS and the possible causes and contributory factors has important implications for assessing speech and defining intervention goals and treatment plans for these populations.

This chapter briefly describes speech development in typical populations; summarizes the prelinguistic vocal development, single-word productions, connected speech, and intelligibility of individuals with DS or FXS; and describes factors that may cause or contribute to speech difficulties in these two latter populations. This chapter also provides guidelines for speech assessment and intervention and parent involvement for individuals with DS or FXS and incorporates suggestions for future research throughout the chapter, concluding with potential research directions.

SPEECH DEVELOPMENT IN TYPICAL POPULATIONS

The foundations for speech in typically developing individuals develop in the first year of life with the emergence of noncommunicative vocalizations, which are

This work was supported in part by Research Grant 5 R01 HD044935 from the National Institute of Child Health and Human Development.

precursors to the production of words and phrases. Of particular importance is the onset, around 6–7 months of age, of canonical (reduplicated) babbling, in which consonant–vowel syllables are repeated (e.g., "baba"). The sounds that infants produce first are perceptually salient sounds that are easily discriminated from each other, such as stops, and their productions increasingly resemble the consonant sounds used by their caregivers (Vihman, 2005). Auditory experiences are critical to the mastery of consonant sounds as children learn to produce the sounds in the language used in their environments. Deaf infants, for example, usually don't produce canonical babbling, as they are unable to use auditory adult models to practice consonant sounds (Oller, Eilers, Bull, & Carney, 1985). As motor control develops, children typically produce more difficult phonemes, continually using comparisons between his or her own production and those of the adult speakers in his or her environment (Kent, 1992; Kent & Miolo, 1995). These consonant–vowel (CV) syllables are phonetically similar, or even identical, to the forms used later in first words. For example, the production of "mama" may be nonmeaningful at 8 months, but it may be an actual word at 14 months when the infant recognizes that sound–meaning relationships form the basis for words. A babbled vocalization becomes a word vocalization and, finally, a word. During the period of early word acquisition, the phonetic characteristics of babble and speech are similar, as both use consonant–vowel syllables and a limited set of consonants (Locke, 1983; Stoel-Gammon, 1998a). By the time children begin to use variegated babbling (babble with CV syllables containing varied consonant sounds) at about 12 months, their babble is phonetically closer to adult-form words.

Not only do babble and early words share phonetic characteristics during the transition to speech, but there is a growing body of evidence linking prelinguistic vocal development to speech and language skills throughout early childhood in both typically developing children and those with speech disorders (Stoel-Gammon, 1998b; Vihman, 1996). Specifically, increased use of complex babble is linked to better performance on speech and language measures after the onset of speech (Stoel-Gammon, 1992). Among typically developing children, substantial individual differences in early word productions have been noted. For example, children appear to pick and choose words for their early lexicon based, in part, on the phonological characteristics of their target words. One child may choose a high proportion of words with fricative consonants while another may choose words with velar sounds (Stoel-Gammon, 1998b). Once a child's vocabulary has reached 250–300 words (at around 24 months), strong commonalities are apparent. Words are produced with relatively simple syllable structures (e.g., CV, CVC, CVCV); predominant sound classes are the same that predominated in babble, namely stops (/p/, /b/, /t/, /d/, /k/, /g/), nasals (/m/, /n/), and glides (/w/, /j/ as in "you"), which emerge between 2 and 4 years of age. Fricatives (/s/, /z/, /f/, /v/), affricates (/č/ of "chair"; /ǰ/ of "jelly"), and liquids (/l/, /r/) generally appear later in development, usually between 4 and 6 years of age.

By the age of 5, children acquiring English can produce nearly all English phonemes, at least in some words (Peña-Brooks & Hegde, 2000). They also can produce multisyllabic words and words with complex consonant sequences (e.g., the three consonants at the beginning of "spring" or "scratch"). In addition, nearly all of a child's speech is fully intelligible to a stranger by the age of 4–5 years. This does not mean that the child's pronunciation is always accurate but that his or her errors do not interfere with a listener's ability to identify the target word. By the age of 8, children's speech patterns closely resemble those of adults: All phonemes are produced accurately, and intonation and stress patterns are appropriate.

SPEECH PRODUCTION OF INDIVIDUALS WITH DOWN SYNDROME

Research on children with DS indicates that their vocalizations in infancy resemble those of their typical developing peers within the form of vocalizations and schedule for emergence. The onset of words, however, is delayed, often by many months, and speech development is extremely slow. When individuals with DS reach a mental age of 8 years, their speech still exhibits delayed production patterns, and their intelligibility is low (Kumin, 1996; Stoel-Gammon, 2001).

The following sections summarize speech development among individuals with DS and present an overview of factors that may contribute to observed impairments.

Prelinguistic Vocal Development and the Transition to Meaningful Speech

Cross-sectional and longitudinal studies of infants with DS have documented strong similarities with typically developing infants in amount of vocalization, developmental timetable (particularly age at onset of canonical babble), and segmental characteristics of canonical and reduplicated babble (Dodd, 1972; Oller & Seibert, 1988; Smith & Oller, 1981; Smith & Stoel-Gammon, 1996; Steffens, Oller, Lynch, & Urbano, 1992). Lynch and colleagues (1995), however, reported that the average age of onset of canonical babbling among infants with DS was about 9 months, approximately 2 months later than that of typically developing infants, and that the proportional occurrence of canonical babbling was less stable for infants with DS. The relative instability in canonical babbling in DS may be a consequence of oral and facial hypotonicity (which can reduce the speed and precision of speech movements), oral structural impairments (e.g., abnormally large tongue), and reduced nasal resonance (due to chronic respiratory infections; Dodd & Thompson, 2001; Stoel-Gammon, 1997). Recurrent otitis media and accompanying hearing loss, which are characteristic of infants with DS, can also affect speech production, as infants are unable to fine tune their own phoneme productions using adult models (Stoel-Gammon, 1997; Stoel-Gammon, 2001). Taken together, research indicates that prelinguistic vocal development is within the normal range for infants with DS, although the babbling period is longer, often extending through the second year of life.

To produce adult-based words, a child must recognize the arbitrary sound-meaning relationships that are the basis of words. Although the relationship between degree of intellectual disability and the onset and use of words is not straightforward, the ability to recognize sound–meaning relationships may be affected by intellectual disability. Limited word use by 18 months has been reported for a few children with DS; however, the majority of affected children first use words between 24 and 60 months (Buckley, 2000; Stray-Gunderson, 1986). Stray-Gunderson noted extreme variability in the age of first-word production for children with DS, citing a chronological age range of 9 months to

7 years. Buckley reported that children with DS had a productive vocabulary of 28 words at 24 months (compared with 250–300 words for a typically developing child of the same age) and 330 words at 6 years (compared with several thousand words for a typically developing child of the same age).

Speech Production in Single Words

Individuals with DS produce words with a small set of consonants and limited variety in syllable structure. The following sections describe speech patterns in terms of phonetic inventory (speech sounds used in word productions) and error patterns.

Phonetic Inventory

The speech sounds used in early word productions of children with DS are similar to early words typically developing children use (Dodd & Leahy, 1989; Smith & Stoel-Gammon, 1983; Van Borsel, 1996). As in babbling, the consonants that occur frequently in early speech sounds are stops (/p/, /b/, /t/, /d/, /k/, /g/), nasals (/m/, /n/), and glides (/w/, and /j/ as in "you"). Consonants acquired later are fricatives (/s/, /z/, /f/, /v/), affricates (/č/ of "chair"; /ǰ/ of "jelly"), and liquids (/l/, /r/). As in typically developing children, consonants that are acquired early often serve as substitutes for consonants that are learned later (Smith & Stoel-Gammon, 1983).

Error Patterns

The speech errors of individuals with DS are generally similar to those seen in younger, typically developing children at similar mental ages; however, children with DS have a greater number of errors that tend to persist for an extended period (Bleile & Schwarz, 1984; Dodd, 1976; Rosin, Swift, Bless, & Vetter, 1988; Stoel-Gammon, 1980). By 8 years of age, the phonology of typically developing children closely resembles that of an adult. In contrast, individuals with DS may achieve a mental age of 7 or 8 years and retain speech errors characteristic of younger children into adulthood (Shriberg & Widder, 1990; Sommers, Patterson, & Wildgen, 1988; Sommers, Reinhart, & Sistrunk, 1988).

Error patterns (often referred to as *phonological processes*) can be grouped into several subtypes. One major error type affects the structure of a word or syllable; a second major error type affects classes of sounds. The following syllable/word structure errors have been documented in individuals with DS: 1) consonant sequences are "reduced" by omission of one or more consonants (the error pattern of cluster reduction; e.g., "bread" is produced as "bed," "snow" is produced as "no"), 2) consonants at the ends of words are omitted (final consonant deletion), and 3) unstressed syllables are often omitted (e.g., "banana" is produced as "nana"). The following substitution patterns are also frequent: 1) fricatives and affricates in the target words are produced as stops (e.g., "sun" is produced "tun," "zoo" and "chew" are produced as "too," and "van" is produced as "ban"), 2) /r/ and /l/ are produced as /w/ (e.g., "red" is produced as "wed" [gliding]), and 3) consonants articulated in the back of the mouth are substituted by front consonants (e.g., "cat" becomes "tat," "go" becomes "doe"). In many instances, words are affected by more than one error pattern, decreasing the likelihood that such a word will be understood. More complete descriptions of these error patterns can be found in studies by Dodd (1976); Kumin, Councill, and Goodman (1994); Mackay and Hodson (1982); Roberts and colleagues (2005); Smith and Stoel-Gammon (1983); Stoel-Gammon (1981); and Van Borsel (1996).

Roberts and colleagues (2005) reported that preschool and school-age boys with DS produced more sounds in error, more error patterns, and different error patterns than younger typically developing boys at the same mental age on a single-word articulation test. The boys with DS were similar to the younger typically developing boys on overall substitution phonological processes but used more processes that reduced word shapes (i.e., omitted syllables, reduced consonant clusters, and deleted consonants). The reduction of word shapes in individuals with speech difficulties may particularly affect their speech intelligibility (Hodson & Paden, 1991).

Error patterns for children with DS are also more variable than for typically developing children (Dodd & Thompson, 2001). Dodd (1976) compared the phonological systems of three groups of children matched for mental age. The three groups consisted of typically developing children, children with intellectual disability without DS, and children with DS. Although there were no statistical differences in the number and type of phonological errors occurring in spontaneous and imitated productions of the three groups, the children with DS had a greater number of inconsistent errors, and their types of errors differed from the typically developing group. Stoel-Gammon (1981) also reported greater variability in errors produced by children with DS. Although typically developing children moved from incorrect to correct phoneme production in a linear manner with a few types of substitution, children with DS had more types of substitutions that varied from one word to another.

In one of the few longitudinal studies of speech patterns in children with DS, Smith and Stoel-Gammon (1983) compared the rate of use of four error types in the speech of children with DS with typically developing children. The average percentage of errors in the group with typically developing children declined 38% in a 12-month period, from 63% at 18–24 months to 25% at 30–36 months. For children with DS, the average percentage of the same error patterns was 61% when the children were 36 months old, declining to 40% at 72 months, an average change per year of 6%.

Production Patterns in Connected Speech

Few studies examine the phonology, fluency, and voice characteristics found within the connected speech of individuals with DS. The few studies that have been conducted found that error rates for individuals with DS were higher for connected speech than for single words, with the same types of errors present in both contexts (Shriberg & Widder, 1990; Sommers et al., 1988; Stoel-Gammon, 1981). Children with DS also exhibit a higher rate of dysfluency in their connected speech than language age–matched typically developing children (Preus, 1973; Willcox, 1988). In a study of speech characteristics of fluent and dysfluent adults with DS, Farmer and Brayton (1979) found that the number of dysfluencies varied considerably across the 13 participants. One subgroup exhibited relatively accurate single-word productions but poor intelligibility in conversational speech. This group also demonstrated a higher rate of dysfluent speech and shorter vowel durations than the participants with higher intelligibility scores.

The authors suggested that these findings may indicate an impairment in segmental timing in some individuals with DS. Other factors, such as deviations in rate, placement of sentence stress, and voice quality (low-pitch, hoarse, harsh voice), have also been reported among individuals with DS (Shriberg & Widder, 1990; Stoel-Gammon, 1997).

Speech Intelligibility

In Chapter 9 in this book, Price and Kent note that decreased intelligibility is a persistent problem for individuals with DS. When compared with children with typical development or other types of intellectual disability matched for mental age, individuals with DS are judged to have lower levels of speech intelligibility. As observed by Price and Kent, a speaker's pronunciation abilities are not the only factor in determining the level of intelligibility. Other factors affecting intelligibility include the listener, the message, and the transmitting environment. In many cases, the latter factors are not considered in research on intelligibility in children.

The speech of many individuals with DS tends to be unintelligible throughout their lives, even though their mental age may exceed 5 years (the age at which typically developing children are judged to be fully intelligible [see Kumin, 1994a; Pueschel & Hoppmann, 1993; Shriberg & Widder, 1990]). Kumin (1994b) reported that 937 parents of individuals with DS (from birth to 40+ years) noted low levels of intelligibility, with nearly 60% of the parents reporting that their children frequently had difficulty being understood, and 37% reporting that their children sometimes had difficulty being understood. Pueschel and Hoppmann (1993) also used a questionnaire to gain information on the parents' views of their children's speech and language skills. Although parents reported that their children were generally capable of making themselves understood, 71%–94% of parents of children with DS (age 4–21 years) noted that their children had speech problems. Chapman, Seung, and Schwartz (2000) reported that 30% of the variability in speech intelligibility in production of narratives was a function of chronological age and hearing status in a group of individuals with DS ages 5–20 years old.

Summary

Speech production patterns in individuals with DS are more delayed than expected for their mental ages and resemble those of younger, typically developing children in terms of most error types. As with younger, typically developing children, substitution error patterns are common in children with DS; unlike typically developing children, however, error patterns that reduce word shapes also occur among individuals with DS. Progress toward adult-like speech patterns is extremely slow, however, and even when an individual with DS reaches a mental age of 8 years, phonemic development is usually not complete, and intelligibility may remain low. The relationship between the phonology of single words and conversational speech is unclear. There is need for a controlled study of these two aspects in the same participants with DS using the same phonological measures. Further, in order to determine what aspects of speech are affecting speech intelligibility, prosodic and segmental aspects of speech, as well as phonological patterns, should be examined. Because some differences in speech may not be audible to a listener, acoustic measures should be used. Future research should use longitudinal studies to describe the changes in speech patterns of individuals with DS over time, particularly in continuous speech. Identifying the specific phonological patterns that affect speech intelligibility in continuous speech is needed. The underlying causes of the marked delays in speech development are not fully understood, but it is believed that factors described in the following section contribute to the delays.

FACTORS AFFECTING SPEECH PRODUCTION IN DOWN SYNDROME

Given the considerable variability in the speech skills of individuals with DS, it is important to describe potential mechanisms underlying their speech difficulties. This section describes factors that may cause or contribute to poor speech intelligibility.

Hearing Loss

Infants and children with DS often experience mild to moderate hearing loss. In 1980, Downs reported that 78% of the children with DS that she tested were found to have hearing problems in one or both ears when the criterion for a problem was a 15 dB loss. Of the children with a hearing problem, 65% displayed significant levels of loss in both ears, 54% evidenced conductive loss, 16% had sensorineural loss in one or both ears, and 8% displayed mixed losses. The incidence of hearing loss reported by Downs in 1980 has not changed much to date. In a study of 47 children with DS, Roizen (2002) reported that about two thirds of the children had conductive or sensorineural hearing losses or both. In a study of 48 preschool-age children with DS, Shott, Joseph, and Heithaus (2001) reported that otitis media, which causes conductive hearing loss, was present in 96% of the children. Otitis media is of concern for children's language development because it is often accompanied by fluid in the middle ear, which can cause a mild to moderate fluctuating hearing loss (American Academy of Pediatrics [AAP], 2004; Roberts, Hunter, et al., 2004). Children with DS (already at risk for speech and language learning difficulties) are thought to be more vulnerable than typically developing children to language difficulties due to hearing loss associated with otitis media with effusion (OME; AAP, 2004; Roberts, Rosenfeld, & Zeisel, 2004). Because no prospective studies exist on the linkage between a history of OME and later language and learning difficulties, longitudinal research is needed to determine if a history of OME and associated hearing loss contributes to later language and learning difficulties in individuals with DS and to specify which aspects of language and learning are affected (AAP, 2004).

Oral Motor Skills

Structural and functional differences in oral structures of individuals with DS are thought to affect speech production (Miller & Leddy, 1998; Stoel-Gammon, 1997). Although variable, oral structure differences may include a small oral cavity; a narrow, high-arched palate; irregular dentition; and a large tongue, which protrudes forward. Facial musculature may have missing, additional, or poorly differentiated muscles; hyperextendable joints; and nerve innervation differences (Miller & Leddy, 1998). These muscular and innervation variances may be associated with some of the observed speech characteristics of individuals with DS, including reduced rate, limited range of motion, and difficulty with coordination of the speech articulators. There are also reports of drooling, open mouth posture, large tongues, hypotonia, velopharyngeal insufficiency, and compromised respiratory support, as well as apraxia (difficulty in execution of the motor programming of speech movements) and dysarthria (weakness or incoordination of the articulators that results in slow, weak, imprecise, or discoordinated speech) (Dodd & Thompson, 2001; Miller & Leddy, 1998).

Leddy (1999; see also Miller & Leddy, 1998) noted that the skeletal system of individuals with DS is characterized by absent or deficient bone growth, a smaller oral cavity, and more posterior tongue carriage. The muscular system is characterized by differences in the facial region and a large, muscular tongue. These differences in structure and in tongue size influence the production of lingual consonants. Furthermore, weak facial muscles limit lip movement, affecting production of labial consonants and rounded vowels. Barnes, Roberts, Mirrett, Sideris, and Misenheimer (2006) reported that boys with DS showed atypical oral structure (of the lips, tongue and velopharyngeal area), oral motor function not involving speech (for the lips), and speech function (of the lips, tongue, velopharynx, larynx, and coordinated speech) compared with typically developing boys. In addition, the boys with DS had more difficulty with speech than nonspeech tasks, indicating that oral function for speech production is especially compromised.

Miller and colleagues (1989) examined the influence of anatomical and physiological characteristics on speech development of children with DS. Using the Robbins and Klee protocol (1987) to assess the speech motor abilities of 43 children with DS, Miller and colleagues found a high correlation between speech motor function and the number of different words produced by children with DS in a spontaneous speech sample. Specifically, the speech function scores obtained at the first data collection session (when the children were 18–60 months of age) accounted for nearly 80% of the variance in predicting the number of different words in samples collected approximately 5 months later. The researchers concluded that speech motor function and phonetic inventory were the best speech predictors of vocabulary diversity 18 months later. Further research is needed to define the oral motor patterns in individuals with DS and to discover how specific oral motor patterns are related to speech development.

Summary

The roles of hearing loss and oral motor difficulties in the speech of individuals with DS are not yet clear. Other factors, such as the presence of developmental apraxia and/or dysarthria and cognitive processing limitations, such as impairments of working memory (see Chapter 4 for more information on this topic), may also contribute to speech difficulties among individuals with DS. Researchers need to examine how these factors explain individual differences in speech production in individuals with DS and whether there are development periods when speech may be more susceptible to these factors.

SPEECH PRODUCTION OF INDIVIDUALS WITH FRAGILE X SYNDROME

It is commonly reported that the conversational speech of males with FXS is very difficult to understand, although there is a spectrum of speech involvement

(Abbeduto & Hagerman, 1997; Madison et al., 1986; Paul, Cohen, Breg, Watson, & Herman, 1984; Spinelli et al., 1995). The speech of males with FXS has also been described as "peculiar," "distinct," and "unusual" (Hanson et al., 1986; Paul et al., 1987). The speech of females with FXS is less affected than that of males with the disorder (Madison et al., 1986; Spinelli et al., 1995), although very little research has been conducted on the speech skills of females (Abbeduto & Hagerman, 1997; Bennetto & Pennington, 2002). The focus of this section is primarily on the speech of males with FXS because there are so few studies of females.

Prelinguistic Vocal Development in Fragile X Syndrome

No studies exist describing the prelinguistic development of vocal skills of children with FXS. Children with FXS begin to use their first words later than their typically developing peers (Brady, Skinner, Roberts, & Hennon, 2006; Roberts, Hatton, & Bailey, 2001). Roberts, Hatton, and Bailey found that parents of 26 boys with FXS reported an average age of 28 months (range from 9–88 months) for use of first spoken words. Similarly, mothers of 55 boys and girls with FXS younger than 3 years of age reported that 29 of the children were nonverbal (mean chronological age of 25 months), 13 had emerging verbal skills (mean chronological age of 28 months), and 13 children were verbal (mean chronological age of 34 months). For more details on prelinguistic vocal and verbal development, see Chapters 3 and 7.

Males with Fragile X Syndrome: Speech Production in Single Words

The following sections describe speech patterns in terms of the phonetic inventory and error patterns in single words.

Phonetic Inventories

In a study of single words, Roberts and colleagues (2005) compared the phonetic inventory (mastery of different consonants as indexed by the percentage of consonants produced correctly) and approximation of phonological word structures (number of consonant and vowel segments and correct consonants) of fifty 3- to 14-year-old boys with FXS with 33 younger, typically developing boys at similar mental ages. They found early developing consonants (e.g., /m/, /b/, /p/), middle-developing consonants (e.g., /t/, /g/, /f/), and later-developing consonants (e.g., /s/, /l/, /r/), as well as a measure of whole-word proximity comparable to younger, typically developing boys at a similar mental age.

Error Patterns

In an examination of error types (sound substitutions, omissions, distortions) in single words, Hanson and colleagues (1986) found frequent sound omissions and substitutions in ten 3- to 9-year-old boys with FXS. Palmer and colleagues (1988) and Prouty and colleagues (1988) also reported developmental errors, most often sound substitutions and a few omissions, in fifteen 3- to 23-year-old males with FXS. Madison and colleagues (1986) reported sound omissions (mostly in consonant clusters with /r/) and substitution errors (most commonly /θ/, /v/, and /r/ targets) for five of six males with FXS who were between 4 and 34 years of age. The phonemes most commonly reported to be produced in error were /l/, /r/, and /s/ in a 5- and 8-year-old (Vilkman, Niemi, & Ikonen, 1988), two 10-year-olds, and one 13-year-old (Paul et al., 1984); these are sounds that typically develop-ing children often produce in error at young ages.

The speech of males with FXS has also been analyzed for phonological processes. Paul and colleagues (1984) reported unstressed syllable deletion, liquid simplification, final consonant deletion, and, occasionally, stopping in three 10- to 14-year-old males with FXS. Palmer and colleagues (1988) studied 15 males with FXS, ages 2 through 22 years, and found occurrences of stopping/stridency dele-tion, liquid simplification, cluster reduction, and cluster simplification. Roberts and colleagues (2005) found that the presence of syllable structure processes (e.g., final consonant deletion, cluster reduction, syllable omissions) and substitution processes (e.g., velar fronting, early stopping, cluster simplification) in fifty 3- to 14-year-old boys with FXS were similar to those in younger typically developing mental age–matched boys.

Production Patterns in Connected Speech

The research on connected speech has focused on prosody; no studies of phono-logical patterns in connected speech exist. Prosody, or aspects of speech that extend beyond sound segments such as rate and stress patterns, have been reported to be affected in individuals with FXS (Belser & Sudhalter, 2001; Han-son et al., 1986; Reiss & Freund, 1992; Spinelli et al., 1995). A rapid and fluctu-ating rate of speech consisting of "bursts" of speech and unpredictable shifts from rapid to slower rates has been described in individuals with FXS in several stud-ies that used parent report or subjective ratings of rate (Belser & Sudhalter, 2001; Hanson et al., 1986; Reiss & Freund, 1992; Spinelli et al., 1995). Reiss and Fre-und found that parents of 34 boys with FXS (ages 3–18 years) reported that their sons used an unusual rate (unusual was not defined) of speech as compared with developmentally delayed boys. Hanson and colleagues (1986) reported that 9 of the 10 boys who were between 3 and 8 years of age used a fast and fluctuating rate of speech with rapid bursts, or cluttering. In other studies, 20 of 23 boys with FXS used a rapid speech rhythm (Borghgraef, Fryns, Dielkens, Pyck, & Van den Bergh, 1987), while five of eight 7- to 26-year-old males had variable rates of speech (Spinelli et al., 1995). Using an objective measure of rate, Zajac and col-leagues (2006) measured speaking rate in syllables per second during intelligible utterances in conversational speech (rather than by perceptual judgments as in previous studies). They reported that thirty-eight 8- to 14-year-old boys with FXS spoke faster than younger, typically developing boys of similar mental ages but did not talk faster than boys of the same chronological age. Because older chil-dren talk faster than younger children (Kent & Forner, 1980; Smith, Kenney, & Hussain, 1996), the authors concluded that the boys with FXS did not have a fast rate of speech when their utterances were intelligible. Dysfluency (rapid repeti-tion of sounds and syllables), which is another aspect of prosody, has also been reported in the conversational speech of young males with FXS (Belser & Sud-halter, 2001; Palmer et al.,1988; Rhoads, 1984).

Speech Intelligibility

The speech of males with FXS has been reported to be difficult to understand in conversation (Abbeduto & Hagerman, 1997; Paul et al., 1984, 1987; Spinelli et al., 1995). Paul and colleagues (1984) reported that the speech of three 10- to 14-year-old males was relatively clear in single words, although conversational speech was often unintelligible. Vilkman and colleagues (1988) reported that the connected speech of one 5-year-old boy and one 8-year-old boy with FXS had many speech errors and was dysfluent, making them highly unintelligible. For a more thorough discussion of speech intelligibility in individuals with FXS, see Chapter 9.

Speech Production in Females with Fragile X Syndrome

In contrast to boys with FXS, there is very little research on the development of speech skills in females with FXS (Abbeduto & Hagerman, 1997; Bennetto & Pennington, 2002). The existing research indicates that females do not have the same speech impairments as males with FXS (Madison et al., 1986; Spinelli et al., 1995). In one of the few studies of females with FXS, Madison and colleagues (1986) reported that the conversational speech of five adult females and one 6-year-old girl was clear and intelligible, and, on a single-word articulation test, the adults had no speech errors, although the child had many speech errors. Spinelli and colleagues (1995) evaluated the speech skills of a 10-year-old girl and a 33-year-old adult female. They reported that, as complexity increased, the 10-year-old had more speech errors and sound omissions, while the adult female had no speech difficulties. Palmer and colleagues (1988) and Prouty and colleagues (1988) studied five females with FXS (ages 7–26 years) and found that all five had speech errors on a single-word articulation test, but the number of errors varied greatly.

Summary

The number and types of single-word speech errors in individuals with FXS is similar to those of younger, typically developing children. Poor speech intelligibility in connected speech has been reported as characteristic of males with FXS in a few studies. Prosodic aspects of speech may be contributing to reduced speech intelligibility in individuals with FXS, although the reports of a rapid rate of speech were not found when objective measures of syllables per second were computed. Overall, very few studies exist describing the speech skills of young boys with FXS, with most studies focused on adolescents and adults with FXS and including a small number of participants. The little research that has been conducted on females with FXS suggests that although variable, speech difficulties are less severe than in males with FXS. Based on the few existing studies, there is some suggestion that the speech errors may be due to a developmental delay.

Future studies should assess speech patterns and speech intelligibility in both single words and in continuous speech in the same group of individuals to determine what aspects of speech are affected and how specific error patterns and prosody affect speech intelligibility in males with FXS. In addition to phonological patterns, prosodic and segmental aspects of speech should be examined, using acoustic measures when possible, in order to determine what aspects of speech are affecting speech intelligibility. Further, longitudinal studies are needed to examine how speech patterns change over time in individuals with FXS. Studies

of the speech development of females with FXS are needed, particularly longitudinal studies that examine the development of speech over time and studies examining speech during different age periods. Possible causes or contributing factors to
these speech difficulties are described in the next section.

FACTORS AFFECTING SPEECH PRODUCTION IN FRAGILE X SYNDROME

Because there is considerable variability in the speech skills of individuals with
FXS, it is useful to examine potential mechanisms underlying speech difficulties,
particularly reduced speech intelligibility in connected speech. Gender is one factor affecting speech production, which is likely due to the degree of intellectual
disability. Most affected males have significant intellectual impairment, whereas
about one quarter to one half of carrier females exhibit mild to moderate intellectual disability (Hagerman, 1991, 1995). Because decreased speech intelligibility has been reported only in males with FXS and studies are lacking on females,
the focus of this section is on males.

Hearing Loss

The hearing loss that occurs with otitis media during early childhood may also
affect later speech intelligibility in individuals with FXS. Otitis media has been
reported to be prevalent among young children with FXS (Hagerman, Altshul-
Stark, & McBogg, 1987). A study of 30 boys with FXS between 2 and 10 years of
age found that they experienced more recurrent otitis media than their typically
developing siblings and typically developing unrelated boys (Hagerman et al.,
1987). Although Roberts and colleagues (2005) found that twenty-three 8- to 14-
year-old boys with FXS had normal middle ear function and hearing sensitivity,
similar to typically developing boys, it is unclear whether there is an increased
incidence of otitis media and hearing loss in individuals with FXS during the first
few years of life when otitis media is most prevalent. Otitis media is of concern for
children's speech development because the fluid in the middle ear or effusion can
cause a mild-to-moderate fluctuating hearing loss (AAP, 2004; Roberts, Hunter, et
al., 2004). Experiencing frequent hearing loss during the first few years of life, a
critical time period for speech acquisition, may hamper later speech development.
Although there is a negligible-to-mild relationship between a history of OME and
later language in typically developing children (AAP, 2004; Roberts, Hunter, et al.,
2004), children with FXS (who are at risk for speech delays) may be more vulnerable to speech difficulties due to persistent OME in early childhood.

Oral-Motor Skills

Oral-motor difficulties including developmental apraxia of speech (DAS) may
also contribute to reduced speech intelligibility in males with FXS (Barnes et al.,
2006; Madison et al., 1986; Paul et al., 1984; Spinelli et al., 1995). Madison and
colleagues (1986) reported that four brothers with FXS between 29 and 34 years
of age had evidence of mild DAS. Spinelli and colleagues (1995) found that eight
males (ages 6–26 years) with FXS had more than five of the following characteristics of DAS: more errors as word length and complexity increased, more errors

in continuous speech than in single words, inconsistent articulatory errors, phonemic transpositions, prosodic disturbances, and articulatory omissions. Paul and colleagues (1984) found that three boys with FXS (ages 10–13 years) had difficulty repeating syllables and deleting and reversing the order of the syllables. Barnes and colleagues (2006) found 59 boys with FXS (ages 3–14 years) scored lower on coordinated speech movements, including rapid syllable repetition, and were less accurate repeating multiple-syllable as compared with single-syllable words than 36 typically developing boys at similar mental ages. Nonspeech oral motor impairments including hypotonia (low muscle tone), oral tactile defensiveness, joint laxity, and drooling have also been cited in several literature reviews of males with FXS (Abbeduto & Hagerman, 1997; Scharfenaker, O'Connor, Stackhouse, Braden, & Gray, 2002).

There is also evidence that some females with FXS may exhibit characteristics of DAS. Madison and colleagues (1986) found that one 6-year-old girl (out of six female participants, ages 6–63 years) exhibited speech characteristics of DAS. Spinelli and colleagues (1995) found that one 10-year-old girl, but not a 33-year-old woman, met two criteria (number of errors increased as word length and complexity increased and phoneme omissions) for DAS. Research is needed to examine the oral motor difficulties found in both males and females with FXS and their relationship to speech patterns and intelligibility.

Sensory Impairments

Impairments in sensory processing, integration, and sensorimotor coordination may also affect speech intelligibility in males with FXS. Tactile sensitivity, increased sensitivity to sensory stimuli, hyper- and hyposensitivity of the oral musculature, and sensory defensiveness have been reported in males with FXS (Baranek et al., 2002; Miller, Reisman, McIntosh, & Simon, 2001; Rogers, Hepburn, & Wehner, 2003). For example, Rogers and colleagues found that 20 children (ages 2–4 years) with FXS had more tactile and auditory sensitivity than typically developing children and were similar to children with autism in their sensory reactivity. Increased arousal due to sensory input may make it difficult for an individual to integrate sensory information in the environment and respond with appropriate motor output. Scharfenaker and colleagues (2002) noted that speech sound production is affected by increased oral sensitivity.

Anxiety

High anxiety/arousal levels may contribute to reduced speech intelligibility in males with FXS. Males with FXS display symptoms of social anxiety, including gaze aversion, overt signs of discomfort, and avoidance, and they tend to have elevated levels of arousal (Cohen, 1995; Hessl et al., 2001; Roberts, Boccia, Bailey, Hatton, & Skinner, 2001), particularly in situations involving social stress. Hessl, Glaser, Dyer-Friedman, and Reiss (2006) studied 32 girls and 58 boys with FXS (ages 6–17 years) and their unaffected siblings and found that during a social challenge protocol in which the children participated in an interview, read silently and aloud, and sang, children with FXS showed more gaze aversion, task avoidance, signs of distress, and poorer vocal quality than their unaffected siblings. The demands of conversation may overstimulate individuals with FXS and lead to a heightened state of arousal, thus causing poorer speech intelligibility. Also, it is possible that the high rate of anxiety in FXS may lead individuals to avoid social interactions. This may then affect speech, which depends on interactions with caregivers, and practice of language.

Summary

Although individuals with FXS can have hearing loss, oral-motor difficulties, sensory impairments, and arousal/anxiety, the role of these factors in affecting speech difficulties is not clear. There is no research specifically examining their impact on speech patterns or intelligibility among individuals with FXS. Furthermore, other factors, such as the amount of FMR1 protein (which appears to be responsible for FXS; see Chapter 2 for more detailed information) or having a diagnosis of autism or cognitive processing impairments in phonological working memory (see Chapter 4 for more information on these topics), could also contribute to speech difficulties. Researchers need to examine the role these factors play in explaining individual differences in speech difficulties among individuals with FXS and whether there are certain periods in development when speech may be more susceptible to these factors.

ASSESSMENT AND INTERVENTION

Although the profile of speech skills in individuals with DS and FXS suggests that some aspects of speech, such as intelligibility in continuous speech, may be particularly affected, there is considerable variability. The profile of each individual's strengths and weaknesses will determine the specific speech skills that should be assessed and targeted in intervention. This section provides assessment and intervention guidelines for individuals with DS and FXS who have speech disorders, based on methods that have been used with individuals from other special populations as well as with typically developing individuals with speech delays. Although this section describes a few studies on speech intervention in individuals with DS, there is no published research on intervention strategies for improving the speech skills of individuals with FXS.

Consider the Role of Factors Contributing to Speech Disorders

When planning for assessment and intervention in individuals with DS and FXS, it is important to consider the role of other factors that may cause or contribute to the speech sound disorders. Efforts should concentrate more on factors contributing to overall speech intelligibility than to individual speech errors. As with all individuals with speech sound disorders, these factors include oral motor and cognitive skills, language, and the communication environment (see Bauman-Waengler, 2004; Bernthal & Bankson, 2004; Williams, 2003). Given what is known about individuals with DS and FXS, this section highlights factors that may need special consideration in speech assessment and intervention with both or either of these populations. The factors that may affect both populations are otitis media and hearing loss, oral motor skills, cognitive and language profile, and presence of autism. For individuals with FXS, sensory impairments and anxiety/arousal may also affect speech production.

Otitis Media and Hearing Loss

The hearing of children with DS and FXS should be routinely screened for middle ear problems and associated hearing loss. Hearing should be tested when OME persists for 3 months or longer (AAP, 2004), as described by the American Speech-Language-Hearing Association (ASHA, 1996). When OME lasts longer than 4 months, tympanostomy tubes for at-risk individuals are recommended (AAP, 2004), as is monitoring of speech and language development. Because of the importance of hearing for speech development, low gain hearing aids or other amplification devices such as FM sound field systems in classrooms (ASHA, 2002) and strategies for optimizing the language learning and listening environment (AAP, 2004; Roberts, Hunter, et al., 2004) may be useful for individuals having hearing loss associated with repeated OME.

Oral Motor Skills

Oral motor difficulties, including DAS, may affect the speech of individuals with DS or FXS (Barnes et al., 2006; Madison et al., 1986; Miller & Leddy, 1998; Stoel-Gammon, 1997). Assessment procedures (Hayden & Square, 1999; Hickman, 1997; Kaufman, 1995) and intervention approaches (Chumpelik, 1984; Kaufman, 1998; Velleman, 2003) have been developed specifically for individuals with DAS. Most of these therapy approaches focus on improving the control of range, rate, and timing of articulatory movements. Several authors have suggested methods to improve oral motor functioning in individuals with DS (see Alcock, 2006; Kumin, 2006; Rosin & Swift, 1999). Scharfenaker and colleagues (2002) describe methods to increase oral motor functioning and speech motor planning in individuals with FXS.

Cognitive and Language Skills

Consideration of strengths and weaknesses in the cognitive and language skills of individuals with DS and FXS can have important implications for speech assessment and intervention plans. For example, individuals with DS are reported to have impairments in attention, working memory, and executive functioning, as well as specific expressive language impairments, particularly in syntax (Chapman, Seung, Schwartz, & Kay-Raining Bird, 1998; Clark & Wilson, 2003; Laws & Bishop, 2003; Sigman & Ruskin, 1999). Males with FXS have been reported to have specific impairments in executive functioning, sequential processing, attention, and working memory (Cornish, Burack, & Rahman, 2005; Cornish, Sudhalter, & Turk, 2004; Dykens, Hodapp, & Leckman, 1989; Munir, Cornish, & Wilding, 2000). Females with FXS have weaknesses in executive functioning, attention, short-term auditory memory, and some visual-spatial tasks (Freund & Reiss, 1991; Mazzocco, Pennington, & Hagerman, 1993; Munir, Cornish, & Wilding, 2000). Knowledge of an individual's cognitive and linguistic profile can assist in tailoring intervention strategies to best meet the needs of each individual with DS and FXS.

Sensory Impairments, Anxiety/Arousal, and Autism

Among individuals with FXS, sensory impairments that may or may not co-occur with increased anxiety/hyperarousal should be considered in speech assessment and intervention. Further, for both individuals with DS and FXS, the presence of autism may potentially affect speech production and the need for specific behavior-management strategies. See Chapter 4 for a more thorough discussion of the implications of having autism for language assessment and intervention in individuals with FXS and DS. Sensory interventions vary greatly, focusing on optimizing arousal levels for learning, decreasing sensory defensiveness, managing the sensory environment, and teaching sensory social routines (such as singing and movement activities) during daily interactions (Hessl, Rivera, & Reiss, 2004; Rogers, 1998; Scharfenaker et al., 2002). Co-treatment using occupational and speech-language therapy, a sensory integration approach, and specific strategies such as calming using deep pressure, eating tactilely satisfying foods (e.g., celery), bouncing on an exercise ball, and minimizing visual and auditory distractions have been suggested for individuals with FXS (Scharfenaker et al., 2002). Although there are many case reports of the value of a sensory integration approach, there have been no systematic studies supporting its efficacy for individuals with FXS or other developmental disabilities (Dawson & Watling, 2000; Schaaf & Miller, 2005).

In addition to sensory issues, high levels of anxiety/hyperarousal and the presence of autism may necessitate specific assessment and intervention strategies, as well as behavior management strategies, when working with individuals with FXS. For example, a requirement for the individual with FXS to make eye contact or look at the clinician's face, both of which are anxiety-provoking in many individuals with FXS (Cohen et al., 1989), could be problematic. Depending on the needs and learning style of each individual, some children with FXS will benefit from a more structured approach for speech intervention (as described in the generalization section below), and others may benefit from a less structured, naturalistic therapy approach that may decrease anxiety/arousal and sensory defensiveness. Interestingly, Koegel, Camarata, Koegel, Ben-Tall, and Smith (1998) found that phonological intervention using a play-based naturalistic approach was more effective in increasing sound accuracy and speech intelligibility in four 3- to 7-year-old children with autism than a drill-based approach.

Assess Single Words and Continuous Speech

Assessment of speech in single words and in continuous speech should be completed to describe the sound pattern accuracy and speech intelligibility in individuals with DS and those with FXS. The assessment should follow the same procedures as used for any individual at risk for or having a speech-sound disorder, keeping in mind that speech intelligibility in continuous speech may be particularly affected. Speech in single words should be assessed using a standardized test and continuous speech assessed in a conversational and, if possible, narrative speech sample. The standardized test and speech sample should be analyzed for consonant and vowel inventories, syllable and word shape inventories, consonant and vowel errors, phonological process usage (e.g., substitutions, syllable structure, assimilation processes), and speech intelligibility (see Hodson, 2006a; Hodson, Scherz, & Strattman, 2002; Smit, 2004; and Williams, 2003, for more details). For individuals who are unintelligible, idiosyncratic phonological processes (patterns of sounds that typically developing children do not use, such as initial consonant deletion) as well as prosody (e.g., phrasing, fluency, rate, stress) and voice characteristics (e.g., resonance, loudness) should also be examined. The speech measures collected in single words and continuous speech should be compared to determine if there are context-dependent variations in speech production. It is also important to examine how specific speech contexts (e.g., narration, conversation, reading), environments (e.g., classroom, one-to-one therapy, home), and conversational partners (e.g., peers, teacher, parents) increase or decrease speech intelligibility. Determining contexts that increase or decrease speech intelligibility has important implications for speech intervention. Measurements of speech intelligibility are described in more detail in Chapter 9. The information collected on speech in single words and continuous speech and the factors contributing to speech difficulties will help determine if an individual has an articulation disorder (impairment in speech sound formation) or a phonological disorder (impairment in representation and organization of sounds) or both.

Provide Intervention to Improve Accuracy and Increase Intelligibility

Speech intervention should be individualized to improve the speech accuracy and speech intelligibility in individuals with DS and those with FXS. The focus should be on improving overall speech intelligibility and, ultimately, the effectiveness of communication. Because speech errors and phonological patterns in many individuals with DS and FXS are similar to those seen in younger typically developing children, speech intervention approaches that have been successful for treatment of individuals with phonological disorders who do not have developmental delays could be used. See Bauman-Waengler (2004), Bernthal and Bankson (2004), Hodson (2006b), and Smit (2004) to review these interventions. Kamhi (2006) reviewed five speech treatment approaches and noted that they all have varying degrees of research support: normative, bottom up, discrete skills, language based, broad based, and complexity based. Given the speech intelligibility difficulties in DS and FXS, cycles training (Hodson, 2006b; Hodson & Paden, 1991), designed for highly unintelligible individuals, may be particularly useful. Cycles training targets several sounds within a cycle, includes auditory bombardment, uses minimal pairs to train production, and cycles phonological targets. The cycles approach has been adapted for children with intellectual disability, for example, by working longer on each sound or error pattern. Of the other approaches, the complexity approach (Gierut, 2001, 2005), which targets more complex sounds than easier sounds and is very programmatic, has considerable research support and may be useful in increasing the phonetic repertoire of individuals with DS and FXS. See Chapter 9 for further discussion of methods to improve speech intelligibility in individuals with DS and FXS.

Promote Generalization of Speech

A lack of generalization of speech skills may occur in many individuals with DS and FXS. Therefore, it is important that intervention plans focus on generalization of speech skills. The lack of generalization to untrained word positions, words, and contexts is the biggest problem in speech intervention for individuals with developmental delays (Smit, 2004). A speech intervention program needs to plan for generalization, including the transfer of learning from a trained sound to other untrained word positions, untrained sounds, and untrained contexts. To facilitate generalization, speech intervention should include approaches that are systematic and structured, teach overlearned patterns, and provide multiple trials and exemplars. For individuals with DS and FXS who are unintelligible, it is important to select targets that are highly functional and important for an individual's functioning in daily interactions. For example, names of family members and pets, daily living needs, and vocabulary frequently used in the child's schedule and behavior-management system would be essential.

Use of augmentative and alternative communication systems, such as a visual schedule, choice board, or speech output device to present, model, and reinforce speech material should be very helpful. (See Chapter 11 for use of alternative and augmentative communication systems.) Materials from the environment, such as storybooks, textbooks, or interactive toys, can also be integrated into intervention. Targets that are successful at the word level should also be targeted in larger discourse units of conversation and narration. As individuals learn particular speech targets, it is important to create opportunities to practice speech in contexts that will facilitate generalization. Practice that occurs in a natural environment, such as the classroom or at home, and with many communication partners, such as teachers, parents, and classmates, should help promote generalization. See Bauman-Waengler (2004), Smit (2004), and Williams (2003) for suggestions for speech intervention strategies when working with individuals with intellectual disability. See Kamhi (2006) for a discussion of how selection of speech intervention methods should be based on treatment efficacy and how research, a clinician's theoretical perspective, and the service delivery model affect intervention treatment decisions.

Consider Specific Speech Interventions Designed for Individuals with Down Syndrome

A few intervention studies have been conducted with the goal of improving the speech skills of individuals with DS. These studies vary greatly in their focus. To encourage the emergence of words in the transition from babble to speech, caregivers should consider the use of phonetically contingent responses to nonmeaningful vocalizations (Stoel-Gammon, 2001). In this approach, caregivers would repeat the babble [ma] and highlight its link to the phonetically similar word "mama," thus increasing the likelihood of [ma] being used as a meaningful utterance. In addition, sound games may be useful to foster an awareness of speech sounds and of sound–meaning relationships and to increase the repertoire of speech sounds and syllable shapes (Kumin, 1994a, 1999).

Most intervention programs for individuals with DS have focused on increasing the phonetic repertoire and reducing the number of errors in single-word productions, using therapy techniques similar to those for children with phonological delays or disorders. Cholmain (1994) described a therapy program for young children with DS (chronological age 4–5.5 years, language ages 1.3–2.8 years) with unintelligible speech. Key elements of the program included listening and production practice focused on particular phonemes and phonological processes, with therapy occurring in the clinic and at home. Although children were at a young language age, they showed change in their phonological systems within the first 2 weeks of therapy initiation, despite minimal change in the previous 3–12 months. Their consonant accuracy increased from 3%–38% pretherapy to 19%–88% 6–14 weeks posttherapy.

Another approach to therapy has focused on the variability of word productions in children with DS (Dodd & Leahy, 1989; Dodd, McCormack, & Woodyatt, 1994). This approach differed from traditional intervention programs in two ways: The unit of treatment was whole words rather than phonemes or phonological processes, and parents provided therapy. Parents were instructed to accept only one pronunciation for a set of words individually selected for their preschool children. Acceptable pronunciations did not necessarily need to be correct. Results indicated that, over the 13-week program, the four children in the study showed exceptional improvement in the number of consonants produced correctly. Moreover, the mean proportion of deviant errors decreased from around 70% to 41% during this period.

The use of electropalatography (EPG) to assess, diagnose, and treat speech disorders in individuals with DS has also been described. EPG requires a speaker to wear an artificial palate under the hard palate in the mouth, which records when and where the tongue hits the hard palate during speech (Gibbon, Stewart, Hardcastle, & Crampin, 1999). Gibbon, McNeill, Wood, and Watson (2003) used EPG to reduce velar fronting of the /k/ sound and make alveolar-velar distinctions for the /k/ and /t/ sounds in a 10-year-old girl with DS. During a 14-week training program, therapy included weekly clinic sessions and a home-based program. Researchers took EPG recordings at the beginning, middle, and end of the program. At the end of training, the young girl demonstrated a substantial improvement in production of the /k/ sound.

The most controversial intervention designed to increase speech accuracy in individuals with DS is surgery for tongue reduction. Parsons, Iacono, and Rozner (1987) reported the results of a study in which 18 children with DS underwent tongue-reduction surgery as a means of increasing articulatory proficiency. The children's articulatory skills were assessed pre- and postoperatively and at a 6-month follow-up visit. No significant differences in the number of articulation errors were found. In addition, the articulation scores of the children undergoing the surgery were not significantly different than the scores of a nonsurgery group of children with DS. In spite of the lack of change in articulatory skills, parents of the children in the surgery group claimed that their children's speech had improved in the 6-month period after surgery.

Summary

A few intervention programs have been conducted with individuals with DS. These programs are diverse in their focus and include a small number of study participants. No published speech intervention studies on individuals with FXS exist. The assessment and intervention guidelines presented in this section are based on the speech literature for either other special populations or typically developing individuals with speech disorders and the phenotypic characteristics of individuals with DS and FXS. Speech intervention for individuals with DS and FXS should focus on improving overall speech intelligibility, considering the role of factors affecting speech development, and planning for generalization of speech. The speech difficulties during the preschool years highlight the need for early intervention, whereas the impact of poor speech intelligibility on communication effectiveness and social functioning (Gierut, 1998; Kent, Miolo, & Bloedel, 1994) and the continued difficulties with speech into adolescence and adulthood emphasize the importance of speech intervention. Well-controlled intervention studies examining the efficacy of interventions to increase speech accuracy and overall speech intelligibility for individuals with DS and for individuals with FXS are needed. Specifically, studies are needed to determine what speech methods cause the most gains in speech accuracy and speech intelligibility and generalize to untreated contexts.

PARENT INVOLVEMENT

Parents can have an important role in the assessment and intervention of speech for individuals with DS and those with FXS. The suggestions for parental involvement in this section are based on the literature and best practice on typically developing children and children with developmental delays. (In this section, we use the term *parents* to refer also to other caregivers.)

First, parents can be interviewed to gain information about whether there are specific contexts or conversational partners for which their children's speech is more or less intelligible. For example, a child may be more intelligible when talking about a topic of his or her choice, speaking in short utterances, talking with a family member, or during a frequent routine (e.g., requesting juice) versus when narrating what happened in school, speaking in longer utterances, talking to an unfamiliar adult, or talking about something about which he or she is excited.

Second, parents can identify words, phrases, and sentences, as well as routines and contexts, in which increased speech intelligibility would increase their children's communication effectiveness during daily activities. Parents can also identify contexts that seem to increase anxiety and arousal and potentially affect speech production.

Third, parents should use strategies to facilitate language development, such as talking often to their children, modeling speech patterns, and repeating and expanding on what their children say (Girolametto & Weitzman, 2006; Pepper & Weitzman, 2004; Snow, Burns, & Griffin, 1998).

Fourth, parents can capitalize on activities in their children's daily environments to reinforce speech patterns. For example, at the supermarket, a child can find fruits that begin with a particular sound, such as /p/. The parent can purposely mislabel the peach and say "Thanks for the carrot" as the child puts the peach in the shopping cart to encourage the child to say "peach."

Fifth, when the speech of individuals with DS or FXS is unintelligible, it is important to examine the strategies parents use to try to understand their children. Although it is not clear which strategies are most effective, the parent can use a variety of strategies in response to a request such as *want* as the individual points to a drink in the refrigerator. Strategies include requesting a clarification ("Did you want the juice or milk?"), giving a confirmation ("You want the juice?"), repeating the utterance ("Want?"), acknowledging the request ("Yes, you want the juice"), giving a cue ("Something to drink?"), or expanding on what was said in attempting to resolve what was meant ("You want apple juice?"). See Yont, Hewitt, and Miccio (2000) and Brinton, Fujiki, Loeb, and Winkler (1986) for further discussion of these strategies.

Sixth, repeated reading of storybooks and using texts that focus on specific sounds as part of the story (as described in Hoffman & Norris, 2005) may be useful. See Williams (2003), Hoffman and Norris (2005), and Smit (2004) for other suggestions for parent involvement in speech development.

Further research is needed to determine the most effective methods for involving parents in facilitating speech development of individuals with DS and FXS.

FUTURE DIRECTIONS

There is continued need for research in several areas examining the speech skills of individuals with DS and FXS. First, research is needed to further determine speech patterns that are specific to DS or FXS. Both individuals with DS and males with FXS often have unintelligible speech, yet it appears that specific phonology and other aspects of speech, as well as the underlying mechanism explaining speech difficulties, may differ in these two populations. Comparisons of individuals with DS with individuals with FXS help to discern whether the speech patterns observed in DS or FXS are due to the syndrome in particular rather than to the general effects of intellectual disability. The speech of both populations should also be compared with that of other groups of individuals with intellectual disability to further the understanding of how the specific phenotype and intellectual disability in general are affecting speech patterns in these syndromes.

Second, research is needed to explain individual differences in speech patterns in children with DS and those with FXS. For example, some individuals with DS or FXS are very intelligible and others are hard to understand. The possible mechanisms that may explain speech difficulties in these both similar and different populations need further study. If the predictors of particular speech impairments in individuals with DS and those with FXS can be identified, then it can be determined who is at greatest risk for speech difficulties and where to focus intervention strategies.

Third, studies of the speech development in females with FXS are markedly lacking. Studies examining the speech phenotype in females with FXS, focusing on both speech accuracy and speech intelligibility, are needed, as well as studies that compare males and females with FXS to understand the role of gender in FXS.

Fourth, few studies of individuals with DS and no studies of individuals with FXS were longitudinal in design, following speech development over time. Future studies should use longitudinal study designs to analyze speech development in the same group of individuals at different ages from childhood through adulthood, particularly during periods in which changes in speech patterns may occur. Determining the rate of growth in speech skills, as well as whether there is continued growth in speech development or a plateau at a certain age, would have important implications for the timing of speech intervention.

Finally, rigorous intervention studies examining the efficacy of interventions to increase speech accuracy and overall speech intelligibility for individuals with DS and FXS are needed. Specifically, studies are needed to determine what speech methods cause the most gains in speech accuracy and speech intelligibility and generalize to untreated contexts.

REFERENCES

Abbeduto, L., & Hagerman, R. (1997). Language and communication in FXS. *Mental Retardation and Developmental Disabilities Research Reviews, 3,* 313–322.

Alcock, K. (2006). The development of oral motor control and language. *Down Syndrome: Research & Practice, 11*(1), 1–8.

American Academy of Pediatrics. (2004). Clinical practice guideline: Otitis media with effusion. *Pediatrics, 113,* 1412–1429.

American Speech-Language-Hearing Association. (2002). Guidelines for fitting and monitoring FM systems. *ASHA Desk Reference.*

American Speech-Language-Hearing Association Audiologic Assessment Panel. (1996). *Guidelines for audiologic screening.* Rockville, MD: 339–341.

Baranek, G.T., Chin, Y.K.H., Hess, L.M.G., Yankee, J.G., Hatton, D.D., & Hooper, S. (2002). Sensory processing correlates of occupational performance in children with fragile X syndrome: Preliminary findings. *American Journal of Occupational Therapy 56*(5), 538–546.

Barnes, E.F., Roberts, J.E., Mirrett, P., Sideris, J., & Misenheimer, J. (2006). A comparison of oral structure and oral motor function in young males with fragile X syndrome and Down syndrome. *Journal of Speech, Language, and Hearing Research, 49*(4), 903–917.

Bauman-Waengler, J. (2004). *Articulatory and phonological impairments.* Washington, DC: American Psychological Association.

Belser, R.C., & Sudhalter, V. (2001). Conversational characteristics of children with fragile X syndrome: Repetitive speech. *American Journal on Mental Retardation, 106*(1), 28–38.

Bennetto, L., & Pennington, B.F. (2002). The neuropsychology of fragile X syndrome. In R.J. Hagerman & A.C. Cronister (Eds.), *Fragile X syndrome: Diagnosis, treatment, and research* (2nd ed., pp. 210–248). Baltimore: The Johns Hopkins University Press.

Bernthal, J.E., & Bankson, N.W. (2004). *Articulation and phonological disorders* (5th ed.). Boston: Allyn & Bacon.

Bleile, K., & Schwarz, I. (1984). Three perspectives on the speech of children with Down syndrome. *Journal of Communication Disorders, 17,* 87–94.

Borghgraef, M., Fryns, J.P., Dielkens, A., Pyck, K., & Van den Bergh, H. (1987). Fragile X syndrome: A study of the psychological profile in 23 prepubertal patients. *Clinical Genetics, 2,* 179–186.

Brady, N., Skinner, D., Roberts, J., & Hennon, E. (2006). Communication in young children with fragile X syndrome: A qualitative study of mothers' perspectives. *American Journal of Speech Language Pathology, 15,* 353–364.

Brinton, B., Fujiki, M., Loeb, D.F., & Winkler, E. (1986). Development of conversational repair strategies in response to requests for clarification. *Journal of Speech and Hearing Research, 2,* 75–81.

Buckley, S. (2000, September). Teaching reading to develop speech and language. Paper presented at the 3rd International Conference on Language and Cognition in Down Syndrome, Portsmouth, England.

Chapman, R.S., Seung, H.-K., & Schwartz, S.E. (2000). Predicting language production in children and adolescents with Down syndrome: The role of comprehension. *Journal of Speech, Language, and Hearing Research, 43*(2), 340–350.

Chapman, R.S., Seung, H.-K., Schwartz, S.E., & Kay-Raining Bird, E. (1998). Language skills of children and adolescents with Down syndrome: II. Production deficits. *Journal of Speech, Language, Hearing Research, 41,* 861–873.

Cholmain, C.N. (1994). Working on phonology with young children with Down syndrome. *Journal of Clinical Speech and Language Studies, 1,* 14–35.

Chumpelik, D. (1984). The prompt system of therapy: Theoretical framework and applications for developmental apraxia of speech. *Seminars in Speech and Language, 5,* 199–215.

Clark, D., & Wilson, G.N. (2003). Behavioral assessment of children with Down syndrome using the Reiss Psychopathology Scale. *American Journal of Medical Genetics Part A, 118A,*(3), 210–216.

Cohen, I.L. (1995). A theoretical analysis of the role of hyperarousal in the learning and behavior of fragile X males. *Mental Retardation and Developmental Disabilities Research Reviews, 1,* 286–291.

Cohen, I.L., Vietze, I.L., Sudhalter, P.M., Jenkins, V., Jenkins, E.C., & Brown, W.T. (1989). Parent–child dyadic gaze patterns in fragile X males and in non-fragile X males with autistic disorder. *Journal of Child Psychology and Psychiatry, 30*(6), 845–856.

Cornish, K., Burack, J.A., & Rahman, A. (2005). Theory of mind deficits in children with fragile X syndrome. *Journal of Intellectual Disability Research, 49*(5), 372–378.

Cornish, K., Sudhalter, V., & Turk, J. (2004). Attention and language in fragile X. *Mental Retardation and Developmental Disabilities Research Reviews, 10*(1), 11–16.

Dawson, G., & Watling, R. (2000). Interventions to facilitate auditory, visual, and motor integration in autism: A review of the evidence. *Journal of Autism and Developmental Disorders, 30*(5), 415–421.

Dodd, B.J. (1972). Comparison of babbling patterns in normal and Down-syndrome infants. *Journal of Mental Deficiency Research, 16,* 35–40.

Dodd, B.J. (1976). A comparison of the phonological systems of mental age matched normal, severely abnormal and Down's syndrome children. *British Journal of Disorders of Communication, 11,* 27–42.

Dodd, B.J., & Leahy, P. (1989). Phonological disorders and mental handicap. In M. Beveridge, G. Conti-Ramsden, & I. Leudar (Eds.), *Language and Communication in Mentally Handicapped People* (pp. 33–56). London: Chapman and Hall.

Dodd, B.J., McCormack, P., & Woodyatt, G. (1994). Evaluation of an intervention program: Relation between children's phonology and parents' communicative behavior. *American Journal on Mental Retardation, 98*(5), 632–645.

Dodd, B.J., & Thompson, L. (2001). Speech disorder in children with Down's syndrome. *Journal of Intellectual Disabilities Research, 45,* 308–316.

Downs, M.P. (1980). The hearing of Down's individuals. *Seminars in Speech, Language, and Hearing, 1,* 25–38.

Dykens, E.M., Hodapp, R.M., & Leckman, J.F. (1989). Adaptive and maladaptive functioning of institutionalized and noninstitutionalized fragile X males. *Journal of the American Academy of Child & Adolescent Psychiatry, 28*(3), 427–430.

Farmer, A., & Brayton, E.R. (1979). Speech characteristics of fluent and dysfluent Down's syndrome adults. *Folia Phoniat, 31,* 284–290.

Freund, L.S., & Reiss, A.L. (1991). Rating problem behaviors in outpatients with mental retardation: Use of the Aberrant Behavior Checklist. *Research in Developmental Disabilities, 12*(4), 435–451.

Gibbon, F.E., McNeill, A.M., Wood, S.E. & Watson, J.M. (2003). Changes in linguapalatal contact patterns during therapy for velar fronting in a 10-year-old with Down's syndrome. *International Journal of Language & Communication Disorders, 38*(1), 47–64.

Gibbon, F., Stewart, F., Hardcastle, W.J, & Crampin, L. (1999). Widening access to electropalatography for children with persistent sound system disorders. *American Journal of Speech-Language Pathology, 8,* 319–334.

Gierut, J.A. (1998). The conditions and course of clinically induced phonological change. *Journal of Speech and Hearing Research, 35,* 1049–1063.

Gierut, J.A. (2001). Complexity in phonological treatment: Clinical factors. *Language, Speech, and Hearing in Schools, 32*(4), 220–241.

Gierut, J.A. (2005). Phonological intervention: The how or the what? In S.F. Warren & M.E. Fey (Series Eds.) & A.G. Kamhi & K.E. Pollock (Vol. Eds.), *Communication and language intervention series. Phonological disorders in children: Clinical decision making in assessment and intervention* (pp. 201–210). Baltimore: Paul H. Brookes Publishing Co.

Girolametto, L., & Weitzman, E. (2006). It Takes Two to Talk: The Hanen Program for Parents. Early intervention through caregiver training. In S.F. Warren & M.E. Fey (Series Eds.) & R.J. McCauley & M.E. Fey (Vol. Eds.), *Communication and language intervention Series: Treatment of language disorders in children* (pp. 77–103). Baltimore: Paul H. Brookes Publishing Co.

Hagerman, R.J. (1991). The physical and behavioral phenotype. In R.J. Hagerman & A.C. Silverman (Eds.), *Fragile X syndrome: Diagnosis, treatment, and research* (pp. 3–68). Baltimore: The Johns Hopkins University Press.

Hagerman, R.J. (1995). Molecular and clinical correlations in fragile X syndrome. *Mental Retardation and Developmental Disabilities Research Reviews, 1,* 276–280.

Hagerman, R.J., Altshul-Stark, D., & McBogg, P. (1987). Recurrent otitis media in boys with the fragile X syndrome. *American Journal of Diseases of Children 141,* 184–187.

Hanson, D.M., Jackson, A.W., & Hagerman, R.J. (1986). Speech disturbances (cluttering) in mildly impaired males with the Martin-Bell/fragile X syndrome. *American Journal of Medical Genetics, 23,* 195–206.

Hayden, D., & Square, P. (1999). *Verbal Motor Assessment for Children.* San Antonio, TX: Harcourt Assessment.

Hessl, D., Dyer-Friedman, J., Glaser, B., Wisbek, J., Barajas, R.G., Taylor, A., et al. (2001). The influence of environmental and genetic factors on behavior problems and autistic symptoms in boys and girls with fragile X syndrome. *Pediatrics, 108*(5), 88–104.

Hessl, D., Glaser, B., Dyer-Friedman, J., & Reiss, A.L. (2006). Social behavior and cortisol reactivity in children with fragile X syndrome. *Journal of Child Psychology and Psychiatry, 47*(6), 602–610.

Hessl, D., Rivera, S.M., & Reiss, A.L. (2004). The neuroanatomy and neuroendocrinology of fragile X syndrome. *Mental Retardation and Developmental Disabilities Research Reviews, 10,* 17–24.

Hickman, L. (1997). *The Apraxia Profile.* San Antonio, TX: Psychological Corporation.

Hodson, B.W. (2006a). Overview of the diagnostic evaluation process for children with highly unintelligible speech. In B.W. Hodson (Ed.), *Evaluating and enhancing children's phonological systems* (pp. 45–64). Greenville, SC: Thinking Publications.

Hodson, B.W. (2006b). Enhancing children's phonological systems: The cycles remediation approach. In B.W. Hodson (Ed.), *Evaluating and enhancing children's phonological systems* (pp. 87–114). Greenville, SC: Thinking Publications.

Hodson, B.W., & Paden, E.P. (1991). *Targeting intelligible speech: A phonological approach to remediation* (2nd ed.). Austin, TX: PRO-ED.

Hodson, B.W., Scherz, J.A., & Strattman, K.H. (2002). Evaluating communicative abilities of a highly unintelligible preschooler. *American Journal of Speech Language Pathology, 11*(3), 236–242.

Hoffman, P.R., & Norris, J.A. (2005). Intervention: Manipulating complex input to promote self-organization of a neuron-network. In S.F. Warren & M.E. Fey (Series Eds.) & A.G. Kamhi & K.E. Pollock (Vol. Eds.), *Communication and language intervention Series: Phonological disorders in children. Clinical decision making in assessment and intervention* (pp. 139–155). Baltimore: Paul H. Brookes Publishing Co.

Kamhi, A.G. (2006). Treatment decisions for children with speech-sound disorders. *Language, Speech, and Hearing Services in Schools, 37,* 271–279.

Kaufman, N. (1995). *Kaufman Speech Praxis Test for Children.* Detroit, MI: Wayne State University Press.

Kaufman, N. (1998). *Kaufman Speech Praxis Treatment Kit.* Gaylord, MI: Northern Speech Services.

Kent, R.D. (1992). The biology of phonological development. In C.A. Ferguson, L. Menn, & C. Stoel-Gammon (Eds.), *Phonological development: Models, research, implications* (pp. 65–90). Parkton, MD: York Press.

Kent, R.D., & Forner, L.L. (1980). Speech segment durations in sentence recitations by children and adults. *Journal of Phonetics, 8,* 157–168.

Kent, R.D., & Miolo, G. (1995). Phonetic abilities in the first year of life. In P. Fletcher & B. MacWhinney (Eds.), *The handbook of child language* (pp. 303–324). Oxford, England: Blackwell Publishing.

Kent, R.D., Miolo, G., & Bloedel, S. (1994). The intelligibility of children's speech: A review of evaluation procedures. *American Journal of Speech Language Pathology, 3,* 81–95.

Koegel, R.L., Camarata, S., Koegel, L.K., Ben-Tall, A., & Smith, A.E. (1998). Increasing speech intelligibility in children with autism. *Journal of Autism and Developmental Disorders, 28*(3), 241–251.

Kumin, L. (1994a). *Communication skills in children with Down syndrome: A guide for parents.* Bethesda, MD: Woodbine House.

Kumin, L. (1994b). Intelligibility of speech in children with Down syndrome in natural settings: Parents' perspective. *Perceptual and Motor Skills, 78,* 307–313.

Kumin, L. (1996). Speech and language skills in children with Down syndrome. *Mental Retardation and Developmental Disabilities Research Reviews, 2,* 109–115.

Kumin, L. (1999). Comprehensive speech and language treatment for infants, toddlers, and children with Down syndrome. In T.J. Hassold & D. Patterson (Eds.), *Down syndrome: A promising future together* (pp. 145–153). New York: Wiley-Liss.

Kumin, L. (2006). Speech intelligibility and childhood verbal apraxia in children with Down syndrome. *Down Syndrome, Research and Practice, 10,* 10–22.

Kumin, L., Councill, C., & Goodman, M. (1994). A longitudinal study of the emergence of phonemes in children with Down syndrome. *Journal of Communication Disorders, 27,* 265–275.

Laws, G., & Bishop, D.V. (2003). A comparison of language abilities in adolescents with Down syndrome and children with specific language impairment. *Journal of Speech, Language, and Hearing Research, 46,* 1324–1339.

Leddy, M. (1999). The biological bases of speech in people with Down syndrome. In J.F. Miller, M. Leddy, & L.A. Leavitt (Eds.), *Improving the communication of people with Down syndrome* (pp. 61–80). Baltimore: Paul H. Brookes Publishing Co.

Locke, J.L. (1983). *Phonological acquisition and change.* New York: Academic Press.

Lynch, M.P., Oller, D.K., Steffens, M.L., Levine, S.L., Basinger, D.L., & Umbel, V.M. (1995). Development of speech-like vocalizations in infants with Down syndrome. *American Journal of Mental Retardation, 100,* 68–86.

Mackay, L., & Hodson, B. (1982). Phonological process identification of misarticulations of mentally retarded children. *Journal of Communication Disorders, 15,* 243–250.

Madison, L.S., George, C., & Moeschler, J.B. (1986). Cognitive functioning in the fragile-X syndrome: A study of intellectual, memory, and communication skills. *Journal of Mental Deficiency Research, 30,* 129–148.

Mazzocco, M.M., Pennington, B.F., & Hagerman, R.J. (1993). The neurocognitive phenotype of female carriers of fragile X: Additional evidence for specificity. *Journal of Developmental Behavioral Pediatrics, 14,* 328–335.

Miller, J.F., & Leddy, M. (1998) Down syndrome: The impact of speech production on language development. In S.F. Warren & J. Reichle (Series Eds.) & R. Paul (Vol. Ed.), *Communication and language intervention series: Vol. 8. Exploring the speech–language connection* (pp. 163–177). Baltimore: Paul H. Brookes Publishing Co.

Miller, J.F., Miolo, G., Sedey, A., Pierce, K., & Rosin, M. (1989). Predicting lexical growth in children with Down syndrome. Poster presented at the annual meeting of the American Speech–Language-Hearing Association, St. Louis, MO.

Miller, L.J., Reisman, J., McIntosh, D.N., & Simon, J. (2001). The ecological model of sensory modulation: Performance of children with fragile X syndrome, autism, ADHD, and SMD. In S. Roley, R. Schaaf, & E. Blanche (Eds.), *Sensory integration and developmental disabilities* (pp. 57–87). San Antonio, TX: Therapy Skill Builders.

Munir, F., Cornish, K.M., & Wilding, J. (2000). Nature of the working memory deficit in fragile-X syndrome. *Brain and Cognition, 44,* 387–401.

Newell, K., Sanborn, B., & Hagerman, R. (1983). Speech and language dysfunction in the fragile X syndrome. In R.J. Hagerman & P.M. McBogg (Eds.), *The fragile X syndrome: Diagnosis, biochemistry, and intervention* (pp. 175–100). Dillon, CO: Spectra.

Oller, D.K., Eilers, R.E., Bull, D.H., & Carney, A.E. (1985). Prespeech vocalizations of a deaf infant: A comparison with normal metaphonological development. *Journal of Speech and Hearing Research, 28,* 47–63.

Oller, D.K., & Seibert, J.M. (1988). Babbling of prelinguistic mentally retarded children. *American Journal on Mental Retardation, 92,* 369–375.

Palmer, K.K., Gordon, J.S., Coston, G.N., & Stevenson, R. (1988). Fragile X syndrome: IV. Speech and language characteristics. *Proceedings of the Greenwood Genetic Center, 7,* 93–97.

Parsons, C.L., Iacono, T.A., & Rozner, L. (1987). Effect of tongue reduction on articulation in children with Down syndrome. *American Journal of Mental Deficiency, 91,* 328–332.

Paul, R., Cohen, D.J., Breg, W.R., Watson, M., & Herman, S. (1984). FXS: Its relation to speech and language disorders. *Journal of Speech and Hearing Disorders, 49,* 326–336.

Paul, R., Dykens, E., Leckman, J.F., Watson, M., Breg, W.R., & Cohen, D.J. (1987). A comparison of language characteristics of mentally retarded adults with fragile X syndrome and those with nonspecific mental retardation and autism. *Journal of Autism and Developmental Disorders, 17,* 457–468.

Peña-Brooks, A., & Hegde, M.N. (2000). *Articulation and phonological disorders in children.* Austin, TX: PRO-ED.

Pepper, J., & Weitzman, E. (2004). *It takes two to talk: A practical guide for parents of children with language delays* (2nd ed.). Toronto, Ontario: The Hanen Centre.

Preus A. (1973). Stuttering in Down's syndrome. In Y. Lebrun & R. Hoops (Eds.), *Neurolinguistic approaches to stuttering* (pp. 90–100). The Hague, Netherlands: Mouton.

Prouty, L.A., Rogers, R.C., Stevenson, R.E., Dean, J.H., Palmer, K.K., Simensen, R.J., et al. (1988). Fragile X syndrome: Growth, development, and intellectual function. *American Journal of Medical Genetics, 30,* 123–142.

Pueschel, S., & Hopmann, M. (1993). Speech and language abilities of children with Down syndrome: A parent's perspective. In S.F Warren & J. Reichle (Series Eds.) & A.P. Kaiser & D.B. Gray (Vol. Eds.), *Communication and language intervention series: Vol. 2. Enhancing children's communication: Research foundations for intervention* (pp. 335–362). Baltimore: Paul H. Brookes Publishing Co.

Reiss, A.L., & Freund, L. (1992). Behavioral phenotype of fragile X syndrome: DSM-III-R autistic behavior in male children. *American Journal of Medical Genetics, 43,* 35–46.

Rhoads, F. (1984). Fragile X syndrome in Hawaii: A summary of clinical experience. *American Journal of Medical Genetics, 17,* 209–214.

Robbins, J., & Klee, T. (1987). Clinical assessment of oropharyngeal motor development in young children. *Journal of Speech and Hearing Disorders, 52,* 271–277.

Roberts, J.E., Boccia, M.L., Bailey, D.B., Jr., Hatton, D.D., & Skinner, M. (2001). Cardiovascular indicators of arousal in boys with fragile X syndrome. *Developmental Psychobiology, 39,* 107–123.

Roberts, J.E., Hatton, D.D., & Bailey, D.B. (2001). Development and behavior of male toddlers with fragile X syndrome. *Journal of Early Intervention, 24*(3), 207–223.

Roberts, J.E., Hunter, L., Gravel, J., Rosenfeld, R., Berman, S., Haggard, M., et al. (2004). Otitis media, hearing loss, and language learning: Controversies and current research. *Developmental and Behavioral Pediatrics, 25*(2), 1–13.

Roberts, J.E., Long, S.H., Malkin, C., Barnes, E., Skinner, M., Hennon, E.A., et al. (2005). A comparison of phonological skills of young boys with fragile X syndrome and Down syndrome. *Journal of Speech, Language, and Hearing Research, 48*(5), 980–995.

Roberts, J.E., Rosenfeld, R.M., & Zeisel, S.A. (2004). Otitis media and speech and language: A meta-analysis of prospective studies. *Pediatrics, 113*(3), 237–247.

Rogers, S.J. (1998). Empirically supported comprehensive treatments for young children with autism. *Journal of Clinical Child Psychology, 27*(2), 138–145.

Rogers, S.J., Hepburn, S., & Wehner, E. (2003). Parent reports of sensory symptoms in toddlers with autism and those with other developmental disorders. *Journal of Autism and Developmental Disorders, 33,* 631–642.

Roizen, N.J. (2002). Down syndrome. In M.L. Batshaw (Ed.), *Children with disabilities* (5th ed.). Baltimore: Paul H. Brookes Publishing Co.

Rosin, M., & Swift, E. (1999). Communication interventions: Improving the speech intelligibility of children with Down syndrome. In J.F. Miller, M. Leddy, & L.A. Leavitt (Eds.), *Improving the communication of people with Down syndrome* (133–154). Baltimore: Paul H. Brookes Publishing Co.

Rosin, M.M., Swift, E., Bless, D., & Vetter, D.K. (1988). Communication profiles of adolescents with Down syndrome. *Journal of Childhood Communication Disorders, 12*(1), 49–64.

Schaaf, R.C., & Miller, L.J. (2005). Occupational therapy using a sensory integrative approach for children with developmental disabilities. *Mental Retardation and Developmental Disabilities, 11*(2), 143–148.

Scharfenaker, S., O'Connor, R., Stackhouse, T., Braden, M.L., & Gray, K. (2002) An integrated approach to intervention. In R.J. Hagerman & P.J. Hagerman (Eds.), *Fragile X syndrome: Diagnosis, treatment, and research* (3rd ed., pp. 363–427). The Johns Hopkins University Press.

Shott, S.R., Joseph, A., & Heithaus, D. (2001). Hearing loss in children with Down syndrome. *International Journal of Pediatric Otorhinolaryngology, 61,* 199–205.

Shriberg, L., & Widder, C.J. (1990). Speech and prosody characteristics of adults with mental retardation. *Journal of Speech and Hearing Research, 33,* 627–653.

Sigman, M., & Ruskin, E. (1999). Continuity and change in the social competence of children with autism, Down syndrome, and developmental delays. *Monographs of the Society for Research in Child Development, 64*(1), v–114.

Smit, A.B. (2004). *Articulation and phonology resource guide for school-age children and adults.* Clifton Park, NY: Delmar Learning.

Smith, B.L., Kenney, M.K., & Hussain, S. (1996). A longitudinal study of duration and temporal variability in children's speech production. *Journal of the Acoustical Society of America, 99,* 2344–2349.

Smith, B.L., & Oller, D.K. (1981). A comparative study of pre-meaningful vocalizations produced by normally developing and Down's syndrome infants. *Journal of Speech and Hearing Disorders, 46,* 46–51.

Smith, B.L., & Stoel-Gammon, C. (1983). A longitudinal study of the development of stop consonant production in normal and Down's syndrome children. *Journal of Speech and Hearing Disorders, 48,* 114–118.

Smith, B.L., & Stoel-Gammon, C. (1996). A quantitative analysis of the reduplicated and variegated babbling in vocalizations by Down syndrome infants. *Clinical Linguistics and Phonetics, 10,* 119–130.

Snow, C.E., Burns, M.S., & Griffin, P. (1998). *Preventing reading difficulties in young children.* Washington, DC: National Academies Press, Committee on the Prevention of Reading Difficulties in Young Children, National Research Council.

Sommers, R.K., Patterson, J.P. & Wildgen, P.L. (1988). Phonology of Down syndrome speakers, ages 13–22. *Journal of Childhood Communication Disorders, 12*(1), 65–91.

Sommers, R.K., Reinhart, R.W., & Sistrunk, D.A. (1988). Traditional articulation measures of Down syndrome speakers, ages 13–22. *Journal of Childhood Communication Disorders, 12*(1), 93–108.

Spinelli, M., de Oliveira Rocha, A.C., Giacheti, C.M., & Richieri-Costa, A. (1995). Word-finding difficulties, verbal paraphasias, and verbal dyspraxia in ten individuals with fragile X syndrome. *American Journal of Medical Genetics, 60,* 39–43.

Steffens, M.L., Oller, D.K., Lynch, M., & Urbano, R.C. (1992). Vocal development in infants with Down syndrome and infants who are developing normally. *American Journal of Mental Retardation, 97,* 235–246.

Stoel-Gammon, C. (1980). Phonological analysis of four Down's syndrome children. *Applied Psycholinguistics, 1,* 31–48.

Stoel-Gammon, C. (1981). Speech development of infants and children with Down's syndrome. In J.K. Darby (Ed.), *Speech evaluation in medicine* (pp. 341–360). New York: Grune and Stratton, Inc.

Stoel-Gammon, C. (1992). Prelinguistic vocal development: Measurement and predictions. In C. A. Ferguson, L. Menn, & C. Stoel-Gammon (Eds.), *Phonological development: Models, research, implications* (pp. 439–456). Timonium, MD: York Press.

Stoel-Gammon, C. (1997). Phonological development in Down syndrome. *Mental Retardation and Developmental Disabilities Research Reviews, 3,* 300–306.

Stoel-Gammon, C. (1998a). The role of babbling and phonology in early linguistic development. In S.F. Warren & J. Reichle (Series Eds.) & A.M. Wetherby, S.F. Warren, & J. Reichle (Vol. Eds.), *Communication and language intervention series: Transitions in prelinguistic communication: Preintentional to intentional and presymbolic to symbolic* (pp. 87–110). Baltimore: Paul H. Brookes Publishing Co.

Stoel-Gammon, C. (1998b). Sounds and words in early language acquisition: The relationship between lexical and phonological development. In S.F. Warren & J. Reichle (Series Eds.) & R. Paul (Vol. Eds.), *Communication and language intervention series: Exploring the speech–language connection* (pp. 25–53). Baltimore: Paul H. Brookes Publishing Co.

Stoel-Gammon, C. (2001). Down syndrome phonology: Developmental patterns and intervention strategies. *Down Syndrome Research and Practice, 7*(3), 93–100.

Stray-Gunderson, K. (1986). *Babies with Down syndrome: A new parents guide.* Rockville, MD: Woodbine House.

Van Borsel, J. (1996). Articulation in Down's syndrome adolescents and adults. *European Journal of Disorders of Communication, 31,* 415–444.

Velleman, S. (2003). *Childhood apraxia of speech resource guide.* Clifton Park, NY: Thompson Delmar Learning.

Vihman, M.M. (1996). *Phonological development: The origins of language in the child.* Cambridge, MA: Blackwell Publishing.

Vihman, M.M. (2005). Early phonological development. In J.E. Bernthal & N.W. Bankson (Eds.), *Articulation and phonological disorders* (5th ed., pp. 63–104). Boston: Allyn & Bacon.

Vilkman, E., Niemi, J., & Ikonen, U. (1988). Fragile X speech phonology in Finnish. *Brain and Language, 34,* 203–221.

Willcox, A. (1988). An investigation into non-fluency in Down's syndrome. *British Journal of Disorders of Communication, 23,* 153–170.

Yont, K.M., Hewitt, L.E., & Miccio, A.W. (2000). A coding system for describing conversational breakdowns in preschool children. *American Journal of Speech-Language Pathology, 9*(4), 300–309.

Zajac, D.J., Roberts, J.E., Harris, A.A., Hennon, E.A., & Barnes, E.F. (2006). Articulation rate and vowel space characteristics of young males with fragile X syndrome: Preliminary acoustic findings. *Journal of Speech, Language, & Hearing Research, 49,* 1147–1155.

Interventions for Individuals with Down Syndrome and Fragile X Syndrome

Prelinguistic and Early Language Interventions for Children with Down Syndrome or Fragile X Syndrome

NANCY C. BRADY, SHELLEY L. BREDIN-OJA, AND STEVEN F. WARREN

Long before children start to speak, they communicate through vocalizations, gestures, and movements that convey meanings to familiar communication partners. For example, infants cry, and caregivers interpret these cries as indicating that the infant is hungry, tired, or angry. Later, children give or point to interesting objects to share experiences with someone. Although most typically developing children quickly pass through this stage and begin communicating with words and sentences, the prelinguistic and early linguistic periods of development extend over several years for many children with developmental disabilities. Hence, several early intervention approaches have been developed that specifically address prelinguistic and early linguistic communication development (McCauley & Fey, 2006). This chapter reviews prelinguistic and early linguistic strategies that have been used with children with Down syndrome (DS) or fragile X syndrome (FXS). Although little research is available to date for children with FXS, information from children with autism may be relevant for the proportion of children with FXS who also meet diagnostic criteria for autism spectrum disorders (ASD).

Before describing the interventions, however, the chapter first presents a brief review of prelinguistic development in typically developing children. This review focuses on the specific developmental transitions and behaviors targeted by many of the intervention approaches discussed in this chapter. (For a more complete review of early communication development in children with DS or FXS, see Chapter 3.)

The authors wish to acknowledge support for the development of this manuscript provided by the National Institute of Child Health and Human Development (Grant HD002528).

PRELINGUISTIC DEVELOPMENT IN TYPICALLY DEVELOPING CHILDREN

A consistent progression in prelinguistic to linguistic development has been noted by researchers studying development in typically developing children (Bates, Benigni, Bretherton, Camaioni, & Volterra, 1979; Volterra, Caselli, Capirci, & Pizzuto, 2005). The key transitions within stages of prelinguistic development include the transition between preintentional and intentional communication and the transition between intentional communication and symbolic, linguistic communication. Prelinguistic interventions focus on the behaviors that constitute intentional communication. Early linguistic interventions focus on the behaviors that signal the transition into linguistic communication.

Transitions from Preintentional to Intentional Communication

The earliest social signals that are indicative of an infant's internal state are cries, smiles, and other reflexive behaviors. Although parents are soon able to differentiate between an infant's different cries (e.g., hunger versus discomfort), the meanings of the cries are assigned by communication partners. Similarly, infants will interact with objects and with caregivers, but these early actions are not coordinated in a purposeful fashion (Adamson & Chance, 1998; Bakeman & Adamson, 1984). For example, when caregivers present toys to infants during the first few months of life, infants gaze at the toys and they gaze at the caregivers, but the infants do not shift their gaze back and forth as if they were trying to direct their caregiver's attention to the toy. Hence, this initial phase of communication has been referred to as *perlocutionary* or *preintentional* (Bates et al., 1979; Sugarman, 1984). During the first few months of life, infants also can differentiate sounds and learn to recognize and respond to sounds of the language that they are exposed to through every day nurturing (Jusczyk, 2002; Kuhl, 1998).

Sometime around 9 months of age, typically developing infants will transition from preintentional into intentional communication, also referred to as *illocutionary communication* (Bates et al., 1979; Volterra et al., 2005). This transition is marked across several behavioral domains, including coordinated attention, gestures, and vocalizations. By about 6 months of age, infants may switch their attention between a caregiver and an object that lies in the same visual field, but it takes several more months for infants to maintain sustained attention to both caregivers and objects (Adamson & Chance, 1998). By about 12 months of age, children begin to employ gaze shifts to draw a caregiver's attention to an interesting object or event (Iverson & Thal, 1997). During this same time period, gesture use becomes a primary means to communicate. Giving, showing, and reaching appear at around 8 months of age, followed by pointing at about 12 months (Bates, 1976; Bates et al., 1979; Iverson & Thal, 1997; Masur, 1983). Pointing has received considerable attention from researchers of prelinguistic development because mature forms of pointing can be used to refer to distant objects and also to communicate social functions, such as directing attention toward objects of interest (Butterworth, 2003; Butterworth & Morisette, 1996;

Dobrich & Scarborough, 1984). Hence, pointing appears key to the transition between communicating about the here and now and communicating about distal events. Vocal behaviors also develop into more word-like forms during this time. At about 6–7 months, infants begin producing canonical babbling (babbling that contains well-formed syllables such as "ba" and "da"), and by 11–12 months, they are producing variegated, word-like vocalizations and often true words (Stoel-Gammon, 1998b).

Although developments in coordinated attention, gestures, and vocalizations each help a communication partner to recognize when an infant is intentionally communicating, communication acts that combine these behaviors provide the most obvious signals to communication partners. Warren and Yoder (1998) reported that communication acts that combined coordinated attention with gestures and/or vocalizations were responded to most often by caregivers. For example, caregivers are likely to respond when a child points toward an object, looks back toward the caregiver, and vocalizes. Synchronized behaviors such as these clearly indicate that the child is intentionally communicating. By about 12 months of age, children use gestures combined with vocalizations and eye gaze to request, protest, greet, show off, and comment (Wetherby & Prizant, 1992).

During this stage, infants also show evidence for comprehending spoken words in context (Miller & Paul, 1995). At first infants understand words used in simple predictable routines, such as when playing peekaboo. Evidence for early understanding can be seen in children's responses when hearing these highly familiar words. They may look at or orient themselves toward the activity associated with the words, or they may demonstrate positive affect when they hear words associated with enjoyable activities. According to parent report measures (Carpenter, Nagell, & Tomasello, 1998), children at 9 months of age generally understand up to 25 words sampled on the MacArthur-Bates Communicative Development Inventories (CDIs; Fenson et al., 1992). Miller and Paul (1995), however, presented a more conservative estimate of an average receptive vocabulary—3 words at 12 months. The discrepancy between these sources may reflect the difficulty in assessing comprehension during early stages of development (Miller & Paul, 1995; Tomasello & Mervis, 1994).

Children's comprehension is also related to joint engagement with primary caregivers. Carpenter and colleagues (1998) reported that infants between the ages of 10–12 months who had more frequent episodes of joint engagement with their mothers comprehended significantly more words than children who did not engage in episodes of joint engagement during this period. It is likely that mothers and other caregivers accompany these periods of joint engagement with vocabulary that labels objects and activities that the child is engaged with (*following-in language*). This increased exposure to vocabulary spoken by caregivers may facilitate comprehension development (Tomasello & Farrar, 1986).

Transition from Intentional to Symbolic Communication

Sometime toward the end of the first year or the beginning of the second, typically developing children begin to communicate with words, although there is wide variability, and some children do not start talking until 18 months of age or later. For hearing children being raised by hearing parents, these words are spoken. Spoken words develop after variegated word-like babbling and typically convey names for familiar people and objects and words spoken in social routines, such as "bye-bye" and peekaboo. According to constructionists' views of language development, children's speech development is based on the communication exchanges developed during stages of prelinguistic communication (Wetherby, Reichle, & Pierce, 1998). Early lexical acquisition grows out of concept formation and increasing mental representation abilities. A limiting factor for early word use may be sound production abilities. That is, children may have difficulty learning to say words composed of sounds that they have not yet mastered.

During the expressive one-word stage, only a small proportion of vocalizations are intelligible speech (Wetherby, Cain, Yonclas, & Walker, 1988). As children progress in speech development, they continue to rely on gestures to supplement or complement their speech (Capirci, Iverson, Pizzuto, & Volterra, 1996; McNeill, 1992; Volterra et al., 2005). The transition from predominantly gestural to predominantly spoken word communication is gradual and takes place during the course of the second year.

During this second year, children also experience a rapid increase in vocabulary called the *vocabulary burst* (Bates, O'Connell, & Shore, 1987). Bloom (1993) reported that the mean age for children to reach the vocabulary burst, defined as learning three new words per week, was 19 months. Bloom reported that children were saying about 50 words at the time of the vocabulary burst. At about the same time or soon after the vocabulary burst, children begin combining words into multiword phrases and simple sentences (e.g., "my mommy," "more juice").

Comprehension during the second year also shows rapid increases. Children demonstrate understanding of people and object names early on but soon are also able to comprehend verbs and more complex semantic relations (Miller, Chapman, Branston, & Reichle, 1980). Late in the second year, most children demonstrate comprehension of possessor–possession ("my shoe"), action–object ("kick ball") and agent–action ("baby drink") relations.

Children use their new words to communicate different pragmatic intents during the 18- to 24-month period. In addition to requesting and commenting, children communicate to answer questions, protest, refuse or deny something, greet, and request social interactions (Chapman, 1981; Prutting & Kirchner, 1983). They also use their language during pretend play. Thus, rapid growth is evidenced during this period in all aspects of language development—vocabulary, semantics, syntax, and pragmatics.

PRELINGUISTIC AND EARLY LINGUISTIC DEVELOPMENT IN CHILDREN WITH DEVELOPMENTAL DISABILITIES

In general, the course of prelinguistic and early linguistic development outlined in the previous section also pertains to children with developmental disabilities, but they usually demonstrate these skills at later ages. Children with milder disabilities may show minimal delays in prelinguistic development and transition into symbolic communication within the first 2 years. Individuals with severe or profound intellectual disability, however, may continue to function at prelinguistic levels of communication into adolescence or even adulthood (Brady, McLean, McLean, & Johnston, 1995; McLean, Brady, McLean, & Behrens, 1998).

Prelinguistic Development in Children with Down Syndrome

Developmental delays are often not detected until a child is past infancy, and delays in speech development are often the first signs of a broader developmental delay, making it difficult to conduct prospective research on prelinguistic development. Children with DS, however, are usually identified at birth, if not before. Hence, a body of research does exist on prelinguistic and early linguistic development in children with DS.

The same communication development that takes place over the first 18 months of life for a typically developing infant occurs for children with DS, but it is extended to 2 or 3 years (Rondal, 2003). Developments in coordinated attention, gestures, and vocalizations appear to follow the same general paths as in typically developing infants. Gesture development even appears to be a relative strength of children with DS. Franco and Wishart (1995) measured production of a number of different gestures and found that children with DS produced nearly twice as many gestures as a comparison group of typically developing children. These researchers measured production of a number of different gestures, but it is notable that the children with DS produced nearly twice as many points as the comparison group. Singer-Harris, Bellugi, Bates, Jones, and Riossen (1997) also reported that children with DS had significantly larger gestural repertoires than typically developing children matched on vocabulary comprehension and production.

Children in both of these studies were in prelinguistic stages of communication development. Even as they become word users, however, children with DS continue to rely on gestures. Iverson, Longobardi, and Caselli (2003) compared gesture use by five children with DS with gesture use by five typically developing language-matched children. All of the children in this study said between 5 and 16 different words during 30 minutes of free play with their mothers. Iverson and colleagues reported roughly equivalent rates of gesture use by the two groups, but the typically developing children used gestures that provided additional information more often than the children with DS. For example, if a child pointed to a cup and said "mommy," the gesture was coded as providing information that supplemented the word.

Differences in the communicative functions conveyed by gestures have been reported by some research teams. A study by Smith and von Tetzchner (1986) found that children with DS displayed impairments in commenting but not in requesting. Mundy, Kasari, Sigman, and Ruskin (1995), however, found impairments in requesting by children with DS compared with language-matched typically developing children, but they found no significant group differences in commenting. Increased rates of both requesting and commenting have been linked to better language outcomes in children with DS (Mundy et al., 1995; Yoder & Warren, 2004). Hence, most prelinguistic interventions target both requesting and commenting.

The pattern of vocal development in children with DS is similar to that of typically developing children but with delayed onset of important milestones. Lynch and colleagues (1995) reported that infants with DS began canonical babbling, on average, 2 months later than typically developing infants. In addition, these authors reported that canonical babbling was less stable over time than in children without DS. The onset of canonical babbling has been viewed as an important milestone because earlier onset has been associated with earlier speech production and better language outcomes (McCathren, Warren, & Yoder, 1996; Stoel-Gammon, 1998a). Delayed onset of canonical babbling in children with DS may be due to general motor delays and differences in the oral structure and hearing losses associated with DS (Stoel-Gammon, 2001). Another possible contributing factor is delayed cognitive development (Lynch et al., 1995). The onset of first spoken words is also delayed in children with DS. Stoel-Gammon (2001) reported that the average age of onset of meaningful speech was 21 months in children with DS. In addition, speech vocabulary increases at a much slower rate than in typically developing children (Mervis & Becerra, 2003).

In summary, vocal development in children with DS is characterized by late onset and unstable development of both canonical babbling and first words. More research is needed regarding prelinguistic vocal development as well as other aspects of prelinguistic development because such research could yield additional clues as to why the onset of conventional language is often markedly delayed in children with DS.

Comprehension is also delayed in children with DS. Lexical comprehension (comprehension for spoken word meanings) was found to exceed mental age equivalents in school-age children with DS (Chapman, Seung, Schwartz, & Kay-Raining Bird, 2000). Comprehension for syntax, however, was more severely impaired.

Prelinguistic Development in Children with Fragile X Syndrome

Little information is available regarding prelinguistic development in children with FXS. Children with FXS show significant delays in language development, including the onset of first words (Abbeduto & Hagerman, 1997; Harris-Schmidt, 2006; Rice, Warren, & Betz, 2005; Roberts, Mirrett, Anderson, Burchinal, & Neebe, 2002). Hence, children with FXS show a protracted period of prelinguistic development. Brady, Skinner, Roberts, and Hennon (2006) synthesized information reported by 55 mothers of young children (younger than 3 years of age) with FXS. Most of the children in this study were reported to be nonverbal or using only a few words to communicate, and a majority of these nonverbal children were reportedly learning some form of augmentative and alternative communication (AAC). Only a couple of the mothers identified prelinguistic intervention targets such as gesture production when asked about current strategies to improve communication. Therefore, it appears important and timely to convey information about the prelinguistic interventions discussed later in this chapter to families of children with FXS.

Many boys with FXS also meet diagnostic criteria for autism or ASD (Bailey et al., 2004); therefore, a brief summary of prelinguistic development in autism follows. It should be noted that only a subset of boys with FXS also meet diagnostic criteria for ASD, and these boys are more severely affected in general.

Disturbances in coordinated attention and in gesture development are core features of prelinguistic children with ASD. These impairments appear specific to social use. For example, young children with autism will rarely use eye gaze or gestures such as pointing to share attention about an interesting event or object, but they may use these same behaviors to request a desirable object that is out of reach (Baron-Cohen, Allen, & Gillberg, 1992; Mundy & Stella, 2000). Vocalizations of prelinguistic children with ASD have been characterized as similar to children with delayed language not associated with autism (Wetherby, Prizant, & Schuler, 2000). McCleery, Tully, Slevc, and Schreibman (2006) analyzed the speech sounds produced during play by 14 children with ASD in the prelinguistic or early one-word stages of communication development. All of the children produced some consonants, but most of the consonants they produced were developmentally early sounds (e.g., /b/, /d/, /m/), although some children produced later developing sounds (e.g., /sh/, /s/).

Summary

The information presented regarding early communication development in children with DS or FXS indicates delays and differences in development for both populations. Interventions that target the specific behaviors described thus far (e.g., gestures, eye gaze, canonical vocalizations, requests, comments) may be of benefit for children with DS or FXS who are at prelinguistic or early linguistic stages of communication development. Studies have found that children with disabilities who use frequent intentional communication develop language abilities earlier than children with less frequent intentional communication (Mundy et al., 1995; Yoder & Warren, 1999). In addition, prelinguistic behaviors may be more appropriate targets than linguistic behaviors for children who have not yet mastered prelinguistic communication. The following sections will further describe such interventions, with special emphasis on ways to intervene with children with DS or FXS.

PRELINGUISTIC AND EARLY LINGUISTIC INTERVENTIONS

A number of different interventions have been developed that specifically target communication behaviors associated with developmental ages between birth and 3 years. Some of these interventions include Responsivity Education/Prelinguistic Milieu Teaching (RE/PMT; Warren et al., 2006), It Takes Two to Talk—The Hanen Program for Parents (Girolametto & Weitzman, 2006), the Picture Exchange Communication System (PECS; Frost & Bondy, 1994), the System for Augmenting Language (SAL; Romski & Sevcik, 1996), Focused Stimulation Approach to Language Intervention (Ellis Weismer & Robertson, 2006), Language is the Key (Cole, Maddox, & Lim, 2006), Enhanced Milieu Teaching (EMT; Hancock & Kaiser, 2006), and Conversational Recast (Camarata & Nelson, 2006). See McCauley & Fey, 2006, for a thorough review of each intervention. Both similarities and differences can be found across many of these interventions. Similarities include a focus on teaching within ongoing naturally occurring communication exchanges. Many include an emphasis on teaching parents either how to implement the intervention themselves (e.g., It Takes Two to Talk, Enhanced Milieu Teaching) or how to support language development through responsive interactions (e.g., RE/PMT, Language is the Key). Common teaching strategies can also be found among these interventions, such as following a child's utterance with a more complex utterance (e.g., Language is the Key, Conversational Recast).

An important difference in these interventions, however, is the set of communicative behaviors targeted. Of the listed interventions, only RE/PMT exclusively targets prelinguistic behaviors. Targeting prelinguistic behaviors and thereby increasing the frequency and complexity of nonverbal communication acts may be an important first step in the treatment of children with language delays, including children with DS or FXS.

Responsivity Education/Prelinguistic Milieu Teaching with Children with Developmental Disabilities, Including Down Syndrome and Fragile X Syndrome

RE/PMT is grounded in the assumption that prelinguistic skills form the foundation for later language development. Prelinguistic milieu teaching (PMT) incorporates prompting along with environmental arrangement in a play-based milieu teaching method designed to teach children to communicate through gestures; nonword vocalizations; directed gaze; and, later, spoken words. When combined with a parent education program designed to teach parents responsive interaction strategies (e.g., following the child's lead, taking turns, adding language to play), the intervention is referred to as Responsivity Education/Prelinguistic Milieu Teaching (Warren et al., 2006). This teaching method has been developed and studied over many years, and several longitudinal studies have analyzed its effectiveness. A substantial portion of the children in these studies had DS, and at least one child was known to have FXS.

In the first longitudinal experimental study of PMT, Yoder and Warren (1998) studied 58 children between the ages of 17 and 32 months. All of the children had fewer than 5 productive words, fell below the 10th percentile on the expressive portion of the CDI (Fenson et al., 1994) and fit the Tennessee definition for developmental delay (i.e., 40% delay in one domain or 25% delay in two or more domains). Children were randomly assigned either to PMT or to Responsive Small Group (RSG). In the RSG group, adults played with the child and commented on what they were doing but did not require the child to produce any communication. Treatment sessions for both groups were 20 minutes per day, 3–4 times per week for 6 months. Results of this study revealed an interaction between treatment condition and pretreatment maternal responsivity. Specifically, children who received PMT increased their production of intentional communication acts *if* their mothers were highly responsive at the start of the intervention. Importantly, the intervention was carried out totally within the confines of a preschool setting by trained interventionists, and there was no parent training component. For those children with unresponsive mothers, the RSG treatment was more effective in increasing their production of intentional communication. Twelve months after completing the intervention, children who received PMT (and had responsive mothers) did significantly better on linguistic measures, as shown by lexical diversity (number of different words produced in a given time period) and scores from a standardized language test (Yoder & Warren, 1999, 2001). Analyses specific to children with DS were not possible in this study because of the low number of participants with DS.

Based on these findings, Yoder and Warren (2002) conducted another longitudinal experimental study that combined PMT with responsivity education (RE) for parents. The inclusion of RE with PMT was designed to ensure that parents would increase their responsiveness to their child's prelinguistic communication bids. Thirty-nine children with developmental delays, including 17 children with DS, and their primary caregivers participated. Children had a median age of 22 months and a median mental age of 14 months. The parent–child dyads were randomly assigned to either an RE/PMT group or a control group. Treatment sessions for RE/PMT were 20 minutes per day, 3–4 times per week for 6 months; the control group received no intervention from the study. Parents in the RE/PMT group were offered up to 12 individualized 1-hour sessions of RE.

Results of this study revealed no main effect of the intervention but did reveal some interesting interactions. Specifically, RE/PMT resulted in more comments and greater lexical density if children began the treatment with very few comments and infrequent canonical vocal communication. That is, children who were relatively low on these important dimensions responded more favorably to the intervention. Furthermore, RE/PMT appeared to slow growth in comments and lexical density if children began the treatment with relatively frequent comments and canonical vocal communication. The authors concluded that children who make frequent comments and use canonical vocal communication regularly are not appropriate candidates for prelinguistic intervention. Rather, these children may make greater gains if linguistic skills are immediately targeted.

There was an unexpected finding in this study specific to children with DS. RE/PMT resulted in more requests if children had etiologies other than DS. For children with DS, the rate of growth in requests was not as great as the control group. Yoder and Warren (2002) noted that this pattern suggests that requests are more difficult than comments for children with DS. In addition, the authors suggested that children with DS may actively resist explicit prompts to request but caution against making treatment decisions based on diagnosis.

In a systematic replication and extension of this study, Fey and colleagues (2006) conducted a longitudinal experimental study of RE/PMT. The investigators changed the intervention in some modest but important ways. Specifically, they accepted a less complex form of requests, such as eye gaze alone in the initial stage of intervention. Accepting this easier form of a request may have benefited children who were prone to resist prompts to produce a more complex request such as eye gaze combined with a gesture and/or vocalizations. Also, the treatment providers in the Yoder and Warren (2002) study would imitate the child's nonverbal vocalization, even when the children's vocalization referenced a specific object or event. Fey and colleagues reasoned that a child might incorrectly associate a nonverbal model with the clear referent using Yoder and Warren's method. Therefore, the treatment providers in a study by Fey and colleagues responded to nonverbal vocalizations that made reference to objects or events by complying and linguistically mapping the referent. For example, after a child vocalized and pointed to a ball, the interventionist might respond by saying, "Yes, that's a ball."

Fifty-one children with developmental delays between the ages of 24 and 33 months participated in this study, 26 of whom were diagnosed with DS. All of the children had mild to moderate intellectual disability, fewer than 10 different expressive words, and a rate of intentional communication that was less than 2 of one act per minute. Children were randomly assigned to either a RE/PMT group or a control group. Treatment sessions for PMT were 20 minutes per day, 3 times per week for 6 months. Parents of children in the RE/PMT group received eight 1-hour individual sessions of RE.

Results following 6 months of intervention showed a main effect for intentional communication acts. Children in the RE/PMT group, regardless of their diagnosis, produced more intentional acts than children in the control group. Therefore, results of this study indicate that RE/PMT leads to increased communication rates by prelinguistic children with and without DS.

RE/PMT has also been successfully implemented for children with ASD. Yoder and Stone (2006) compared the efficacy of RE/PMT with PECS on nonimitative spoken communication. PECS is an intervention program that teaches children to ask for objects or food items, initially by handing a picture of the desired item to a recipient. (For a more complete description of PECS, see Chapter 11.) Yoder and Stone found a treatment by object exploration interaction in this study. Specifically, if children began the treatment with high object exploration during play, PECS was the better treatment for number of nonimitated words. Conversely, if children began the treatment with low object exploration, RE/PMT facilitated development of different nonimitated words faster than PECS. Effects of this interaction were maintained 6 months after the end of the treatment.

Although no studies have specifically focused on RE/PMT with children with FXS, one of the children who participated in the Fey and colleagues (2006) study had FXS. The child was a 2-year-old boy, and his results were consistent with the main effect of treatment—that is, he increased his communication rate during the 6 months of intervention. Teaching strategies used in RE/PMT and milieu therapy match well to the behavioral characteristics associated with FXS. For example, RE/PMT teaches children to communicate within social routines, and adherence to routines appears to facilitate learning and decrease anxiety in children with FXS (Abbeduto & Murphy, 2004). Once a routine is established, an interventionist may prompt a communication response. Although direct prompts such as "Show me" or "Tell me" can be used to prompt communication behaviors, less direct prompts may be more effective for some children with FXS, as direct approaches may increase arousal levels and cause anxiety. For example, moving a toy that a child is visually tracking directly in front of the adult's face may be a more effective means of prompting eye contact than telling a child "Look at me." Gradually, the adult should be able to increase the distance he or she moves his or her head, until finally, the child regularly seeks adult eye contact when commenting about or requesting an object, event, or service.

Cumulatively, these studies on RE/PMT suggest that targeting prelinguistic skills serves to increase targeted behaviors such as gestures, joint attention, and eye gaze shifts. The data to date—with the exception of the Yoder and Warren (1998) study, which included very few children with DS—does not indicate that these approaches result in enhanced language development later in life. It is important to note, however, that all of these studies have been implemented at relatively low intensity levels—typically about 1 hour per week of direct intervention with the child, plus a modest amount of parent training over a 6-month period. From this perspective the modest effects achieved are promising. Perhaps stronger results would be obtained at a higher intensity level (e.g., perhaps several hours per week of direct intervention) for 1 or 2 years. Autism interventions, for example, have generally been provided at much higher intensity levels (25–40 hours per week) and for much longer periods of time (e.g., 2 years; Smith, Eikeseth, Klevstrand, & Lovaas, 1997).

Other Prelinguistic and Early Linguistic Interventions

A number of studies have demonstrated gains in prelinguistic communication by children with developmental disabilities using methods other than RE/PMT. These studies have focused on prelinguistic skills such as gestures and eye gaze but have not measured any long-term effects on language outcomes. Salmon, Rowan, and Mitchell (1998) compared the use of explicit prompts with a condition using no explicit prompts for teaching prelinguistic requests and comments. Their study involved three children ages 17, 24, and 30 months who participated in a single-participant alternating treatment design. Two children were diagnosed with DS and one was diagnosed with agenesis of the corpus callosum. The results indicated that the children's discourse pattern depended on the condition. Children had higher rates of intentional communication in the explicit prompt condition, but these communications were predominantly requests and were in response to an adult initiation. In the absence of explicit prompts, children produced more comments than requests, and both of these pragmatic functions were more evenly distributed between initiations and responses.

Several studies have focused on teaching prelinguistic skills to children with ASD. For example, Kasari, Freeman, and Paparella (2006) employed a combination of applied behavior analysis (ABA) procedures (i.e., discrete trial training with positive reinforcement) and more child-directed interactive procedures to teach joint attention to a group of children diagnosed with ASD between the ages of 3 and 4 years. Joint attention skills observed in children in the intervention group improved significantly more than joint attention skills in the control group. Behavioral teaching strategies were also used by Whalen and Schreibman (2003) to teach children with autism to initiate and respond to gaze shifts and gestures, including pointing. Hwang and Hughes (2000) taught three children with autism to engage in more eye contact, joint attention, and motor imitation using a teaching approach called *social interaction training.* This approach was developed by Klinger and Dawson (1992) and is similar to PMT. The teaching package includes contingent imitation, use of an expectant look, environmental arrangement, and naturally occurring reinforcement.

Similar teaching strategies are recommended for teaching early lexical skills to children with DS. Mervis and Becerra (2003) recommended that interventions focus on developing interaction patterns that will facilitate coordinated joint attention because episodes of coordinated joint attention are conducive to learning new words (Tomasello & Farrar, 1986). Mervis and Becerra contended that maintaining the child's attention is particularly important with children with DS because the focused attention may help encoding and retention of new words.

Once children are engaged in an activity with an interaction partner, the partner can provide frequent and consistent input of target vocabulary, consistent with a focused stimulation approach. For example, an interventionist may provide multiple models of the word *hat* while engaged in a dress-up activity. The input may be through speech or sign language or both (as in total communication). Research by Clibbens, Powell, and Atkinson (2002) has suggested that using displaced signs may help children learn new words while maintaining attention to the referent object. These authors observed that deaf mothers of deaf children often moved the location of their signs so that the signs occurred within the child's visual field. For example, if the child was playing with a doll and the mother wanted to sign "crying," the mom would sign on the doll's face—to which the child was attending—rather than on the mother's face. Mothers of children with DS who participated in this study rarely performed these dislocated signs, but the authors suggested that this procedure could facilitate sign learning. (For additional information about signing to children, please see Chapter 11.)

Although the intervention studies described in this chapter have not specifically measured comprehension as an outcome, it is important for interventions to incorporate comprehension goals, and most intervention techniques lend themselves easily to this task. During the prelinguistic stage, finger plays, songs, or games such as Peekaboo provide repetitive, predictable routines that facilitate a child's understanding. Including gestures during these communication games is an additional way to support a child's understanding of the routine. Consistently and frequently labeling the objects and events that are the child's focus of attention also facilitates language comprehension of these labels.

Parent-Focused Prelinguistic/Early Linguistic Interventions for Children with Down Syndrome or Fragile X Syndrome

Parent-focused interventions attempt to affect child communication indirectly by teaching parents to interact in specific ways designed to promote communication and language. It Takes Two to Talk (Girolametto & Weitzman, 2006) is perhaps the best known intervention approach that focuses directly on parent-implemented interventions for prelinguistic and early linguistic behaviors. In this program, speech-language pathologists teach groups of up to eight families a series of interaction skills designed to promote interaction, create opportunities for communication, and model language at a level appropriate for the children. The Hanen program also teaches parents ways to increase their children's comprehension skills. Parents are taught to add language to everyday situations not only by labeling those objects that their children are attending to but also by using a greater variety of words (e.g., verbs, adjectives, prepositions, possessives, question words). Parents are given strategies to expand their children's single-word utterances to two- and three-word combinations to express a number of semantic–syntactic relations such as existence (e.g., child says "ball"; parent expands this to "that ball"), recurrence (e.g., child says "more"; parent expands this to "more juice"), and possession (e.g., child says "mine"; parent expands this to "your ball/my ball"), to list just a few. Depending on a child's level of communication development, goals include improved lexical, morphological, syntactic, and prelinguistic communication behaviors.

Girolametto (1988) conducted a study of the Hanen program that involved 20 children ages 15–59 months, and their mothers, including 11 children with DS. The mother–child dyads were randomly assigned to a treatment or a control group. Mothers in the treatment group attended eight group sessions and three individual sessions where they received training to increase their awareness of their children's communication bids and to use social interaction and language facilitating techniques, such as establishing joint focus, balancing turns, responding contingently, and providing clear linguistic models.

Pre- and posttesting included standardized language tests as well as a 20-minute mother–child interaction that was videotaped in a test room. Results for child outcomes revealed that children in the treatment group initiated more topics, took more turns in the conversation, and had a more diverse vocabulary than children in the control group. However, standardized language test results revealed no differences in language development.

McCauley and Fey (2006) observed that most recent versions of the Hanen program included more focused stimulation on specific words or structures. According to these authors, the inclusion of focused stimulation appears to produce somewhat stronger effects for children with milder delays specifically in speech or language. An adapted version of the original curriculum has been developed specifically for parents of children with autism. The adapted version is called More Than Words and stresses social interaction skills, such as how to develop predictable routines within everyday activities. Information on all of the Hanen programs is available at http://www.hanen.org/.

Other early language interventions, such as EMT (Hemmeter & Kaiser, 1994; Kaiser, Hancock, & Nietfeld, 2000) differ somewhat in focus from It Takes Two to Talk—The Hanen Program for Parents. In EMT, parents are taught to use teaching principles such as modeling, mand-model, time delay, and incidental teaching prompts to teach their children to produce specific early language targets. Studies have demonstrated positive gains in both parents' instructional behaviors and their children's language outcomes using EMT (Hancock & Kaiser, 2006).

An approach similar to EMT was implemented in a study conducted with mothers and their children with ASD (Kashinath, Woods, & Goldstein, 2006). Five children, ages 33–65 months, and their mothers participated. The mothers were taught two of six teaching strategies to implement during the course of existing daily routines. Teaching strategies included arranging the environment, using natural reinforcement, using time delay, imitating contingently, modeling, and gestural/visual cuing. The teaching strategies selected for each mother varied and were based on the mothers' existing use of the facilitating techniques. Communication goals for each child were also selected for the mothers to target; these ranged from gestures and vocalizations to the use of single words. Results indicated that all mothers were able to implement the teaching strategies and to generalize these strategies across routines. Children's communication targets also increased in accordance with their mothers' use of the new strategies.

Special Considerations for Caregivers of Children with Down Syndrome or Fragile X Syndrome

Characteristics of caregiver–child interactions observed in dyads with children with DS or FXS may require special considerations for the interventionist working specifically with parents. The interventions reviewed previously are based on the transactional model of development that assumes that both the child and the environment change over time in a reciprocal manner (McLean & Snyder-McLean, 1978). Changes in the child elicit changes in the social milieu that the child inhabits: A social child who initiates interaction with his or her parent will receive cumulatively more language facilitating input from his or her parents than a child who infrequently engages his or her parent.

Children with disabilities such as DS and FXS may make significantly fewer communication bids and may, in turn, partake in fewer reciprocal social interactions, and therefore receive less input from their parents. In addition, some of the behaviors associated with these disorders may lead to fewer interactions. For example, children with FXS often demonstrate gaze avoidance or atypical eye gaze, hypersensitivity to sensory input, social anxiety and shyness, perseveration, stereotypical and challenging behaviors, unintelligible speech, and problems with conversational discourse—all of which may affect responsivity (Abbeduto & Hagerman, 1997; Bailey, Hatton, & Skinner, 1998).

Characteristics of mothers of children with FXS may also have an impact on mother–child interactions. Biological mothers of children with FXS either carry the premutation or have the full mutation themselves. Mothers with the full mutation may have cognitive impairments, increased social anxiety, and depression (Abbeduto, Wyngaarden Krauss, Orsmond, & Murphy, 2004). Although less is known about women who carry the premutation, some reports indicate increased rates of affective disorders (Hagerman & Hagerman, 2002). Abbeduto and colleagues (2004) found that mothers of adolescents with FXS were more pessimistic and had more depressive symptoms than did mothers of adolescents with DS.

Mothers of children with DS do not share the gene mutation that affects their children, but research indicates that mothers of children with disabilities, including mothers of children with DS, appear more directive toward their children than mothers of children without disabilities (Mahoney, 1988). For example, mothers of children with DS may refocus their children's attention to what the mother is attending to more often than mothers of children without disabilities. Closer examination of these interactions, however, reveals that mothers adapt to the lower language level in the children with disabilities (Legerstee, Varghese, & Beek, 2002). That is, the amount of maternal directiveness is negatively related to the developing language skills in their children (Marfo, 1990). Mothers of children with relatively low language levels (e.g., primarily prelinguistic) appear to try to actively engage their children in teaching-like episodes, and these attempts at active engagement may be coded as directive behaviors by some coding systems.

CONCLUSION AND IMPLICATIONS FOR FURTHER RESEARCH

This chapter has described interventions aimed at improving prelinguistic and early linguistic communication. In terms of research with children with developmental disabilities and associated language delays, the evidence to date suggests that intervention is effective in increasing rates of prelinguistic communicative behaviors such as gesturing and vocalizing. This is important because improved prelinguistic communication will enable prelinguistic children to communicate more effectively with their partners. Clearer, more effective communication can lead to decreases in less desirable forms of communication, such as tantrums or aggressive behaviors (Mirenda, 1997; Reichle & Wacker, 1993). In addition, targeting communication behaviors that are within or just in advance of a child's current development may be less frustrating for both child and parent than targeting forms that are well above the child's present functioning level.

Clear evidence linking these increases in prelinguistic behaviors to improved language outcomes is lacking, however. Thus far, the evidence suggests that at low intensity levels, PMT or RE/PMT may improve language outcomes for some children with certain characteristics (e.g., responsive parents, low initiators, low object explorations), but longitudinal main effects have not been found. Ongoing research is exploring whether a more intensively delivered version of RE/PMT will have demonstrable benefits to language gains. In addition, it should be noted again that several recent research studies on RE/PMT used rigorous, randomly assigned comparison group designs. Although significant main effects for language gains were not found, many participants who experienced RE/PMT did show substantial language growth. Further comparisons of children who did show improved language outcomes (responders) with those who did not show improved language outcomes (nonresponders) are warranted.

An unexpected finding that is relevant to the topic addressed in this chapter is that children with DS, as a group, did not show increases in language after participating in RE/PMT in the Yoder and Warren (2002) study. In fact, children with DS showed greater increases in requesting behaviors if they were in the control group than if they were in the treatment group. Recent findings by Fey and colleagues (2006), however, found increases in prelinguistic requesting and commenting behaviors following RE/PMT. Further research is needed to clarify the role of DS in prelinguistic interventions, but one may speculate about the possible contributors to poorer outcomes for children with DS. One possibility is that the children with DS were more cognitively and/or linguistically impaired than the children without DS. Post hoc analyses, however, indicated that there were not any significant group differences in measured intelligence, chronological age, or parent-reported vocabulary size at the start of intervention (Yoder & Warren, 2004).

Another possibility is that these results point to early signs of an expressive language-learning difficulty that persists for many individuals with DS. Several researchers have presented findings indicating that language development in children with DS lags behind other areas, such as visual discriminations (Chapman et al., 2000; Miller, 1999). The amount of prelinguistic intervention delivered thus far may not be enough to overcome a persistent language-learning problem. All of the additional benefits already mentioned for targeting prelinguistic communication (e.g., improved interactions, decreased frustrations), however, also pertain to families with a child with DS. Therefore, RE/PMT or similar interventions are not contraindicated for this group.

Further research is also needed comparing interventions targeting prelinguistic communication behaviors with the other primary form of early communication intervention—specifically AAC intervention. (Early applications of AAC are described in Chapter 11.) The study by Yoder and Stone (2006) is the only attempt reported to date to directly compare RE/PMT (or similar interventions) to any form of AAC. Young children with DS or FXS are frequently taught to sign or use visual symbols such as in PECS. No information is available at the time of this writing that would indicate whether one of these forms of AAC or prelinguistic interventions, or some combination of the two approaches, would be optimally beneficial for a given child.

The need for further research on communication development and interventions during the prelinguistic and early linguistic periods for children with DS or FXS is clear. Communicative behaviors that occur prior to word development and use are key for both diagnostics and intervention planning. In addition, further research is needed about the prognostic value of particular early communication behaviors for specific etiologies. In general, the rate of prelinguistic communication, the variety of communication functions expressed (e.g., requests, comments), and the use of consonants in prespeech vocalizations predict language outcomes for children with developmental disabilities (Brady, Marquis, Fleming, & McLean, 2004; McCathren et al., 1996; Yoder & Warren, 2004). More information about how these and other behaviors interact with phenotypic profiles of children with particular disabilities would benefit families and practitioners. Studies aimed at identifying behaviors that are specifically prognostic for children with DS or FXS, and that are potential targets for future early interventions, are required.

REFERENCES

Abbeduto, L., & Hagerman, R. (1997). Language and communication in fragile X syndrome. *Mental Retardation and Developmental Disabilities Research Reviews, 3*(4), 313–322.

Abbeduto, L., & Murphy, M. (2004). Language, social cognition, maladaptive behavior, and communication in Down syndrome and fragile X syndrome. In M.L. Rice & S.F. Warren (Eds.), *Developmental language disorders: From phenotypes to etiologies* (pp. 77–97). Mahwah, NJ: Lawrence Erlbaum Associates.

Abbeduto, L., Wyngaarden Krauss, M., Orsmond, G., & Murphy, M. (2004). Psychological well-being and coping in mothers of youths with autism, Down syndrome, or fragile X syndrome. *American Journal on Mental Retardation, 109*(3), 237–254.

Adamson, L.B., & Chance, S.E. (1998). Coordinating attention to people, objects, and language. In S.F. Warren & J. Reichle (Series Eds.) & A.M. Wetherby, S.F. Warren, & J. Reichle (Vol. Eds.), *Communication and language intervention series: Vol. 7. Transitions in prelinguistic communication* (pp. 15–39). Baltimore: Paul H. Brookes Publishing Co.

Bailey, D., Hatton, D., & Skinner, M. (1998). Early developmental trajectories of males with fragile X syndrome. *American Journal on Mental Retardation, 103*(1), 29–39.

Bailey, D.B., Roberts, J.E., Hooper, S.R., Hatton, D.D., Mirrett, P.L., Roberts, J.E., et al. (2004). Research on fragile X syndrome and autism: Implications for the study of genes, environments, and developmental language disorders. In M.L. Rice & S.F. Warren (Eds.), *Developmental language disorders: From phenotypes to etiologies* (pp. 121–150). Mahwah, NJ: Lawrence Erlbaum Associates.

Bakeman, R., & Adamson, L.B. (1984). Coordinating attention to people and objects in mother-infant and peer-infant interaction. *Child Development, 55,* 1278–1289.

Baron-Cohen, S., Allen, J., & Gillberg, C. (1992). Can autism be detected at 18 months? The needle, the haystack, and the CHAT. *British Journal of Psychiatry, 161,* 839–843.

Bates, E. (1976). *Language and context.* New York: Academic Press.

Bates, E., Benigni, L., Bretherton, I., Camaioni, L., & Volterra, V. (1979). *The emergence of symbols: Cognition and communication in infancy.* New York: Academic Press.

Bates, E., O'Connell, B., & Shore, C. (1987). Language and communication in infancy. In J.D. Osofsky (Ed.), *Handbook of infant development* (pp. 149–203). New York: John Wiley & Sons.

Bloom, L. (1993). *The transition from infancy to language.* New York: Cambridge University Press.

Brady, N., Marquis, J., Fleming, K., & McLean, L. (2004). Prelinguistic predictors of language growth in children with developmental disabilities. *Journal of Speech, Language and Hearing Research, 47*(3), 663–667.

Brady, N., McLean, J., McLean, L., & Johnston, S. (1995). Initiation and repair of intentional communication acts by adults with severe to profound cognitive disabilities. *Journal of Speech and Hearing Research, 38,* 1334–1348.

Brady, N., Skinner, M., Roberts, J., & Hennon, E. (2006). Communication in young children with fragile X syndrome: A qualitative study of mothers' perspectives. *American Journal of Speech-Language Pathology, 15,* 353–364.

Butterworth, G. (2003). Pointing is the royal road to language for babies. In S. Kita (Ed.), *Pointing: Where language, culture, and cognition meet* (pp. 9–33). Mahwah, NJ: Lawrence Erlbaum Associates.

Butterworth, G., & Morisette, P. (1996). Onset of pointing and the acquisition of language in infancy. *Journal of Reproductive and Infant Psychology, 14,* 219–231.

Camarata, S.M., & Nelson, K.E. (2006). Conversational recast intervention with preschool and older children. In S.F. Warren & M.E. Fey (Series Eds.) & R.J. McCauley & M.E. Fey (Vol. Eds.), *Communication and language intervention series: Treatment of language disorders in children* (pp. 237–264). Baltimore: Paul H. Brookes Publishing Co.

Capirci, O., Iverson, J.M., Pizzuto, E., & Volterra, V. (1996). Gestures and words during the transition to two-word speech. *Journal of Child Language, 23,* 645–673.

Carpenter, M., Nagell, K., & Tomasello, M. (1998). Social cognition, joint attention, and communicative competence from 9 to 15 months of age. *Monographs of the Society for Research in Child Development, 63*(4), Serial No. 255.

Chapman, R. (1981). Exploring children's communicative intents. In J. Miller (Ed.), *Assessing language production in children* (pp. 111–138). Baltimore: University Park Press.

Chapman, R., Seung, H., Schwartz, S., & Kay-Raining Bird, E. (2000). Predicting language production in children and adolescents with Down syndrome: The role of comprehension. *Journal of Speech and Hearing Research, 43*(2), 340–350.

Clibbens, J., Powell, G., & Atkinson, E. (2002). Strategies for achieving joint attention when signing to children with Down's syndrome. *International Journal of Language and Communication Disorders, 37*(3), 309–323.

Cole, K.N., Maddox, M., & Lim, Y.S. (2006). Language is the key: Constructive interactions around books and play. In S.F. Warren & M.E. Fey (Series Eds.) & R.J. McCauley & M.E. Fey (Vol. Eds.), *Communication and language intervention series: Treatment of language disorders in children* (pp. 149–173). Baltimore: Paul H. Brookes Publishing Co.

Dobrich, W., & Scarborough, H.S. (1984). Form and function in early communication: Language and pointing gestures. *Journal of Experimental Child Psychology, 38,* 475–490.

Ellis Weismer, S., & Robertson, S. (2006). Focused stimulation approach to language intervention. In S.F. Warren & M.E. Fey (Series Eds.) & R.J. McCauley & M.E. Fey (Vol. Eds.), *Communication and language intervention series: Treatment of language disorders in children* (pp. 175–201). Baltimore: Paul H. Brookes Publishing Co.

Fenson, L., Dale, P., Reznick, J.S., Bates, E., Thal, D.J., & Pethick, S.J. (1994). Variability in early communicative development. *Monographs of the society for research in child development, 59*(5), 1–173.

Fenson, L., Dale, P.S., Reznick, J.S., Thal, D., Bates, E., Hartung, J.P., et al. (1992). *MacArthur-Bates Communicative Development Inventories user's guide and technical manual.* Baltimore: Paul H. Brookes Publishing Co.

Fey, M.E., Warren, S., Brady, N., Finestack, L., Bredin-Oja, S., & Fairchild, M. (2006). Early effects of prelinguistic milieu teaching and responsivity education for children with developmental delays and their parents. *Journal of Speech, Language and Hearing Research, 49*(3), 526–547.

Franco, F., & Wishart, J.G. (1995). Use of pointing and other gestures by young children with Down syndrome. *American Journal on Mental Retardation, 100,* 160–182.

Frost, L., & Bondy, A. (1994). *The Picture Exchange Communication System: Training manual.* Cherry Hill, NJ: Pyramid Educational Consultants, Inc.

Girolametto, L. (1988). Improving the social-conversational skills of developmentally delayed children: An intervention study. *Journal of Speech and Hearing Disorders, 53,* 156–167.

Girolametto, L., & Weitzman, E. (2006). It takes two to talk: The Hanen program for parents: Early language intervention through caregiver training. In S.F. Warren & M.E. Fey (Series Eds.) & R.J. McCauley & M.E. Fey (Vol. Eds.), *Communication and language intervention series: Treatment of language disorders in children* (pp. 77–104). Baltimore: Paul H. Brookes Publishing Co.

Hagerman, R.J., & Hagerman, P.J. (2002). The fragile X permutation: Into the phenotypic fold. *Current Opinion in Genetics and Development, 12,* 278–283.

Hancock, T.B., & Kaiser, A.P. (2006). Enhanced milieu teaching. In S.F. Warren & M.E. Fey (Series Eds.) & R.J. McCauley & M.E. Fey (Vol. Eds.), *Communication and language intervention series: Treatment of language disorders in children* (pp. 203–236). Baltimore: Paul H. Brookes Publishing Co.

Harris-Schmidt, G. (2006). *Characteristics of speech language disorders in children with fragile X syndrome.* Retrieved February 6, 2006, from http://www.fragilex.org/html/cognitive.htm

Hemmeter, M.L., & Kaiser, A.P. (1994). Enhanced milieu teaching: Effects of parent-implemented language intervention. *Journal of Early Intervention, 18*(3), 269–283.

Hwang, B., & Hughes, C. (2000). Increasing early social-communicative skills of preverbal preschool children with autism through social interactive training. *JASH, 25*(1), 18–28.

Iverson, J., Longobardi, E.L., & Caselli, M.C. (2003). Relationship between gestures and words in children with Down's syndrome and typically developing children in the early stages of communicative development. *International Journal of Language and Communication Disorders, 38*(2), 179–197.

Iverson, J.M., & Thal, D.J. (1997). Communicative transitions: There's more to the hand than meets the eye. In S.F. Warren & J. Reichle (Series Eds.) & A.M. Wetherby, S.F. Warren, & J. Reichle (Vol. Eds.), *Communication and language intervention series: Transitions in prelinguistic communication* (pp. 59–87). Baltimore: Paul H. Brookes Publishing Co.

Jusczyk, P. (2002). Language development: from speech perception to first words. In A. Slater & M. Lewis (Eds.), *Introduction to infant development* (pp. 147–166). Oxford: Oxford University Press.

Kaiser, T., Hancock, T., & Nietfeld, J. (2000). The effects of parent-implemented enhanced milieu teaching on the social communication of children who have autism. *Early Education and Development, 11*(4), 423–446.

Kasari, C., Freeman, S., & Paparella, T. (2006). Joint attention and symbolic play in young children with autism: A randomized controlled intervention study. *Journal of Child Psychology and Psychiatry, 47*(6), 611–620.

Kashinath, S., Woods, J., & Goldstein, H. (2006). Enhancing generalized teaching strategy use in daily routines by parents of children with autism. *Journal of Speech, Language and Hearing Research, 49*(3), 466–485.

Klinger, L.G., & Dawson, G. (1992). Facilitating early social and communicative development in children with autism. In S.F. Warren & J. Reichle (Series and Vol. Eds.), *Communication and language intervention series: Vol. 1. Causes and effects in communication and language intervention* (pp. 157–186). Baltimore: University Park Press.

Kuhl, P. (1998). Language, culture and intersubjectivity: The creation of shared perception. In S. Braten (Ed.), *Intersubjective communication and emotion in early ontogeny: Studies in emotion and social interaction* (2nd series, pp. 297–315). New York: Cambridge University Press.

Legerstee, M., Varghese, J., & Beek, Y. (2002). Effects of maintaining and redirecting infant attention on the production of referential communication in infants with and without Down syndrome. *Journal of Child Language, 29*, 23–48.

Lynch, M., Oller, D.K., Steffens, M., Levine, S., Basinger, D., & Umbel, V. (1995). Onset of speech-like vocalizations in infants with Down syndrome. *American Journal on Mental Retardation, 100*(1), 68–86.

Mahoney, G. (1988). Maternal communication style with mentally retarded children. *American Journal on Mental Retardation, 92*, 352–359.

Marfo, K. (1990). Maternal directiveness in interactions with mentally handicapped children: An analytical commentary. *Journal of Psychology and Psychiatry, 31*, 531–549.

Masur, E.F. (1983). Gestural development, dual-directional signaling, and the transition to words. *Journal of Psycholinguistic Research, 12*, 93–109.

McCathren, R.B., Warren, S.F., & Yoder, P.J. (1996). Prelinguistic predictors of later language development. In S.F. Warren & J. Reichle (Series Eds.) & K.N. Cole, P.S. Dale, & D.J. Thal (Vol. Eds.), *Communication and language intervention series: Vol. 6. Assessment of communication and language* (pp. 57–76). Baltimore: Paul H. Brookes Publishing Co.

McCauley, R.J., & Fey, M.E. (Vol. Eds.) & S.F. Warren & M.E. Fey (Series Eds.). (2006). *Communication and language intervention series: Treatment of language disorders in children.* Baltimore: Paul H. Brookes Publishing Co.

McCleery, J., Tully, L., Slevc, R., & Schreibman, L. (2006). Consonant production patterns of young severely language-delayed children with autism. *Journal of Communication Disorders, 39*, 217–231.

McLean, J., & Snyder-McLean, L. (1978). *A transactional approach to early language training.* Columbus, OH: Charles E. Merrill.

McLean, L., Brady, N., McLean, J., & Behrens, G. (1998). Communication forms and functions of children and adults with severe mental retardation in community and institutional settings. *Journal of Speech and Hearing Research, 42*, 231–240.

McNeill, D. (1992). *Hand and mind: What gestures reveal about thought.* Chicago: University of Chicago Press.

Mervis, C., & Becerra, A. (2003). Lexical development and intervention. In J. Rondal & S. Buckley (Eds.), *Speech and language intervention in Down syndrome* (pp. 63–85). London: Whurr Publishers.

Miller, J.F. (1999). Profiles of language development in children with Down syndrome. In J.F. Miller, M. Leddy, & L.A. Leavitt (Eds.), *Improving the communication of people with Down syndrome* (pp. 11–39). Baltimore: Paul H. Brookes Publishing Co.

Miller, J., Chapman, R., Branston, M., & Reichle, J. (1980). Language comprehension in sensorimotor stages V and VI. *Journal of Speech and Hearing Research, 23,* 284–311.

Miller, J.F., & Paul, R. (1995). *The clinical assessment of language comprehension.* Baltimore: Paul H. Brookes Publishing Co.

Mirenda, P. (1997). Supporting individuals with challenging behavior through functional communication training and AAC: Research review. *Augmentative and Alternative Communication, 13,* 207–224.

Mundy, P., Kasari, C., Sigman, M., & Ruskin, E. (1995). Nonverbal communication and early language acquisition in children with Down syndrome and in normally developing children. *Journal of Speech and Hearing Research, 38,* 157–167.

Mundy, P., & Stella, J. (2000). Joint attention, social orienting, and communication in autism. In S.F. Warren & J. Reichle (Series Eds.) & A.M. Wetherby & B.M. Prizant (Vol. Eds.), *Communication and language intervention series: Vol. 9. Autism spectrum disorders: A transactional developmental perspective* (pp. 55–79). Baltimore: Paul H. Brookes Publishing Co.

Prutting, C.A., & Kirchner, D.M. (1983). Applied pragmatics. In T.M. Gallagher & C.A. Prutting (Eds.), *Pragmatic assessment and intervention issues in language* (pp. 29–64). San Diego: College-Hill Press.

Reichle, J., & Wacker, D.P. (Vol. Eds.) & S.F. Warren & J. Reichle (Series Eds.). (1993). *Communication and language intervention series: Vol. 3. Communicative alternatives to challenging behavior: Integrating functional assessment and intervention strategies.* Baltimore: Paul H. Brookes Publishing Co.

Rice, M.L., Warren, S., & Betz, S. (2005). Language symptoms of developmental language disorders: An overview of autism, Down syndrome, fragile X, specific language impairment, and Williams syndrome. *Applied Psycholinguistics, 26,* 7–27.

Roberts, J., Mirrett, P., Anderson, K., Burchinal, M., & Neebe, E. (2002). Early communication, symbolic behavior, and social profiles of young males with fragile X syndrome. *American Journal of Speech-Language Pathology, 11,* 295–304.

Romski, M.A., & Sevcik, R.A. (1996). *Breaking the speech barrier: Language development through augmented means.* Baltimore: Paul H. Brookes Publishing Co.

Rondal, J. (2003). Prelinguistic training. In J. Rondal & S. Buckley (Eds.), *Speech and language intervention in Down syndrome* (pp. 11–30). London: Whurr.

Salmon, C.M., Rowan, L.E., & Mitchell, P.R. (1998). Facilitating prelinguistic communication: Impact of adult prompting. *The Transdisciplinary Journal, 8*(1), 11–27.

Singer-Harris, N., Bellugi, U., Bates, E., Jones, W., & Riossen, M. (1997). Contrasting profiles of language development in children with Williams and Down syndromes. *Developmental Neuropsychology, 13,* 345–370.

Smith, L., & von Tetzchner, S. (1986). Communicative, sensorimotor and language skills of young children with Down syndrome. *American Journal of Mental Deficiency, 91,* 57–66.

Smith, T., Eikeseth, S., Klevstrand, M., & Lovaas, O.I. (1997). Intensive behavioral treatment for preschoolers with severe mental retardation and pervasive developmental disorder. *American Journal on Mental Retardation, 102*(3), 238–249.

Stoel-Gammon, C. (1998a). Role of babbling and phonology in early linguistic development. In S.F. Warren & J. Reichle (Series Eds.) & A.M. Wetherby, S.F. Warren, & J. Reichle (Vol. Eds.), *Communication and language intervention series: Vol. 7. Transitions in prelinguistic communication* (pp. 87–111). Baltimore: Paul H. Brookes Publishing Co.

Stoel-Gammon, C. (1998b). Sounds and words in early language acquisition: The relationship between lexical and phonological development. In S.F. Warren & J. Reichle (Series Eds.) & R. Paul (Vol. Ed.), *Communication and language intervention series: Vol. 8. Exploring the speech–language connection* (pp. 25–53). Baltimore: Paul H. Brookes Publishing Co.

Stoel-Gammon, C. (2001). Down syndrome phonology: Developmental patterns and intervention strategies. *Down Syndrome Research and Practice, 7*(3), 93–100.

Sugarman, S. (1984). The development of preverbal communication: Its contribution and limits in promoting the development of language. In R.L. Schiefelbusch & J. Pickar (Eds.), *The acquisition of communicative competence* (pp. 23–67). Baltimore: University Park Press.

Tomasello, M., & Farrar, M.J. (1986). Joint attention and early language. *Child Development, 57,* 1454–1463.

Tomasello, M., & Mervis, C. (1994). The instrument is great, but measuring comprehension is still a problem. *Monographs of the Society for Research in child Development, 59*(5), 242.

Volterra, V., Caselli, M.C., Capirci, O., & Pizzuto, E. (2005). Gesture and the emergence and development of language. In M. Tomasello & D. Slobin (Eds.), *Beyond nature-nurture: Essays in honor of Elizabeth Bates* (pp. 3–41). Mahwah, NJ: Lawrence Erlbaum Associates.

Warren, S.F., Bredin-Oja, S.L., Fairchild, M., Finestack, L.H., Fey, M.E., & Brady, N.C. (2006). Responsivity education/Prelinguistic milieu teaching. In S.F. Warren & M.E. Fey (Series Eds.) & R.J. McCauley & M.E. Fey (Vol. Eds.), *Communication and language intervention series: Treatment of language disorders in children* (pp. 47–77). Baltimore: Paul H. Brookes Publishing Co.

Warren, S.F., & Yoder, P.J. (1998). Facilitating the transition from preintentional to intentional communication. In S.F. Warren & J. Reichle (Series Eds.) & A.M. Wetherby, S.F. Warren, & J. Reichle (Vol. Eds.), *Communication and language intervention series: Vol. 7. Transitions in prelinguistic communication* (pp. 365–385). Baltimore: Paul H. Brookes Publishing Co.

Wetherby, A., Cain, D.H., Yonclas, D.G., & Walker, V.G. (1988). Analysis of intentional communication of normal children from the prelinguistic to the multiword stage. *Journal of Speech and Hearing Research, 31,* 240–252.

Wetherby, A.M., & Prizant, B.M. (1992). Profiling young children's communicative competence. In S.F. Warren & J. Reichle (Series and Vol. Eds.), *Communication and language intervention series: Vol. 1. Causes and effects in communication and language intervention* (pp. 217–255). Baltimore: Paul H. Brookes Publishing Co.

Wetherby, A.M., Prizant, B.M., & Schuler, A.L. (2000). Understanding the nature of the communication and language impairments. In S.F. Warren & J. Reichle (Series Eds.) & A.M. Wetherby & B.M. Prizant (Vol. Eds.), *Communication and language intervention series: Vol. 9. Autism spectrum disorders: A transactional developmental perspective* (pp. 109–143.). Baltimore: Paul H. Brookes Publishing Co.

Wetherby, A., Reichle, J., & Pierce, P. (1998). The transition to symbolic communication. In S.F. Warren & J. Reichle (Series Eds.) & A.M. Wetherby, S.F. Warren, & J. Reichle (Vol. Eds.), *Communication and language intervention series: Vol. 7. Transitions in prelinguistic communication* (pp. 197–230). Baltimore: Paul H. Brookes Publishing Co.

Whalen, C., & Schreibman, L. (2003). Joint attention training for children with autism using behavior modification procedures. *Journal of Child Psychology and Psychiatry, 44*(3), 456–468.

Yoder, P., & Stone, W. (2006). Randomized comparison of two communication interventions for preschoolers with autism spectrum disorders. *Journal of Consulting and Clinical Psychology, 74*(3), 426–435.

Yoder, P., & Warren, S. (1998). Maternal responsivity predicts the prelinguistic communication intervention that facilitates generalized intentional communication. *Journal of Speech, Language and Hearing Research, 41,* 1207–1219.

Yoder, P., & Warren, S. (1999). Maternal responsivity mediates the relationship between prelinguistic intentional communication and later language. *Journal of Early Intervention, 22*(2), 126–136.

Yoder, P., & Warren, S. (2001). Intentional communication elicits language-facilitating maternal responses in dyads with children who have developmental disabilities. *American Journal on Mental Retardation, 106*(4), 327–335.

Yoder, P., & Warren, S. (2002). Effects of prelinguistic milieu teaching and parent responsivity education on dyads involving children with intellectual disabilities. *Journal of Speech, Language and Hearing Research, 45*(6), 1158–1175.

Yoder, P., & Warren, S. (2004). Early predictors of language in children with and without Down syndrome. *American Journal of Mental Retardation, 109*(4), 285–300.

CHAPTER 8

Language Intervention to Encourage Complex Language Use

A Clinical Perspective

LIBBY KUMIN

N o single pattern of speech and language skills is found in individuals with Down syndrome (DS; Chapman & Hesketh, 2000) or fragile X syndrome (FXS; Bailey & Nelson, 1995). As such, it follows that there cannot be a universal speech and language intervention program for individuals with either condition. Rather, there is a wide range of abilities and difficulties in communication related to speech, language, hearing, and cognitive abilities (Rice, Warren, & Betz, 2005), as well as coexisting conditions, such as sensory processing disorders, autism, and childhood apraxia of speech (Kumin, 1996, 2002a). Intervention planning for speech-language pathology services for individuals with DS and FXS begins with a comprehensive evaluation to identify the specific communication needs and strengths of each individual using information gathered from the case history; prior evaluations; parent feedback; and, for the school-age child, teacher evaluations (Kumin, 2001a, 2003). The intervention program should be comprehensive, functional, and flexible, reflecting needs observed at home, at school, and in therapy (Kumin, 1999, 2002a). Because very few interventions are designed specifically for individuals with DS or FXS, the language interventions described in this chapter are generally techniques that have been successful with other populations. This chapter focuses on intervention methods to develop complex language, that is, language at the three-word stage and beyond, in individuals with DS and those with FXS. Interventions for different language ages and stages and domains of language are discussed for both groups of individuals from a clinical perspective.

SPEECH AND LANGUAGE INTERVENTION FOR INDIVIDUALS WITH DOWN SYNDROME

Many different approaches to speech and language intervention can be used as part of a comprehensive, individually designed program. There is very little research on evidence-based speech and language intervention for individuals with DS, and there is even less for individuals with FXS. Therefore, most therapy tech-

Table 8.1.   Speech and language phenotype of individuals with Down syndrome

Delayed development of expressive language

Language below cognitive level

Receptive–expressive language gap

Morphosyntax difficulty

Relative strength in vocabulary

Relative strength in pragmatics

Poor auditory memory

Difficulties with verbal short-term memory

Difficulty with topicalization (introducing, maintaining, and changing topic)

Short mean length of utterance

Short conversations

Reduced speech intelligibility

Difficulty with oral-motor skills

Childhood apraxia of speech

niques are adapted from successful strategies used with other populations that target the areas of intervention. Techniques can be adapted to take into account the relative visual processing strengths and auditory processing difficulties found in individuals with DS (Hopmann & Wilen, 1993; Kanno & Ikeda, 2002; Kay-Raining Bird & Chapman, 1994; Limongi & Carvallo, 2000). Visual cues and supports in the form of pictures or writing can be used. Visualization, chunking, and verbal rehearsal are other strategies that can be used (Kumin, 2001a) to help with language. Many individuals with DS learn to read effectively, and this can help in learning language concepts (Buckley, 1993, 1995; Buckley & Bird, 1993, 2001a, 2001b). See Table 8.1 for more information about the speech and language profile of individuals with DS.

Language Intervention at Different Ages and Stages of Language Development

Individuals with DS demonstrate both strengths and challenges at different ages and stages of language development (Berglund, Eriksson, & Johansson, 2001; Kumin, 2003).

Preschool and Kindergarten Years

Many preschool-age children with DS speak in multiword phrases and short sentences, but some children with DS are not yet using speech at this age. Children with DS in preschool and kindergarten are usually relatively more advanced in receptive language skills than in expressive language skills (Jenkins, 1993; Kumin, 2003; Kumin, Councill, & Goodman, 1995; Miller, Leddy, Miolo, & Sedey, 1995), but both areas are targeted in therapy. There are wide variations in communication skills among preschool-age children with DS; some children rely primarily on assistive technology such as sign language to communicate, and others speak with large vocabularies and are able to have conversations and read aloud.

During this stage, receptive language intervention may focus on auditory memory and on following directions, which are important skills for the early school years (Jarrold & Baddeley, 2002). Intervention may also focus on concept development such as colors, shapes, directions (top and bottom), and prepositions through practice and play experiences (Kumin, Goodman, & Councill, 1991). Reading is often introduced during this stage and can facilitate vocabulary development and complex language use (Buckley, 1996, 2000; Buckley & Bird, 2001a; Laws, Buckley, Bird, MacDonald, & Broadley, 1995). Expressive language therapy focuses on semantics and on expanding the mean length of utterance and begins to focus on grammatical structures (word order) and word endings (e.g., plurals, possessives) (Fowler, 1990, 1995). Work on conversational skills can be advanced beyond turn taking to increasing the number of conversational turns (MacDonald, 1989). Conversational skills can also be addressed by training parents, teachers, and/or classroom aides how to use prompting to facilitate interactions (Girolametto, Weitzman, & Greenberg, 2003, 2004; Weitzman & Greenberg, 2002). Pragmatics skills such as requests (e.g., asking for help, requesting information, responding to requests) and use of greetings may be addressed.

Often, language and speech are both targeted in intervention programs for individuals with DS (Buckley & Bird, 2001c). The long-term goal of the speech component is to maximize speech intelligibility (Horstmeier, 1988). Short-term goals can target the factors affecting reduced intelligibility for a specific child (e.g., articulation, phonological processes, resonance, prosody, fluency) (Heselwood, Bray, & Crookston, 1995; Kumin, 2001b, 2002b, 2002c; Kumin & Adams, 2000; Rosin & Swift, 1999; Swift & Rosin, 1990). For more details on speech intervention for individuals with DS, see Chapters 4 and 9.

For language therapy, language experience activities such as cooking, crafts, and field trips that are based on a child's experiences are often used to help teach concepts and enhance vocabulary development (Kumin, 1994, 2003; Kumin, Councill, & Goodman, 1996; Kumin et al., 1991). Most language intervention programs provide direct intervention to children with DS. It Takes Two to Talk—The Hanen Program for Parents (Girolametto & Weitzman, 2006) is different, however, in that it works with the important people in a child's environment (but not directly with the child) to modify the environment to facilitate language development and language interactions. This parent training program includes a preprogram assessment, a minimum of 16 hours of parent training in groups of eight families, and three videotaping and feedback sessions (Girolametto & Weitzman, 2006). The program teaches parents strategies to use to promote child-centered language interactions. The program also teaches specific language modeling strategies such as labeling and expanding. There is also an in-service training program for preschool teachers and other early childhood educators (Girolametto & Weitzman, 2006).

Language activities can be planned around an event such as a class trip or a family trip to the bakery. All of the vocabulary for these activities, such as "oven," "bread," and "baker," can be introduced before the trip. Photographs may be used, as visual aids assist learning in individuals with DS. For older children who are reading, a word bank may be developed. On the trip, vocabulary would be reinforced because a child would have the opportunity to see a bread oven, a dough mixer, cookies, a cake, and a cash register. After the trip, the child and the child's speech-language pathologist (SLP) could develop and write a story about the trip.

In subsequent therapy sessions, the SLP and the child might reread the story or act out the trip to the bakery. Semantic therapy that targets concept development can also focus on early school concepts and concepts that are typically tested in educationally based testing programs, such as *in front of–behind, circle–square, top–bottom, forward–backward, over–under–through, first–last, beginning–end, whole–part,* and *front–back.*

Children's books also can be used to develop vocabulary (Kumin, 1994, 2003; Kumin et al., 1996). For example, books related to the autumn season combined with language experience activities (e.g., collecting leaves, crafts projects with leaves, baking cookies shaped like leaves) can be the basis for therapy sessions. The craft activity can be used as a goal-oriented activity with goals for pragmatics (e.g., requesting paint or glue), goals for articulation for the /l/ sound (e.g., leaf, collecting leaves, yellow leaf, say leaf whenever you pick a leaf up), and goals for semantics involving autumn season vocabulary. SLP–family collaboration and a home–school communication system can facilitate concept and vocabulary development (Kumin, 1994, 2003; Kumin et al., 1996; Kumin et al., 1991). The Language is the Key: Constructive Interactions Around Books and Play program focuses on using language facilitation techniques during shared book reading experiences (Cole, Maddox, & Lim, 2006).

Another method for teaching vocabulary is curriculum based. In this approach, the SLP collaborates with the classroom teacher to combine language therapy with the curriculum. For example, if a child's class were working on a unit on weather or the seasons, the vocabulary taught in therapy would be directly related to the concepts taught in the unit (e.g., clouds, rain, winter, cold, snow; Kumin, 2001a). See the following section on the elementary school years for more information on curriculum-based intervention. See Table 8.2 for a summary of intervention areas for individuals with DS in the preschool and kindergarten years.

Elementary School Years

During the elementary school years, a great deal of growth in language and speech is often observed in children with DS. Receptive language therapy should become more detailed and advanced at this stage (Kumin, 2001a; Miller, 1988, 1992), including following directions with multiple parts, similar to the instructions given in school. Receptive language might include comprehension exercises using vocabulary from the language arts, science, or social studies curriculum. Reading activities and experiential activities such as playing language bingo using vocabulary from the curriculum can be helpful. Worksheets are often used for language arts, which targets comprehension of nouns, pronouns, verbs, adverbs, and adjectives. These worksheets are often part of the general education curriculum but may require modifications when used with individuals with DS. Computer software can be used to provide colorful, animated comprehension exercises. Expressive language therapy at this stage focuses on more advanced topics in vocabulary; similarities and differences; morphology; syntax; and increasing a child's mean length of utterance (MLU) through pattern practice, language experience activities, and the use of children's literature. Pacing boards (described later in this chapter), rehearsal, scaffolds, and scripts have been found helpful in facilitating longer speech utterances.

Table 8.2. Assessment and treatment planning for complex language skills

Skills	Preschool and kindergarten	Early elementary	Later elementary	Middle school
Receptive				
Comprehension	X	X	X	X
Vocabulary/concepts	X	X	X	X
Auditory memory	X	X	X	X
Following simple directions	X	X		
Following complex directions		X	X	X
wh- questions		X	X	X
Literacy	X	X	X	
Expressive				
Vocabulary	X	X	X	X
Expanding MLU	X	X	X	
Morphology	X	X	X	X
Syntax	X	X	X	X
Encoding/sentence formulation			X	X
Answering questions	X	X	X	X
Literacy/reading aloud		X	X	X
Pragmatics				
Requests	X	X	X	X
Greetings	X	X		
Social interactive skills	X	X	X	X
Conversational skills	X	X	X	
Advanced conversational skills				X
Topicalization (introducing, maintaining, and changing topic)			X	X
Clarifications and repairs			X	X
Narrative discourse			X	X
School language skills				
Language of the curriculum	X	X	X	X
Language of instruction	X	X	X	X
Language of the hidden curriculum		X	X	X
Language of testing	X	X	X	X
Language of classroom routines	X	X	X	X

Speech-language pathology intervention may involve collaboration with the teacher and may be based in the classroom. Often, the curriculum becomes the material used for therapy. This method for teaching vocabulary is especially useful in the later elementary school grades and as part of an inclusion model because then the material used in therapy teaches and reinforces the material used in the classroom. In the therapy sessions, the vocabulary taught is directly drawn from the various textbooks and workbooks the child may be using in classroom learning. The parts of a plant or the categories of animals, for example, can be included in therapy sessions. Terms that are being taught in the social studies curriculum, such as *revolution, frontier,* and *westward expansion,* can be pretaught in the therapy sessions. For math, the SLP might work on explaining word problems and translating them into simpler vocabulary (Kumin, 2001a). Information on curriculum-based language intervention, collaboration with classroom teachers, and language consultation in the classroom can be applied to facilitate complex language intervention for individuals with DS who are included in general education classrooms. Intervention is a team effort, with the child, teacher, family, special educator, and SLP working together (Montgomery, 1992; Simon, 1991). For individuals with DS in programs focusing on life skills, the "unit" approach might focus on the language and speech used in food shopping and preparation and in housekeeping rather than units on mammals or insects, which might be units of study in the general education class.

In addition to the language of the curriculum, other school-based language skills include the language of instruction, language of the hidden curriculum, language of testing, and the language of classroom routines. The language of instruction focuses on the vocabulary used to teach and learn within the classroom, such as "underline," "which came first," and "place in order, with the most recent first." The language of the hidden curriculum involves what children need to do in a specific class with a specific teacher to be a successful student. The hidden curriculum may include organizational skills, as well as a teacher's expectations. The language of testing involves the child's ability to respond to decontextualized language (i.e., there are no environmental clues on tests; the language stands alone). Classroom routines involve following directions and using appropriate classroom behavior. Difficulties comprehending directions, asking for help, or making a request are sometimes mislabeled as behavior difficulties. The underlying problem should be explored by a behavioral specialist, with input and observation by the SLP, to determine if assistive technology (e.g., picture communication cards, visual schedules and instructions) would help a child respond more appropriately and improve the "behavior" (Kumin, 2001a). Because the language of classroom routines is closely related to classroom behavior, whenever a functional behavioral analysis is done, the SLP should be consulted. It is important to determine whether behavior difficulties are related to a child's communication difficulties. The SLP can provide input to design appropriate positive behavior intervention plans. Curriculum-based intervention and classroom-based service delivery methods are often adapted from intervention strategies designed for individuals with specific language impairment.

Therapy may be proactive, teaching in advance the language skills that the child will need for the curriculum, or reactive, targeting areas of difficulty as they occur and providing assistance with study skills and strategies to meet classroom expectations or to overcome difficulties when they occur. During the elementary school years, speech-language intervention may also be programmed based on linguistic skills—that is, there may be individual goals for semantics (vocabulary), morphosyntax (language structure), pragmatics (social language interaction and conversation), and phonology (sounds of the language). Therapy may also focus on different channels. The goals for therapy may target auditory processing skills, speech and oral-motor skills, or encoding or producing a language message. One channel, such as reading, may be used to assist another channel, such as expressive or written language. The whole language approach, in which reading, understanding, writing, and expressive language are taught holistically, is often based on the literature in the individual's curriculum. Thematic activities are used in conjunction with books (e.g., a book about weather might be used in conjunction with weather reporting, building a weather station, drawing pictures, or taking photographs of different weather conditions). The whole language approach does not teach in discrete linguistic units, such as focusing on plurals or verb tenses. Rather, it teaches in larger themes using meaningful multisensory experiences to teach concepts. The SLP can also suggest adaptive and compensatory strategies, such as being seated in front of the room or using a peer tutor, visual cue sheets, and organizers (Kumin, 2001a). Visual organizers can be successfully used to help individuals with DS with a variety of language needs (Voss, 2006).

Pragmatics becomes very important during this stage; using real-life communication skills at school, at home, and in the community is the goal. Communication demands in elementary school are more complex than they were in preschool, and the child is communicating with many more people during the day. In preschool, children could play side by side, but in elementary school, it is expected that children work well individually and also interact well and collaborate on group projects. Therapy might address social interactive skills with teachers and peers, conversational skills (discourse), how to make requests, how to ask for help when the child does not understand material in school, and how to clarify what the child said when teacher or other students do not understand what the child means (clarifications and repairs). Using classroom facilitators (teachers and aides) and peer facilitators has been effective in improving individuals' conversational skills (Girolametto, 2004; Girolametto et al., 2004). Speech skills with emphasis on articulation and intelligibility also would be targeted in therapy during this period. For more information on speech intervention for school-age children with DS, see Chapter 4.

In later elementary school years, narrative discourse skills, including analyzing and retelling stories or curricular material, become important. Parents frequently report that their later elementary school and middle school children have difficulty retelling what happened at school during the day. Several intervention approaches used for individuals with specific language impairment can be adapted for intervention with older elementary school children with DS. The *Story Grammar Marker* (Moreau, 2006) is an example of a manipulative cuing system that helps children organize their retelling of a story. The *Story Grammar Marker* has items the children can touch to remind them to include the important parts of the story, including characters, setting, initiating event, plan, actions in the plot, and resolution. Although the *Story Grammar Marker* is probably too complicated for most children with DS until at least middle school, the concept of using a manipulative cuing system to assist with narrative discourse is helpful. For a book report, some of the information that a child needs to retell might include title, author, main characters, setting, plot, and ending. When retelling a story, a cuing board can be developed to establish the questions that need to be answered in the retelling, such as *Who? What happened? Where did it happen? When did it happen?* This type of organizer can help a child retell the events of a story. Other therapy materials, such as the *Narrative Toolbox* (Hutson-Nechkash, 2001), can be used in intervention to help children with DS master narrative skills.

Auditory and visual cues can assist children in elementary school in answering questions, speaking, and following directions for class and home assignments.

In the beginning, it may seem awkward or cumbersome to include these cues, but over time it becomes very natural to use them. Those who will be assisting a child in school—whether a classroom aide, a peer buddy, a communication aide, or a classroom volunteer—need training to use these cues, and systematic use of the cues with several individuals is useful (Kumin, 2001a). Some examples of cues include

- *Initial phonemic cues:* Provide the first sound of the word. For example, if you want the child to say "colonial," say "k-k-k" as an initial phonemic cue.

- *Rhyming word cues:* Provide a rhyming cue to help the child remember a word. To cue "phone" say, for example, "Not tone, but ___."

- *Associated word cues:* Provide a word connected in some way by meaning. For example, you might say "pen and _____" to help the child remember "paper." Opposites are often used as cues as well; for example, "up and ___," "cold and _____."

- *Sequential word cues:* Provide a word that would appear in sequence; it may be similar to a fill-in question. To cue "phone," for example, say "Talk on the ___" or "the cell ___."

- *Visual cues:* These can take the form of

  1. Written cues (using the word, part of the word, or the initial consonant sound to provide a print cue)

  2. Picture cues (a picture or photograph associated with the word or a picture of the object)

  3. Icon cues (a symbol that will provide a cue for the word or concept, such as eyes to remind the child to look at the speaker, or the icons used in the *Story Grammar Marker* to remind the child what needs to be included in retelling a story)

  4. Color code cues (color coding the material to be learned in different colors, using colored highlighters or highlighter tape, to assist the child in learning)

- *Gestural cues:* Provide a hand signal or pointing signal that will cue the word or concept, such as holding up a finger for silence or holding up two hands when you need to find your buddy.

- *Initial sound placement cues:* Place the articulator in the position to say the first sound in the word, or point to the articulator.

Middle School Years

The major difference between inclusion in elementary school and middle school is the need in middle school to adjust to different teachers, their expectations, and their teaching styles. An individualized education program (IEP) can include assistance with these tasks. Reading and writing skills need to be sufficient to help a student learn the curriculum material. SLPs can be helpful in consulting or collaborating with the classroom teachers relating to the language used in the classroom. Together they can determine what kinds of adaptations, scaffolds, and learning assistance will enable the adolescent to learn most effectively.

The middle school student must be able to follow teacher instructions that may vary from subject to subject (language of instruction) and must be able to adapt to different expectations of teachers in different subject areas (language of the hidden curriculum). He or she must be able to understand the language used in the classroom and the language of the curriculum, shift language tasks, and decode teachers' cues and other students' cues (Chapman, Schwartz, & Kay-Raining Bird, 1991). The student must be able to succeed with class assignments. And, he or she must be able to ask questions, seek clarification, answer questions, and make repairs. A child in an inclusive setting needs higher level language skills to meet the educational demands of the general curriculum. If this is not possible, alternative goals or skills must be included in the IEP that are appropriate for the student (e.g., the student can be asked to find the state capitals on a map rather than to memorize them).

The teenage years are a time of social growth. Adolescents need to be able to talk about teen topics and to understand idiomatic and abstract language and jokes (Bray & Woolnough, 1988). One focus in therapy during this time may be to practice conversational skills and to role play various social situations. Many interactions during the day are repetitive, such as greetings and social conversations and can be learned and practiced as scripts. Clarity and understandability of speech become more critical for social needs and for preemployment and community activities. See Table 8.2 for a summary of areas that can be addressed in language intervention at the middle school level.

Interventions Directed at Language Domains

In addition to intervention strategies for different ages and stages, intervention should focus on areas of difficulty. Language difficulties have been documented in individuals with DS in the areas of syntax, vocabulary, and pragmatics skills. Because of relative difficulties in syntax among individuals with DS, this section primarily focuses on syntax.

Syntax

In general, individuals with DS have more trouble with morphology (word segments) and syntax (grammar) than with semantics (vocabulary) (Fowler, 1999), and discrepancies increase with age as grammar becomes more complex. Still, individuals with DS learn grammatical structures in the same order as typically developing individuals. Syntax is a difficult area for individuals with DS because it is abstract and complex. Some researchers have shown that individuals with DS reach a period during adolescence in which there is a slowdown in morphosyntactic development and that there is little spontaneous progress beyond that period (Fowler, 1999; Rondal & Edwards, 1997), but others find no evidence of a critical period for syntax development or of a syntactic ceiling (Chapman, Seung, Schwartz, & Kay-Raining Bird, 1998; Thordardottir, Chapman, & Wagner, 2002). Research has found that syntax development continues until at least late adolescence and is not limited to simple syntax (Thordardottir et al., 2002). For more information on syntactic development in individuals with DS, see Kumin (2003).

When individuals consistently use two-word phrases, development progresses in two directions. There is horizontal growth as an individual continues to learn new vocabulary words, and there is also vertical growth as he or she combines known words into longer multiword utterances (Kumin, 2003). Rondal, Ghiotto, Bredart, and Bachelet (1988) found that MLU is highly correlated with chronological age in individuals with DS up to MLU 3, and MLU is a predictor of grammatical complexity from MLU 1–3.5. Most approaches for training assume that children will begin producing multiword utterances after hearing them and modeling them in therapy. Many individuals with DS, however, do not imitate or spontaneously produce multiword utterances without therapeutic intervention. If a child does not begin to produce multiword utterances, then cues or prompts can be used to elicit the specific semantic relation being targeted in the multiword utterance. Contingent imitation, direct drill work, syntactic reduction, modeling and expansion of the child's utterance (imitation with expansion), and parallel talk are all techniques that can be used to encourage a longer MLU.

The pacing board technique (Kumin et al., 1995) provides a multisensory scaffold that can help children imitate a longer utterance, make the transition from imitation to spontaneous production, increase metalinguistic awareness of the number of words in an utterance, and that provides sensorimotor (visual and motor) cues to a child while speaking. The pacing board is a visual representation of the units of language that can be used at the point at which a child has a sign or verbal vocabulary of at least 50 words and is ready to combine those single words into two-word combinations. The pacing board can be used at home and in the classroom, as well as in speech-language pathology sessions. A beginning pacing board for a child consistently using two-word combinations could be one sided, consisting of three dots, or two sided. When a two-sided board is used, one side would have two dots; that side would be used as the child is speaking. The other side would have three dots; that side would be used when the SLP is speaking. (See Figure 8.1 for illustrations of pacing boards.) Written words can be included above the dots, but this would necessitate a separate pacing board for each two-word phrase. The pacing board is expanded as the child's MLU expands; for example, a six-dot pacing board can be used for the child practicing the carrier phrase "May I have some cheese, please?" The child would point to

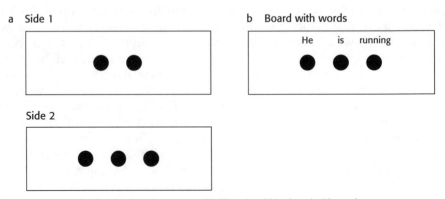

Figure 8.1.   Example of pacing boards: a) a two-sided board and b) a board with words.

each dot as he or she says the word. The pacing board is used with modeling and imitation with expansion by the SLP or parent. In the beginning, the SLP or parent would guide the child's hand to point to the dot as the SLP or parent says the words (e.g., the child says "out now," and the SLP or parent repeats "out now" and expands the phrase to "go out now" as he or she guides the child in pointing to the three dots). The goal is for the child to be able to point to the dots while saying the words him- or herself. The dots serve to cue the child to use the three-word phrase. The pacing board is used as a visual-motor cuing system by the child as he or she encodes phrases and sentences. Pacing boards can be helpful for children with DS because the boards make use of the children's visual strengths.

The process of moving from using single-word to multiword utterances usually takes place from ages 2–8 years in individuals with DS. In a study of 115 individuals with DS, two thirds of the 2-year-olds were not yet combining words, but all of the children were combining words into multiword utterances by age 8 (Kumin, Councill, & Goodman, 1998). In the three-word stage, children are learning to use a variety of semantic and syntactic structures. See Table 8.3 for examples of three-word combinations that can be targeted in intervention. Some specific types of carrier phrases and prepositional phrases can be targeted using specific methodology in intervention.

Carrier phrases consist of words such as "I want____, please" that often occur together in a particular order. They can be taught and then practiced as a unit because children typically use them as a unit in daily conversation. For instance in the phrase "I want cereal, please," the individual words do not have to be retrieved and encoded word by word each time a child wants to use the phrase. Carrier phrases are very useful for children because there is a limited amount of encoding, but carrier phrases transmit a great deal of information. Carrier phrases can be practiced as part of play using models and role playing. A child can go around school or can accompany his or her parents on errands and interview people they meet. While the child is asking questions, he or she is using pattern practice to learn the carrier phrases (Kumin, 2003). A pacing board can be used to provide cues, and the carrier phrase can be written above the dots for individuals who can read (Kumin et al., 1995).

Table 8.3.   Three-word phrases to target in intervention

Phrase structure	Examples
Agent–action–object	Dad throw ball Brother eat pudding
Agent–action–locative	Mom drive away Sister come here
Action–object –locative	Drink milk car Throw apple out
Phrases with prepositions	Put sock on Hide behind tree
Phrases with modifiers	Want more cookie Get my coat
Carrier phrases	I want cheese I see truck

During the stage in which a child is using three-word combinations, he or she usually knows prepositions (at least receptively) and is ready to expand his or her use of prepositional phrases in expressive language. To determine whether the child has receptive and expressive knowledge of prepositions, informal evaluation using motor play on the playground is an effective method. The SLP can observe the child's skill at following verbal directions using motor play and then can ask the child to describe what he or she is doing. In the clinical setting, a motor room setup can be used (Kumin, 2003). If the SLP is able to take photographs of the child at play, they can be used in intervention sessions for MLU expansion activities and work with prepositional phrases. In the two-word period, the child is already using phrases such as "in box" or "under table." In the three-word stage, the phrases can be expanded to "ball in box" and "dog under table." Then, using a pacing board, articles and verbs can be added, such as "The ball is in the box" or "The dog is under the table." Most playgrounds are ideally suited to teaching prepositional phrases. Children can go across the monkey bars, down the slide, under the swing, and up the ladder, and they can describe what they are doing.

Based on clinical experience, the areas of morphosyntax that are especially difficult for individuals with DS are the use of past tense, agreement of pronoun and verb, the use of personal pronouns, active versus passive construction, correct use of negatives and interrogatives, and the use of articles. Once morphosyntax difficulties are identified for a specific child, intervention can target those areas. The methods used for intervention are primarily based on morphosyntactic development in typically developing individuals. Modeling, imitation, and pattern practice techniques are used. The research on phonological processes in individuals with DS has found that the most frequently used phonological process is final consonant deletion (Dodd, 1976; Smith & Stoel-Gammon, 1983; Sommers, Patterson, & Wildgen, 1988; Stoel-Gammon, 1980, 1997). Perhaps that is why past tense, plurals, and possession are not being marked in expressive output. Using correct morphology and being able to formulate appropriate sentences using syntax are skills that are critical for complex language use. The inability to use correct morphosyntax results in short, telegraphic language.

Vocabulary

Although vocabulary is an area of relative strength among individuals with DS, specific areas of vocabulary may need to be targeted in intervention, such as concrete words and labels, basic words, relational words (e.g., time and space terms), categories, convergent/divergent skills, synonyms and antonyms, associated meanings, and subordinate/superordinate words. Being able to use a wide variety of vocabulary words contributes to developing complex language skills. One of the best ways to teach new vocabulary is through real-world experiences. Researchers have found that individuals with DS produced more vocabulary words than typically developing individuals when they were matched by linguistic stage (Rondal, 1978) or MLU (Miller, 1987). Several researchers have matched individuals with DS and typically developing individuals by mental age. In one study, the two groups produced similar levels of different vocabulary words in a language sample (Cardoso-Martins, Mervis, & Mervis, 1985). Another researcher originally found that when individuals with DS were matched with typically developing individuals by mental age, individuals with DS produced fewer different words than typically developing individuals (Miller, 1987), but when they were also matched by socioeconomic status, there were no significant differences (Miller, 1992). In yet another study, the same researcher found that most individuals with DS have smaller vocabularies compared with typically developing individuals matched for mental age but found that 35% percent of the individuals studied with DS had rates of vocabulary growth consistent with mental age (Miller, 1995). A survey of parents of 115 children with DS between the ages of 2 and 5 years (Kumin et al., 1998) using the MacArthur-Bates Communicative Development Inventories (Fenson et al., 1992), found a great deal of variability among individuals, but found that most 5-year-olds could express significantly more words than 2-, 3-, and 4-year-olds.

Pragmatics

Pragmatic therapy addresses social interaction, including conversational skills. Pragmatics is a relative strength for individuals with DS because they have strong communicative intent and good nonverbal social interaction skills. However, individuals with DS often require help in learning and using language strategies for complex conversation (Kumin, 2003; Leifer & Lewis, 1984; Loveland & Tunali, 1991; Miller, 1987; Miller, Leddy, & Leavitt, 1999) and for requesting skills (Duker, van Driel, & van de Bercken, 2002; Mundy, Sigman, Kasari, & Yirmiya, 1988). Although research has shown delays in acquiring conversational skills, young individuals with DS who were matched with typically developing individuals by language level, not chronological age, showed greater response abilities than the typically developing children (Leifer & Lewis, 1984). Pragmatics includes communicative intent, eye contact, facial expression, kinesics, proxemics, requests, conversational skills, topicalization (introducing, maintaining, and changing topics), stylistic variations, contingent queries and repairs, and presuppositions.

Individuals with DS have more difficulty with requesting than with other pragmatic skills (Mundy et al., 1988). Because pragmatics involves social interaction, these skills are best taught in small group therapy sessions. MacDonald (1989) believed that the key to language success is a great deal of practice in social interactions in real situations. Thus, home practice must support the pragmatic skills being worked on in therapy. In teaching pragmatics, role playing, including the use of scripts, simulations, games, and activities, is used.

Questions and Responses

Play activities and reading activities are excellent ways to teach a child to use questions and responses. In school, the child will particularly need to understand *wh-* questions such as *where, why, when,* and *who.* As parents play and read with their child, they can ask the child *wh-* questions. Model the answer—teach, do not test the child. Ask, "Where are your shoes?" and say "On your feet." When reading a book, ask "Where is the car?" and say "In the garage." Many literature books (Kumin, 2003; Kumin et al., 1996) and other published materials that teach about questions and responses focus on *wh-* questions. Another source that can be used for question/answer practice is newspaper sale inserts. They are ideal because they have a similar format but different items from day to day or week to week. Questions such as *what, where, who,* and *when* lend themselves well to practice with newspaper advertising material (Kumin, 2003).

At a simple level, young individuals with DS understand the concept of communicative intent (i.e., the realization that communication brings help and companionship). At the complex language user's level, children with DS are not always successful in communicating their intent through speech. When a child with DS is at a complex language level, the best way to help him or her more clearly formulate intent is to work on requests and communication breakdowns and repairs.

Nonverbal Communication   Individuals with DS often look away from the listener while speaking (Mundy et al., 1988). Usually, this just needs to be brought to an individual's attention, then it can be addressed in therapy and at home and can be improved through practice (Kumin, 2003). Eye contact generally improves when individuals are included in school and the community. Facial expression is usually appropriate in individuals and adults with DS and tends to reinforce the language message. Kinesics, the use of gestures, is not a problem area (Attwood, 1988) for the child in terms of production. Individuals with DS sometimes have difficulty verbalizing what they are feeling or what others are feeling, although they are sensitive to feelings on a nonverbal level. Intervention can help teach the vocabulary of feelings and emotions. Materials designed to be used with individuals with Asperger syndrome who have difficulty with emotions and social skills can be used.

Proxemics, the use of bodily space and distance, is often difficult for individuals with DS (Kumin, 2003). Individuals with DS tend to want to be close to people they meet and to hug them. Once the use of appropriate space is brought into awareness, individuals with DS often are able to modify their behavior. Different cultures, and even people in different areas of the country, may use space differently. This is a skill that will need to be taught based on what is considered appropriate in an individual's local community.

Conversational Skills   Advanced conversational skills are generally learned over time through experience and can be targeted in therapy (Laws & Bishop, 2004a, 2004b). These include initiating the conversation; responding; keeping a conversation going; terminating a conversation; and knowing when to pause, how to interrupt, and how to provide feedback to the speaker. Although research demonstrates that individuals with DS acquire conversational skills at a later age, young individuals with DS who were matched with typically developing individuals by language level demonstrated significantly greater conversational skills than the matched controls (Leifer & Lewis, 1984). Research shows that individuals with DS learn and respond well to social scripts (Loveland & Tunali, 1991). Because many conversational interactions are repeated over and over again in daily life (e.g., greetings, answering a telephone), individuals with DS can learn and practice these skills as social scripts.

Individuals with DS often have very short conversations. They will respond to questions, but often they will not ask any questions to keep the conversation going. They will not continue to take turns to keep the conversation active. Mac-Donald (1989) believes that learning to take enough turns in conversation is one of the areas that is most important for communication success. Conversational length may be related to difficulties in topicalization, vocabulary (semantic), grammatical (syntax), and verbal skills, but turn-taking skills also play a role in the tendency toward short conversations. Often, turn taking and topicalization must be practiced together because they are so intertwined. Areas of topicalization that can be targeted in intervention include choosing a topic, introducing a topic, maintaining a topic, staying on topic, and changing a topic (Kumin, 2001a).

Individuals with DS have difficulty introducing new topics, maintaining a topic, and staying on topic. These difficulties may result from the level of cognitive impairment as well as a lack of conversational experience. When individuals have difficulty maintaining a topic, conversations are short because the individuals do not know what else to say about the topic. And, when individuals have difficulty staying on topic, the conversation may seem rambling, and listeners may lose interest in what is being said.

Clarification and Repairs   The SLP can work with a child to increase awareness of different types of communication breakdown and can suggest how to make various types of repairs. First, however, the speaker or the listener, or both, needs to recognize that a communication breakdown has occurred. There are three general types of requests for more information:

1. Clarification (e.g., "What did you say?")

2. Specification (e.g., "Can you tell me what you mean?")

3. Confirmation (e.g., "Is this what you are saying?")

The speaker will make repairs to provide the information that the listener has requested. Even when the listener does not ask for more information, the speaker can make repairs. Many different types of repairs exist because repairs are very specific to a given situation. Repairs include the ability to

• Recognize when a communication breakdown has occurred

• Understand what caused the breakdown

• Provide the information needed to repair the misunderstanding

To work on communication breakdowns and repairs, barrier games can be used. Abbeduto and Murphy (2004) studied discourse abilities in individuals with DS using a barrier task. In barrier tasks, a physical barrier, such as a portable screen or even a large file folder, is placed between the communicating partners. One provides instructions and the other tries to follow the instructions without any visual cues. Cooking and craft activities lend themselves well to this type of practice. For example, both children—the speaker (#1) and the listener (#2) who is following the directions—are provided with yellow cupcakes; vanilla and chocolate frosting; yellow, pink, and green sprinkles; dark chocolate and white chocolate mini chips; peanuts; and coconut. The speaker needs to provide instructions to the listener regarding how to frost and decorate the cupcakes. The speaker decorates his or her own cupcake while giving the instructions. The listener's responsibility is to follow the instructions and to ask questions if he or she does not understand the instructions. After the decorated cupcakes are finished, the barrier is removed. Then, the SLP and the two children compare the cupcakes. Why doesn't the listener have yellow sprinkles and white chocolate? Why does he have white frosting? The discussion follows the barrier removal and is an important part of the barrier activity.

Abbeduto and Murphy found that the individuals initially had difficulty in considering the informational needs of their listeners but were able to shift over time to more specific descriptions. Barrier games work well to bring listener informational needs into awareness and to help individuals improve their descriptive skills for clarification. Barrier games provide very potent demonstrations of the need for clear directions and the need to ask for information. They are a perfect activity for home–school collaboration because they can easily be practiced at home.

Presuppositions

Presuppositions are the background information a speaker assumes the listener already knows without having to say anything. Young children often have difficulty with presuppositions because young children are egocentric and they do not possess a great deal of language with which to explain things to a listener. Individuals with DS have difficulty with presuppositions and need more practice, coaching, and reminders to learn about what the listener needs to know. School and community inclusion experiences help individuals learn about presuppositions, and the skill continues to develop throughout childhood and can continue to develop into adulthood. Giving directions is one way to practice presuppositions. Loveland, Tunali, McEvoy, and Kelley (1989) found that individuals with DS were able to learn a board game and then teach the rules to another person well. The individuals used gestures and responded to requests for clarification. For older individuals, asking them to describe something that they see through a View-Master device (in which the listeners cannot see what the individuals are seeing) is a good activity.

Social skills and conversational skills usually need to be addressed in intervention for the complex language user. Materials are available that can be used clinically to address this area.

SPEECH AND LANGUAGE INTERVENTION FOR INDIVIDUALS WITH FRAGILE X SYNDROME

Individuals with FXS have a wide variety of speech and language challenges that are affected by coexisting conditions (Abbeduto & Hagerman, 1997; Hagerman, 2000; Hagerman & Cronister, 1996; Hagerman & Hagerman, 2002; Rogers, Wehner, & Hagerman, 2001). The severity of intellectual disability that occurs in most males with FXS, and that can be present in females with FXS, can affect speech and language difficulties. If autism co-occurs with FXS, individuals may have more difficulty in the social and conversational use of language (Bailey, Hatton, & Skinner, 2001; Bailey & Nelson, 1995; Feinstein & Reiss, 1998). If learning disabilities are evident, language organization and executive planning skills can be affected. There have been no studies of evidence-based intervention in individuals with FXS. As in individuals with DS, intervention for individuals with FXS is based on the specific difficulties that the individuals are experiencing, and an individualized comprehensive intervention plan is developed. The methods used to treat individuals with FXS are based on speech and language development in typically developing individuals and speech and language interventions that have been found effective for individuals with other speech and language disorders.

Many individuals with FXS have sensory modulation and sensory integration difficulties (i.e., they have difficulty organizing sensory input from the environment) (Weber, 2000). This may affect the sensory information they receive through hearing, vision, touch, movement, and balance—the channels through which individuals learn language. Sensory processing needs and challenges should be addressed in planning for intervention (Schopmeyer & Lowe, 1992). Males with FXS frequently have difficulty with sensory input and feedback. Hagerman and Hagerman (2002) included tactile defensiveness in their list of FXS characteristics. Occupational therapists (OTs) usually work on sensory processing problems with children with FXS and their families, but there is a need to coordinate the services of the OT and SLP in order for the child to make progress. If the child has difficulty attending to the environment and processing language input, then he or she will have difficulty learning language. In working with individuals with FXS, especially males, sensory processing needs should be addressed. Co-treatment by the OT and SLP that integrates communication and sensory issues has been shown to be effective (Scharfenaker, O'Connor, Stackhouse, Braden, & Gray, 2002).

Some individuals with FXS use sign language or an augmentative and alternative communication system to communicate, but most communicate by using speech. Speech and language development is often severely delayed among individuals with FXS, especially in males. Speech is often difficult to understand because of a rapid rate of speaking, cluttered speech, poor eye contact, and difficulty with staying on topic. Perseveration and echolalia may be present. Speech-language pathology intervention will target the specific areas of communication difficulty for the individual. For many individuals with FXS, intervention materials that have been developed for individuals with autism spectrum disorders or language learning disabilities may be used. A comprehensive evaluation should assess the areas that have been identified as areas of difficulty for individuals with FXS (see Table 8.4). The intervention program may address all or some of the areas, as determined by findings of the evaluation for the individual.

A comprehensive, individually designed intervention program should be developed that will promote functional speech and language skills. This may include oral-sensory, oral-motor, and/or oral-motor planning skills; receptive language skills; expressive language skills; conversational skills; nonverbal communication skills; cluttering; excessive rate; perseveration; and echolalia. The ability to develop complex language use is related to the degree of intellectual disability. Models that coordinate speech-language pathology and occupational therapy interventions include co-treatment, consultation, group intervention, and sequential scheduling (Scharfenaker et al., 2002). The OT can address goals relating to attention, arousal, sensory issues (e.g., tactile defensiveness, hyper and hyposensitivity, postural control, support), and transitions. The SLP can address goals relating to oral sensitivity and oral-motor function, articulation, childhood apraxia of speech, receptive language, expressive language, auditory memory, echolalia, perseveration, rate of speech, prosody of speech, conversational language skills, and narrative discourse skills. The intervention team may include different specialists at different ages and stages of the child's development. A com-

Table 8.4.   Speech and language phenotype of individuals with fragile X syndrome

Males
Delayed onset of expressive language
Syntax difficulty
Relative strength in vocabulary
Receptive-expressive language gap
Childhood apraxia of speech
Cluttering
Poor language organization skills
Reduced speech intelligibility
Fast, uneven rate of speech
Echolalia
Perseveration
Disturbed speech rhythm
Hoarse and breathy voice
Pragmatic difficulties
Difficulty with topic maintenance
Turn-taking difficulties
Females
Speech and language symptoms tend to be milder and may include
   Expressive language difficulties
   Auditory memory difficulties
   Use of tangential language
   Difficulty staying on topic

prehensive language intervention program would involve collaboration among the SLP, OT, special educator or developmental specialist, assistive technology specialist, pediatrician, and family.

The next sections describe interventions to increase receptive and expressive language in individuals with FXS. Because less is known about FXS than DS, the sections are not divided by language domains as in the DS section; rather, they are divided by overall receptive and expressive language. Because the focus of this chapter is on complex language, speech is not discussed. For more information on speech issues in individuals with FXS, see Chapter 6.

Intervention to Increase Receptive Language Skills

Problems with auditory processing are common in males with FXS. This also may be related to attention, so activities that elicit and maintain attention may be helpful. An SLP can assist recall with visual cues or musical cues. Materials that have been developed for individuals with specific language impairment may be useful for auditory processing work. Individuals may have more success answering questions if they can choose from a multiple picture choice, or if questions are phrased in either/or or fill-in modes. Following instructions may be particularly difficult for children with FXS (Lowe, 1992). In school, instructions may need to be given in short units using less complex language, and visual assists such as pictures and photographs may need to be used. *Teaching by Design* (Voss, 2006) is a resource that can help in designing visual material to assist with learning language. Males with FXS have a relatively strong vocabulary, but generalization of information is often difficult (Scharfenaker et al., 2002), especially for males with more severe intellectual disability.

Interventions to Increase Expressive Language Skills

Difficulty with syntax but a relatively strong vocabulary is the typical pattern for individuals with FXS that is cited in the literature (Scharfenaker et al., 2002; Schopmeyer, 1992; Sudhalter, Scarborough, & Cohen, 1991). Some researchers also cite expressive semantics as an area of difficulty (Sudhalter, Maranion, & Brooks, 1992). Many of the same techniques that have been described in the sections on syntax and vocabulary in intervention for individuals with DS can be used for individuals with FXS, but adaptations may be needed based on sensory processing differences. Synonyms, antonyms, associations, analogies, inferences, cause and effect, and proverbs and figurative language can be addressed in intervention for children who are using more complex language. Visual organizers can be helpful in this practice (Voss, 2006). Difficulties with word retrieval and poor sequencing skills may make it difficult for a child with FXS to express him- or herself clearly. Often, the child will rely on automatic phrases to answer direct questions and for conversational turns because of these difficulties.

Conversational skills are often difficult for males with FXS (Newell, Sanborn, & Hagerman, 1983). Difficulties have been found in initiating topics and maintaining topics (Lachiewicz & Mirrett, 2000). Conversation often contains tangential comments, automatic phrases, and perseveration on earlier topics (Madison & Moeschler, 1986; Sudhalter, Cohen, Silverman, & Wolf-Schein, 1990), which interfere with conversational flow and coherence. Role playing and conversational scripts can be used to address these areas in intervention. Topic maintenance can be addressed through games, role-playing activities, and brainstorming activities. Activities such as planning a theme party or developing scrapbooks or special interest books can be used to develop skills in topic maintenance.

Tangential language use affects expressive language and topicalization (Sudhalter & Belser, 2001). Techniques such as conversational recasts can be used to assist a child to master conversational skills (Camarata & Nelson, 2006). Language organization skills can be taught and practiced through activities such as retelling a story, talking about a family vacation or celebration, or using photographs to facilitate sequencing. Materials using written or picture cues can be used to practice conversational skills and discourse skills. A rubric can be developed to remind a child to use precise vocabulary, consider what the listener needs to know (use names, explain who people are), use detail, and discuss the event or story using a clear logical sequence. For younger children, a trip to the supermarket might be a good venue to begin teaching language categorization skills focusing on which foods and products are in which sections of the store. The SLP can point out the bananas, apples, and oranges in the produce section and the Cheerios, Frosted Flakes, and Life in the cereal aisle. Adolescents may enjoy planning a party, taking photographs, and then using the photographs as cues to discuss the party. At any age, food preparation activities using recipes are good ways to teach sequencing and organization. Photographs or lists of steps can be used as aids for retelling the experience. Older children and adolescents can use teen magazines or fan web site information as the basis for discussion when retelling a story.

Social interactive language activities are difficult for many males with FXS because of coexisting social anxiety and sensory modulation difficulties that may contribute to a sensory overload (Belser & Sudhalter, 2001). Social communication skills such as greetings, turn taking, making requests, communication breakdown, making repairs, presuppositions, and topical skills should be addressed in therapy for the complex language user, as these skills have an impact on successful interactions at home, in school, and later in employment settings and in the community. Nonverbal communication skills may be affected in individuals with FXS. Reduced eye contact is common in males with FXS (Cohen, Vietze, Sudhalter, Jenkins, & Brown, 1991). Activities to promote eye contact may include positioning and cuing to remind the child to look people in the eye. Difficulty with turn taking, eye contact, proxemics, and gestures have been identified and can be addressed in intervention.

Excessive verbalization, including perseveration and echolalia, and repetitive speech is a common difficulty among individuals with FXS (Belser & Sudhalter, 2001). Techniques and materials that have been developed for use with individuals with autism spectrum disorders can be used with individuals with FXS who are experiencing similar difficulties.

A small percentage of males with FXS do not develop functional speech. Researchers do not agree on the number; a range from 1%–2% to 10%–15% has been cited in the literature (Lachiewicz & Mirrett, 2000). The need for augmentative and alternative communication systems may be related to childhood apraxia of speech and the subsequent reduced speech intelligibility and/or the severity of intellectual disability. For more information on augmentative and alternative communication system assessment and intervention, see Chapter 11. Assistive technology can also be used to develop visual organizers and schedules in language therapy and to facilitate language learning through specially designed software.

DIRECTIONS FOR RESEARCH

There is a need for research that can result in evidence-based intervention guidelines for individuals with DS and FXS. Very few studies compare intervention methods or evaluate the changes seen with intervention compared with nonintervention for individuals with DS or individuals with FXS. Most of the intervention methods used are those that have been developed for individuals with other language difficulties (e.g., specific language impairment, autism spectrum disorders). The methods are adapted for individuals with DS or FXS who have the same language characteristics (e.g., difficulty staying on topic). For individuals with DS, researchers need to further investigate the relationship among various speech and language skills, including receptive and expressive language, semantics, syntax and pragmatics skills, and phonological processes and morphosyntactic markers. Research should examine the use of pragmatics and conversational abilities in daily living. Few research studies provide evidence-based practice guidelines, and intervention research is needed in all areas of language in order to develop appropriate evidence-based assessment and intervention methods.

For individuals with FXS, there is a need to develop more information on the effects of sensory processing difficulties on receptive and expressive language skills. Assessment methods need to be improved so that co-occurring conditions such as autism spectrum disorders can be identified early and considered in intervention planning. Studies that compare semantics, morphology, and syntax within the same child would provide valuable information. There is very limited information on developmental changes in language in individuals with FXS, and longitudinal studies are needed. Evidence-based assessment and intervention methods also are greatly needed.

CONCLUSION

A body of research exists that describes the speech and language phenotypes for individuals with DS, and studies are increasing in individuals with FXS. Evidence-based research that documents effective intervention strategies or that compares intervention approaches for individuals with DS and FXS who are complex language users are lacking. At present, the best practice is to perform a comprehensive language assessment. Based on test results and family input, a comprehensive, individually designed intervention program can be developed to address a child's communication strengths and needs. Because generalization is often a problem, it is essential to include a two-way home–school/clinic communication plan. The family needs to know the topics and methods being used in therapy sessions so that they can reinforce the learning and provide practice at home. The SLP needs to know about current and upcoming events in the child's life to be able to talk about them in therapy sessions. The SLP also needs to know whether the child is using the skills learned in therapy sessions at home and in the community (i.e., whether the skills are carrying over into daily life). When planning a comprehensive communication intervention program, the child's present needs and future needs should be considered. For younger children, the plan needs to take into account the family's vision for their child's future, and for older children and adolescents, their own vision of their future should be considered.

Speech and language intervention is complex and can include different approaches, a variety of goals, and many different activities for individuals with DS and FXS. The goal is to find intervention approaches and methods that will enable each child with DS and FXS to reach his or her communicative potential.

REFERENCES

Abbeduto, L., & Hagerman, R. (1997). Language and communication in fragile X syndrome. *Mental Retardation and Developmental Disabilities Research Reviews, 7*, 45–55.

Abbeduto, L., & Murphy, M. (2004). Language, social cognition, maladaptive behavior, and communication in Down syndrome and fragile X syndrome. In M.L. Rice & S.F. Warren (Eds.), *Developmental language disorders: From phenotypes to etiologies.* Mahwah, NJ: Lawrence Erlbaum Associates.

Attwood, A. (1988). The understanding and use of interpersonal gestures by autistic and Down's syndrome individuals. *Journal of Autism and Developmental Disorders, 18*, 241–257.

Bailey, D.B., Hatton, D.D., & Skinner, M. (2001). Autistic behavior, FMR1 protein, and developmental trajectories in young males with fragile X syndrome. *Journal of Autism and Developmental Disorders, 31*, 165–174.

Bailey, D.B., & Nelson, D. (1995). The nature and consequences of fragile X syndrome. *Mental Retardation and Developmental Disabilities Research Reviews, 1*, 238–244.

Belser, R.C., & Sudhalter, V. (2001). Conversational characteristics of individuals with fragile X syndrome: Repetitive speech. *American Journal on Mental Retardation, 106*, 28–38.

Berglund, E., Eriksson, M., & Johansson (2001). Parental reports of spoken language skills in individuals with Down syndrome. *Journal of Speech, Language and Hearing Research, 44,* 179–191.

Bray, M., & Woolnough, L. (1988). The language skills of individuals with Down's syndrome aged 12 to 16 years. *Child Language Teaching and Therapy, 4,* 3–11.

Buckley, S. (1993). Language development in individuals with Down's syndrome: Reasons for optimism. *Down's Syndrome: Research and Practice, 1,* 3–9.

Buckley, S. (1995). Teaching individuals with Down syndrome to read and write. In L. Nadel & D. Rosenthal (Eds.), *Down syndrome: Living and learning in the community* (pp. 158–169). New York: Wiley-Liss.

Buckley, S. (1996). *Reading before talking: Learning about mental abilities from individuals with Down's syndrome.* Paper presented at the University of Portsmouth Inaugural Lectures, Portsmouth, United Kingdom.

Buckley, S. (2000). *Speech and language development for individuals with Down syndrome (0–5 years): An overview.* Portsmouth, United Kingdom: The Down Syndrome Educational Trust.

Buckley, S., & Bird, G. (1993). Teaching individuals with Down's syndrome to read. *Down's Syndrome: Research and Practice, 1,* 34–39.

Buckley, S., & Bird, G. (2001a). *Reading and writing development for individuals and infants with Down syndrome (0–5 yrs).* Portsmouth, United Kingdom: The Down Syndrome Educational Trust.

Buckley, S., & Bird, G. (2001b). *Reading and writing development for individuals with Down syndrome (5–11 yrs).* Portsmouth, United Kingdom: The Down Syndrome Educational Trust.

Buckley, S., & Bird, G. (2001c). *Speech and language development in individuals with Down syndrome (5–11 years): An overview.* Portsmouth, United Kingdom: The Down Syndrome Educational Trust.

Camarata, S.M., & Nelson, K.E. (2006). Conversational recast intervention with preschool and older children. In S.F. Warren & M.E. Fey (Series Eds.) & R.J. McCauley & M.E. Fey (Vol. Eds.), *Communication and language intervention series: Treatment of language disorders in children* (pp. 237–264). Baltimore: Paul H. Brookes Publishing Co.

Cardoso-Martins, C., Mervis, C.B., & Mervis, C.A. (1985). Early vocabulary acquisition by individuals with Down syndrome. *American Journal of Mental Deficiency, 90,* 177–184.

Chapman, R.S., & Hesketh, L.J. (2000). Behavioral phenotype of individuals with Down syndrome. *Mental Retardation and Developmental Disabilities Research Reviews, 6,* 84–95.

Chapman, R., Schwartz, S., & Kay-Raining Bird, E. (1991). Language skills of individuals and adolescents with Down syndrome, I: Comprehension. *Journal of Speech and Hearing Research, 34,* 1106–1120.

Chapman, R., Seung, J., Schwartz, S., & Kay-Raining Bird, E. (1998). Language skills of individuals and adolescents with Down syndrome, II: Production deficits. *Journal of Speech, Language and Hearing Research, 41,* 861–873.

Cohen, I.L., Vietze, P.M., Sudhalter, V., Jenkins, E.C., & Brown, W.T. (1991). Effects of age and communication level on eye contact in fragile X males and non-fragile X autistic males. *American Journal of Medical Genetics, 38,* 498–502.

Cole, K.N., Maddox, M., & Lim, Y.S. (2006). Language is the key: Constructive interactions around books and play. In S.F. Warren & M.E. Fey (Series Eds.) & R.J. McCauley & M.E. Fey (Vol. Eds.), *Communication and language intervention series: Treatment of language disorders in children* (pp. 149–173). Baltimore: Paul H. Brookes Publishing Co.

Dodd, B. (1976). A comparison of the phonological systems of mental age matched, normal, severely subnormal and Down's syndrome individuals. *British Journal of Disorders of Communication, 1,* 27–42.

Duker, P.C., van Driel, S., van de Bercken, J. (2002). Communication profiles of individuals with Down's syndrome, Angelman syndrome and pervasive developmental disorder. *Journal of Intellectual Disability Research, 46*(Pt. 1), 35–40.

Feinstein, C., & Reiss, A.L. (1998). Autism: The point of view from fragile X studies. *Journal of Autism and Developmental Disorders, 28,* 499–508.

Fenson, L., Dale, P.S., Reznick, J.S., Thal, D., Bates, E., Hartung, J.P., et al. (1992). *The MacArthur-Bates Communicative Development Inventories.* Baltimore: Paul H. Brookes Publishing Co.

Fowler, A. (1990). Language abilities in individuals with Down syndrome: Evidence for a specific syntactic delay. In D. Cicchetti & M. Beeghly (Eds.), *Individuals with Down syndrome: A developmental perspective* (pp. 302–328). Cambridge: Cambridge University Press.

Fowler, A. (1995). Linguistic variability in persons with Down syndrome. In L. Nadel & D. Rosenthal (Eds.), *Down syndrome: Living and learning in the community* (pp. 121–131). New York: Wiley-Liss.

Fowler, A.E. (1999). The challenge of linguistic mastery in Down syndrome. In T.J. Hassold (Ed.), *Down syndrome: A promising future, together* (pp. 165–182). New York: Wiley-Liss.

Girolametto, L. (2004). Services and programs supporting young individuals' language development. In *Encyclopedia on early childhood development.* Toronto: Center for Excellence for Early Childhood Development.

Girolametto, L., & Weitzman, E. (2006). It Takes Two to Talk—The Hanen Program for Parents: Early language intervention through caregiver training. In S.F. Warren & M.E. Fey (Series Eds.) & R.J. McCauley & M.E. Fey (Vol. Eds.), *Communication and language intervention series: Treatment of language disorders in children* (pp. 77–103). Baltimore: Paul H. Brookes Publishing Co.

Girolametto, L., Weitzman, E., & Greenberg, J. (2003). Training day care staff to facilitate individuals' language. *American Journal of Speech-Language Pathology, 12,* 299–311.

Girolametto, L., Weitzman, E., & Greenberg, J. (2004). The effects of verbal support strategies on small group peer interactions. *Language, Speech, and Hearing Services in Schools, 35,* 254–268.

Hagerman, R.J. (2000). Medical concerns and treatment for individuals with fragile X syndrome. In J.D. Weber (Ed.), *Individuals with fragile X syndrome: A parents' guide* (pp. 93–120). Bethesda, MD: Woodbine House.

Hagerman, R.J., & Cronister, A. (1996). *Fragile X syndrome: Diagnosis, treatment and research* (2nd ed). Baltimore: The Johns Hopkins University Press.

Hagerman, R.J., & Hagerman, P.J. (2002). *Fragile X syndrome: Diagnosis, treatment and research* (3rd ed.). Baltimore: The Johns Hopkins University Press.

Heselwood, B., Bray, M., & Crookston, I. (1995). Juncture, rhythm and planning in the speech of an adult with Down's syndrome. *Clinical Linguistics and Phonetics, 9,* 121–138.

Hopmann, M.R., & Wilen, E. (1993). *Visual and auditory processing in individuals with Down syndrome: Individual differences.* Paper presented at the Society for Research in Child Development, New Orleans.

Horstmeier, D. (1988). "But I don't understand you"—The communication interaction of youth and adults with Down syndrome. In S.M. Pueschel (Ed.), *The young person with Down syndrome* (pp. 53–64). Baltimore: Paul H. Brookes Publishing Co.

Hutson-Nechkash, P. (2001). *Narrative toolbox.* Eau Claire, WI: Thinking Publications.

Jarrold, C., & Baddeley, A.D. (2002). Verbal short-term memory in Down syndrome. *Journal of Speech, Language and Hearing Research, 45,* 531–544.

Jenkins, C. (1993). Expressive language delay in individuals with Down's syndrome: A specific cause for concern. *Down's Syndrome: Research and Practice, 1,* 10–14.

Kanno, K., & Ikeda, Y. (2002). Word length effect in verbal short-term memory in individuals with Down's syndrome. *Journal of Intellectual Disability Research, 46,* 613–618.

Kay-Raining Bird, E., & Chapman, R.S. (1994). Sequential recall in individuals with Down syndrome. *Journal of Speech and Hearing Research, 37,* 1369–1381.

Kumin, L. (1994). *Communication skills in individuals with Down syndrome: A guide for parents.* Bethesda, MD: Woodbine House.

Kumin, L. (1996). Speech and language skills in individuals with Down syndrome. *Mental Retardation and Developmental Disabilities Research Reviews, 2,* 109–116.

Kumin, L. (1999). Comprehensive speech and language treatment for infants, toddlers, and individuals with Down syndrome. In T.J. Hassold & D. Patterson (Eds.), *Down syndrome: A promising future, together* (pp. 145–153). New York: Wiley-Liss.

Kumin, L. (2001a). *Classroom language skills for individuals with Down syndrome: A guide for parents and teachers.* Bethesda, MD: Woodbine House.

Kumin, L. (2001b). Speech intelligibility in individuals with Down syndrome: A framework for targeting specific factors in assessment and treatment. *Down Syndrome Quarterly, 6,* 1–6.

Kumin, L. (2002a). Maximizing speech and language in individuals and adolescents with Down syndrome. In W. Cohen, L. Nadel, & M. Madnick (Eds.), *Down syndrome: Visions for the 21st century* (pp. 403–415). New York: Wiley-Liss.

Kumin, L. (2002b). Why can't you understand what I am saying: Speech intelligibility in daily life. *Disability Solutions,* 5(1),1–15.

Kumin, L. (2002c). You said it just yesterday, why not now? Developmental apraxia of speech in individuals and adults with Down syndrome. *Disability Solutions,* 5(2),1–16.

Kumin, L. (2003). *Early communication skills for individuals with Down syndrome: Guide for parents and teachers.* Bethesda, MD: Woodbine House.

Kumin, L., & Adams, J. (2000). Developmental apraxia of speech and intelligibility in individuals with Down syndrome. *Down Syndrome Quarterly, 5,* 1–6.

Kumin, L., Councill, C., & Goodman, M. (1995). The pacing board: A technique to assist the transition from single word to multiword utterances. *Infant-Toddler Intervention, 5,* 23–29.

Kumin, L., Councill, C., and Goodman, M. (1996). Comprehensive communication intervention for school-aged individuals with Down syndrome. *Down Syndrome Quarterly, 1,* 1–8.

Kumin, L., Councill, C., & Goodman, M. (1998). Expressive vocabulary development in individuals with Down syndrome. *Down Syndrome Quarterly, 3,* 1–7.

Kumin, L., Goodman, M., & Councill, C. (1991). Comprehensive communication intervention for infants and toddlers with Down syndrome. *Infant-Toddler Intervention, 1,* 275–296.

Lachiewicz, A.M., & Mirrett, P.L. (2000). The development of individuals with fragile X syndrome. In J.D. Weber (Ed.), *Individuals with fragile X syndrome* (pp. 199–242). Bethesda, MD: Woodbine House.

Laws, G., & Bishop, D. (2004a). Pragmatic language impairment and social deficits in Williams syndrome: A comparison with Down's syndrome and specific language impairment. *International Journal of Language and Communication Disorders, 39,* 45–64.

Laws, G., & Bishop, D. (2004b). Verbal deficits in Down's syndrome and specific language impairment. *International Journal of Language and Communication Disorders, 39,* 423–451.

Laws, G., Buckley, S.J., Bird, G., MacDonald, J., & Broadley, I. (1995). The influence of reading instruction on language and memory development in individuals with Down's syndrome. *Down's Syndrome Research and Practice, 3,* 59–64.

Leifer, J.S., & Lewis, M. (1984). Acquisition of conversational response skills by young Down syndrome and nonretarded young individuals. *American Journal of Mental Deficiency, 88,* 610–618.

Limongi, S.C.O., & Carvallo R.M.M. (2000). Auditory processing and language in Down syndrome. *Journal of Medical Speech-Language Pathology,* 8(1), 27–34.

Loveland, K.A., & Tunali, B. (1991). Social scripts for conversational interactions in autism and Down syndrome. *Journal of Autism and Developmental Disorders, 21,* 177–186.

Loveland, K.A., Tunali, B., McEvoy, R.E., & Kelley, M. (1989). Referential communication and response adequacy in autism and Down's syndrome. *Applied Psycholinguistics, 10,* 301–313.

Lowe, F. (1992). Speech and language therapy with the fragile X child. In B. Schopmeyer & F. Lowe (Eds.), *The fragile X child* (pp. 173–195). San Diego: Singular Publishing Group.

MacDonald, J. (1989). *Becoming partners with children: From play to conversation.* Chicago: Riverside.

Madison, L.C., & Moeschler, J. (1986). Cognitive functioning in the fragile X syndrome: A study of intellectual memory and communication skills. *Journal of Mental Deficiency Research, 30,* 129–148.

Miller, J.F. (1987). Language and communication characteristics of individuals with Down syndrome. In S.M. Pueschel, J.E. Rynders, A.C. Crocker, & D.M. Crutcher (Eds.), *New perspectives in Down syndrome* (pp. 233–262). Baltimore: Paul H. Brookes Publishing Co.

Miller, J.F. (1988). Developmental asynchrony of language development in individuals with Down syndrome. In L. Nadel (Ed.), *Psychobiology of Down syndrome* (pp. 167–198). New York: Academic Press.

Miller, J.F. (1992). Lexical development in young individuals with Down syndrome. In R. Chapman (Ed.), *Processes in language acquisition and disorders* (pp. 202–216). St. Louis: Mosby Year Book.

Miller, J.F. (1995). Individual differences in vocabulary acquisition in individuals with Down Syndrome. *Progress in Clinical and Biological Research, 393,* 93–103.

Miller, J.F., Leddy, M., & Leavitt, L.A. (Eds.). (1999). *Improving the communication of people with Down syndrome.* Baltimore: Paul H. Brookes Publishing Co.

Miller, J.F., Leddy, M., Miolo, G., & Sedey, A. (1995). The development of early language skills in individuals with Down syndrome. In L. Nadel & D. Rosenthal (Eds.), *Down syndrome: Living and learning in the community* (pp. 115–119). New York: Wiley-Liss.

Montgomery, J.K. (1992). Perspectives from the field. *Language, Speech and Hearing Services in Schools, 23,* 363–364.

Moreau, M. (2006). *Story grammar marker.* Greenville, SC: SuperDuper.

Mundy, P., Sigman, M., Kasari, C., & Yirmiya, N. (1988). Nonverbal communication skills in Down syndrome individuals. *Child Development, 59,* 235–249.

Newell, K., Sanborn, B., & Hagerman, R. (1983). Speech and language dysfunction in the fragile X syndrome. In R.J. Hagerman & P. McBogg (Eds.), *The fragile X syndrome: Diagnosis, biochemistry, and intervention* (pp. 175–200). Denver, CO: Spectra.

Rice, M.L., Warren, S.F., & Betz, S.K. (2005). Language symptoms of developmental language disorders: An overview of autism, Down syndrome, fragile X, specific language impairment, and Williams syndrome. *Applied Psycholinguistics, 26,* 7–27.

Rogers, S.J., Wehner, D.E., & Hagerman, R. (2001). The behavioral phenotype in fragile X: Symptoms of autism in very young individuals with fragile X syndrome, idiopathic autism, and other developmental disorders. *Journal of Developmental Pediatrics, 22,* 409–417.

Rondal, J.A. (1978). Maternal speech to normal and Down's syndrome individuals matched for mean length of utterance. In C.E. Myers (Ed.), *Quality of life in severely and profoundly mentally retarded people: Research foundations for improvement* (pp. 193–265). Washington, DC: American Association on Mental Deficiency.

Rondal, J.A., & Edwards, S. (1997). *Language in mental retardation.* London: Whurr.

Rondal, J.A., Ghiotto, M., Bredart, S., & Bachelet, J.F. (1988). Mean length of utterance of individuals with Down syndrome. *American Journal on Mental Retardation, 93,* 64–66.

Rosin, P., & Swift, E. (1999). Communication interventions: Improving the speech intelligibility of children with Down syndrome. In J.F. Miller, M. Leddy, & L.A. Leavitt (Eds.), *Improving the communication of people with Down syndrome* (pp. 133–159). Baltimore: Paul H. Brookes Publishing Co.

Scharfenaker, S., O'Connor, R., Stackhouse, T., Braden, M., & Gray, K. (2002). An integrated approach to intervention. In R.J. Hagerman & P.J. Hagerman (Eds.), *Fragile X syndrome: Diagnosis, treatment and research* (3rd ed., pp. 363–427). Baltimore: The Johns Hopkins University Press.

Schopmeyer, B. (1992). Speech and language characteristics in Fragile X syndrome. In B. Schopmeyer & F. Lowe (Eds.), *The fragile X child* (pp. 71–90). San Diego: Singular Publishing Group.

Schopmeyer, B., & Lowe, F. (1992). *The fragile X child.* San Diego: Singular Publishing Group.

Simon, C. (1991). *Communication skills and classroom success: Therapy methodologies for language learning disabled students.* San Diego: College-Hill Press.

Smith, B.L., & Stoel-Gammon, C. (1983). A longitudinal study of the development of stop consonant production in normal and Down's syndrome individuals. *Journal of Speech and Hearing Disorders, 48,* 114–118.

Sommers, R.K., Patterson, J.P., & Wildgen, P.L. (1988). Phonology of Down syndrome speakers, ages 13–22. *Journal of Childhood Communication Disorders, 12,* 65–91.

Stoel-Gammon, C. (1980). Phonological analysis of four Down's syndrome individuals. *Applied Psycholinguistics, 1,* 31–48.

Stoel-Gammon, C. (1997). Phonological development in Down syndrome. *Mental Retardation and Developmental Disabilities Research Reviews, 3,* 300–306.

Sudhalter, V., & Belser, R.C. (2001). Conversational characteristics of individuals with fragile X syndrome: Tangential language. *American Journal on Mental Retardation, 106,* 389–400.

Sudhalter, V., Cohen, I., Silverman, W., & Wolf-Schein, E. (1990). Conversational analyses of males with fragile X, Down syndrome and autism: Comparison of the emergence of deviant language. *American Journal of Mental Retardation, 94,* 431–441.

Sudhalter, V., Maranion, M., & Brooks, P. (1992). Expressive semantic deficit in the productive language of males with fragile X syndrome. *American Journal of Medical Genetics, 43*, 65–71.

Sudhalter, V., Scarborough, H., & Cohen, I.L. (1991). Syntactic delay and pragmatic deviance in the language of fragile X males. *American Journal of Medical Genetics, 38*, 493–497.

Swift, E., & Rosin, P. (1990). A remediation sequence to improve speech intelligibility for students with Down syndrome. *Language, Speech and Hearing Services in Schools, 21*, 140–146.

Thordardottir, E.T., Chapman, R.S., & Wagner, L. (2002). Complex sentence production by adolescents with Down syndrome. *Applied Psycholinguistics, 23*, 163–183.

Voss, K. (2006). *Teaching by design.* Bethesda, MD: Woodbine House.

Weber, J.D. (Ed.). (2000). *Individuals with fragile X syndrome: A parent's guide.* Bethesda, MD: Woodbine House.

Weitzman, E., & Greenberg, J. (2002). *Learning language and loving it: A guide to promoting individuals' language and literacy development in early childhood settings* (2nd ed.). Toronto: The Hanen Centre.

CHAPTER 9

Increasing Speech Intelligibility in Down Syndrome and Fragile X Syndrome

JOHANNA R. PRICE AND RAY D. KENT

S peech intelligibility is often considered the most important indicator of communicative competence (Kent, Miolo, & Bloedel, 1994; Subtenly, 1977). Comments on reduced speech intelligibility are frequently encountered in clinical reports and research articles on Down syndrome (DS) and fragile X syndrome (FXS; Abbeduto & Chapman, 2005; Kumin, 1994; Rosin, Swift, Bless, & Vetter, 1988; Spinelli, Rocha, Giacheti, & Richieri-Costa, 1995). This chapter explores the general topic of intelligibility, including methods of measurement, and then reviews the literature on speech intelligibility in children with DS or FXS.

INTRODUCTION

Several related terms have been used in respect to the capability of listeners to understand a talker. *Intelligibility* is the extent to which a listener can receive the message intended by a sender. Similarly, Schiavetti (1992) defined intelligibility as "the match between the intention of the speaker and the response of the listener to the speech passed through the transmission system" (p. 13). It is important to note that speech intelligibility can take on somewhat different connotations in different applications, such as with the effects of hearing loss (in which auditory impairment is the major obstacle to intelligibility), the influence of transmission systems (in which channel bandwidth and noise are typically of major concern), and the consequences of speech-language disorders or language differences (in which characteristics of the speaker are of paramount importance). In these various applications of the construct of intelligibility, it is recognized that intelligibility is not an absolute quantity. Rather, it is a relative measure that is a function of multiple parameters including talkers, test material, judges, training (or familiarity), and testing procedures (Flanagan, 1972; Grant & Seitz, 2000; Kent, Weismer,

This work was supported in part by Research Grant 5 R01 DC 00319 from the National Institute on Deafness and Other Communication Disorders, Training Grant T32-HD40127 from the National Institute of Child Health and Human Development, and the Charles J. Epstein Award from the National Down Syndrome Society.

Kent, & Rosenbek, 1989). To think of intelligibility as an absolute measure can be misleading. Nonetheless, there is a clinical need for a measure of intelligibility that has a certain degree of cross-listener and cross-environment coherence. This is a fundamental challenge of clinical intelligibility assessment.

Comprehensibility is a measure of message content received by a listener, which embraces the entire communicative environment, including acoustic signal, familiarity with the message and speaker, gestures and signs, topic knowledge, interfering factors (noise, reverberation), and lighting (Barefoot, Bochner, Johnson, & vom Eigen, 1993; Yorkston, Strand, & Kennedy, 1996). The distinction between *intelligibility* and *comprehensibility* is somewhat blurred, given that classic and contemporary studies of intelligibility have included some of the same factors that are used to define comprehensibility.

Efficiency is typically assessed as the rate of either intelligible or comprehensible speech, with rate being measured in units such as intelligible words per minute (Yorkston & Beukelman, 1981). Accordingly, a measure of efficiency depends on a prior measure of either intelligibility or comprehensibility. It should be noted that any given measurement of efficiency (e.g., 30 words per minute) does not distinguish a slow but intelligible talker (e.g., a person who produces 30 words in one minute, with all words intelligible) from a faster but relatively unintelligible talker (e.g., a person who produces 200 words in one minute, but only 30 of them are identifiable). When a measure of efficiency is accompanied by a measure of fail rate (number of words correctly identified out of total words attempted), a more accurate assessment of communicative capacity is achieved.

The ambiguity in terminology is accompanied by differences in approach to measurement. No single measure of intelligibility is a "gold standard" against which all others can be compared. The ultimate choice of a measure depends on the goal of measurement, time and environmental limitations, and characteristics of the speaker. (For a general discussion of issues in testing the speech intelligibility of children, see Kent et al., 1994.)

METHODS FOR THE MEASUREMENT OF SPEECH INTELLIGIBILITY

Whenever intelligibility is to be assessed or treated, an immediate question arises: What method should be used to measure a talker's intelligibility? Several possibilities are discussed in this section.

Rating Scales

Rating scales have widespread application, and they take several different forms. One of the most common rating scales is the Likert scale, which is often used to gauge an attitude or perception. An example of this is

• Statement: This course presented a great amount of new information.

• Response choices

   Strongly disagree

   Somewhat disagree

   Somewhat agree

   Strongly agree

Rating scales are used for various purposes, including surveys of products and services, judging the intensity of pain (often with "pain face" scales in which different facial expressions are selected to represent the degree of pain that a person feels), and estimating the quality or quantity of a certain stimulus. It is the last of these that is most relevant here. Whether the intelligibility of speech is considered a quality or a quantity, it can be rated by listeners with a scale like the one shown next.

1. The person's speech is completely unintelligible.

2. The person's speech is mostly unintelligible.

3. The person's speech is occasionally unintelligible.

4. The person's speech is mostly intelligible.

5. The person's speech is completely intelligible.

Simple rating scales of this kind often have been used to rate intelligibility for clinical or research purposes, and data derived from this method make up a large part of the published data on intelligibility across the spectrum of speech-language disorders. Because rating scales have both strengths and limitations, it is important to discuss these scales and how they have been applied to the task of intelligibility assessment. If it is assumed in the example just given that the five response choices represent equal distances in perceptual judgment, then the scale can be considered to be an *equal-appearing interval scale* (EAIS).

The procedure for EAIS is that a listener assigns "a number to each stimulus sample in order to place the stimulus along a linear partition of the continuum to be scaled" (Schiavetti, 1992, p. 19). The most common partitions are 5- or 7-point scales, but 9- or 11-point scales probably are preferable to attain maximum sensitivity. As shown in the example just given, a popular scale for intelligibility is a 5-point scale in which the end-point descriptors are 1 = *Speech is completely unintelligible* and 5 = *Speech is completely intelligible.* Schiavetti (1992) concluded that though this kind of scale is used more frequently than any other scale in intelligibility studies, EAIS is a quantitative measure and is not an appropriate scaling method for the qualitative construct of speech intelligibility.

In *direct magnitude estimation* (DME), listeners assign to each stimulus sample a number that is proportional to the perceived ratios of all of the stimuli to be judged. The procedure has two major variants, depending on whether a modulus (standard) is used. In free-modulus DME, the listener is free to assign any number to the first stimulus sample to be judged. Subsequent stimulus samples are assigned numbers that correspond to the ratios of the perceived magnitudes of the samples. In the other variant, the listener assigns a number to each stimulus sample relative to a standard sample that the experimenter defines as a modulus or standard subjective value. For example, the experimenter may select a stimulus from the middle of the stimulus range to be judged and assign to it a modulus of 100. The listener would then scale all stimuli relative to that modulus. As noted previously, Schiavetti (1992) concluded that speech intelligibility is a qualitative dimension, for which DME is preferred over EAIS as a scaling procedure.

The *visual analog scale* (VAS) is designed to present to the rater a rating scale with minimal constraints. The scale is simply a straight line of specified length, with verbal descriptors at each end. The line is usually 100 mm long and may be either vertical or horizontal. Listeners are asked to place a mark on the line to report their judgment of the speaker's intelligibility. Verbal descriptors may be *Not intelligible at all* at one end and *Completely intelligible* at the other end. VAS is frequently used in health care research for purposes such as scaling of pain.

Transcription Tests

In the usual application of the transcription test method, one or more listeners transcribe the words (or less commonly, the phonetic sequences) produced by a talker. The speech material can take several forms, including single words, reading passages, sentence lists, or conversation. Single words are typically taken as the unit of analysis so that intelligibility can be scored as the percentage of words correctly identified by the listener(s). This method can be problematic with some conversational samples in which the talker's intent is not known. That is, when a talker has low intelligibility, it can be very difficult to know what words were intended. For this reason, transcription tests are most successful when used with known speech samples, such as passage reading.

Single-word intelligibility tests use one or more sets of words that the talker is asked to produce. Usually, recordings of the words are presented to listeners who try to identify the words. Various criteria can be used in construction of the word lists. For example, words can be chosen to represent different syllable lengths (e.g., one-, two-, or three-syllable words), or words can be selected according to phonetic criteria (e.g., to be sure that certain phonetic contrasts are represented). One advantage of this type of test is that it can be used with individuals across a fairly wide range of speech production capability, including talkers who may be limited to very short utterances. The Preschool Speech Intelligibility Measure (PSIM) is a single-word, multiple-choice intelligibility measure developed by Morris, Wilcox, and Schooling (1995) based on an intelligibility test developed for adults with dysarthria (Yorkston & Beukelman, 1981). More recently, Hodge and Daniels (2005) introduced the Test of Children's Speech Plus (TOCS+), which includes software to record, play back, judge, and analyze speech recordings to measure children's speech intelligibility at the word and sentence level. (For detailed information on this software, visit http://www.tocs.plus.ualberta.ca.)

Sentence intelligibility tests have also been constructed. Considerations include the length of sentences, syntactic structure and vocabulary, and how an intelligibility measure will be derived (e.g., by transcription of the entire sentence, by identification of a target word embedded in the sentence, by determining if listeners get the meaning of the sentence). Sentences offer the advantage of control over the linguistic and phonetic properties of the test utterances, and they also afford the opportunity to examine multisyllabic patterns, with potential manipulation of speaking rate and some aspects of prosody. Prosody is also known by the term *suprasegmentals*. As the name suggests, suprasegmentals are properties of speech that extend across the segmental boundaries of vowels and consonants. Prosodic features include intonation (pitch rises and falls) and the pattern of stress across utterances. The way in which a speaker controls these prosodic features can affect the quality and intelligibility of speech. But care should be taken that the sentences do not exceed the cognitive, linguistic, and motoric capabilities of the individual to be examined.

Conversation may lend itself to more valuable results than other kinds of tests because it is most similar to ordinary speaking situations. Scoring of intelligibility, however, necessarily rests on the assumption that the speaker's message is known. For severely unintelligible speakers, this assumption may not be satisfied. A typical approach in determining the intelligibility is for listeners to write the words that they hear (glossing). Intelligibility can be scored as the number of words correctly identified, the number of consonants correctly produced, or some other measure.

General Remarks

No matter what approach is used to measure speech intelligibility, it is virtually inevitable that any measurement is a joint product of at least four primary factors: the speaker, the message, the transmitting environment, and the listener. It is no surprise, then, that concerns about validity and reliability have plagued the study of intelligibility. As noted previously, no gold standard exists; that is, there is no intelligibility test that meets with universal acceptance and is free from contaminating or biasing factors. For all its importance in clinical practice and in everyday discourse, intelligibility defies measurement that is efficient, unquestionably valid, and reliable within and across judges. This dismaying conclusion is not a statement of futility but rather a caution to be recognized in any effort to put a number on how well a talker is understood by one or more listeners.

To gain a better understanding of the properties of speech with varying degrees of intelligibility, efforts have been made to determine the acoustic correlates of speech intelligibility. Research on intrinsic intelligibility differences among individual talkers points to some general relationships between acoustic measures and talker intelligibility. Bradlow, Torretta, and Pisoni (1996) concluded that intelligibility does not correlate with global characteristics such as speaking rate and average pitch but does correlate with fine-grained acoustic characteristics relating to formant patterns and pitch change. In a study of normally speaking adult and child talkers, Hazan and Markham (2004) reported that although some correlates of intelligibility can be identified, it appears that high levels of intelligibility can be achieved through a combination of different acoustic-phonetic characteristics. The inverse of Hazan and Markham's conclusion is probably true as well: Low levels of intelligibility can be related to different combinations of acoustic-phonetic characteristics. Nonetheless, it is possible that fairly reliable combinations of acoustic-phonetic characteristics can be identified for well-defined clinical groups, such as those of primary interest in this book. Particularly if certain anatomic or motor control impairments are common to individuals with clinical syndromes, then particular patterns of acoustic-phonetic features may be typical. In fact, overlapping and generally confirmatory results have been reported in studies of dysarthria that have established fine-grained acoustic characteristics relating to differences in speaker intelligibility and/or severity of speech disorder (Kent et al., 1989; Turner, Tjaden, & Weismer, 1995; Weismer, Jeng, Laures, Kent, & Kent, 2001; Weismer & Martin, 1992).

INTELLIGIBILITY IN DOWN SYNDROME AND FRAGILE X SYNDROME

Decreased intelligibility appears to be a significant problem for children with DS and FXS. Children with DS demonstrate lower levels of speech intelligibility than mental age–matched control groups of typically developing children and children with intellectual disability of unknown etiology (Abbeduto & Murphy, 2004; Rosin et al., 1988). In a survey of 937 parents of individuals with DS, Kumin (1994) reported that more than 95% of parents indicated that their children frequently or sometimes had difficulty being understood. Little research has directly investigated speech intelligibility in children with FXS; however, reduced intelligibility has been noted by a number of authors (Abbeduto & Chapman, 2005; Abbeduto & Hagerman, 1997; Lachiewicz & Mirrett, 2000; Madison, George, & Moeschler, 1986; Paul, Cohen, Breg, Watson, & Herman, 1984; Rice, Warren, & Betz, 2005; Spinelli et al., 1995).

Given that research on speech intelligibility in DS and FXS is rather limited, information presented in this chapter also draws from literature on related populations, such as individuals with unspecified types of intellectual disability and individuals with developmental apraxia of speech. The speech of children and adults with intellectual disability may be unintelligible and has been described as slurred and indistinct, with a lack of articulatory precision, inappropriate pauses, inconsistent errors, and high rates of deletion errors (Shriberg & Widder, 1990; Weiss, Gordon, & Lillywhite, 1987). Developmental apraxia of speech, a disorder in which motor planning for speech is impaired, can also result in unintelligible speech and is characterized by difficulty sequencing sounds, persistent and inconsistent speech errors, and inappropriate use of stress (Shriberg, Aram, & Kwiatkowski, 1997; Velleman, 2003).

Speech Intelligibility Treatment in Down Syndrome

Biological characteristics and cognitive characteristics—including oral-motor impairments, hypotonicity, impairment in fine motor coordination, chronic otitis media, difficulty planning motor sequences, general cognitive delay, and a specific linguistic impairment—have been hypothesized to contribute to decreased intelligibility in individuals with DS (Dodd, McCormack, & Woodyatt, 1994; Kumin & Adams, 2000; Leddy, 1999; Miller, 1988; Miller & Leddy, 1999; Stoel-Gammon, 2003). A variety of approaches have been recommended to increase speech intelligibility in children with DS, ranging from surgical intervention to phonological treatment. The effectiveness of only some of these approaches, however, is supported by empirical data.

Tongue reduction surgery has been performed on hundreds of children with DS, as noted by Swift and Rosin (1990). Investigations of children's pre- and post-surgery speech production do not support the use of this approach to increase children's speech intelligibility. In one study (Parsons, Iacono, & Rozner, 1987), the phonological skills of nine children with DS were assessed pre- and postoperatively and 6 months after surgery; however, the number of errors in consonant production was not significantly different across the three assessment points. In addition, when the study participants' production of consonants was compared with that of a group of nine children with DS who had not undergone surgery, no differences were found. In a similar vein, randomized pre- and post-operative samples of words and connected speech of children with DS who had undergone partial glossectomies were judged for intelligibility, and no significant differences in intelligibility were found pre- and postoperatively (Klaiman, Witzel, Margar-Bacal, & Munro, 1988; Margar-Bacal, Witzel, & Munro, 1987).

Several authors have recommended exercises for children with DS to strengthen oral muscles used in the production of speech (Kumin, 2003; Kumin,

Councill, & Goodman, 1994; Rosin & Swift, 1999; Swift & Rosin, 1990; Yarter, 1980). For example, Kumin and colleagues suggested techniques such as lip massage and bubble and whistle blowing to strengthen the facial muscles used in speech production. Swift and Rosin suggested using tubes to practice sucking, tongue resistance work to increase tongue strength and awareness, and bite blocks to increase jaw stabilization. No empirical evidence exists, however, to demonstrate that oral-motor techniques improve speech intelligibility.

Others have suggested that treating hearing loss associated with otitis media, a condition that frequently occurs in children with DS, may improve intelligibility (Balkany, 1980; Downs, 1980; Kumin, 2003; Roizen, 2001; Rosin & Swift, 1999). The use of tubes, low-amplification hearing aids, and medication for otitis media have been recommended. Though no evidence directly links the treatment of hearing loss to improved speech intelligibility in children with DS, Chapman, Seung, Schwartz, and Kay-Raining Bird (2000) found that hearing status directly affected the intelligibility of individuals with DS.

Palatal plate therapy has been recommended for children with DS whose speech intelligibility is negatively influenced by hypernasality (Swift & Rosin, 1990). Carlstedt, Henningsson, and Dahllof (2003) reported that articulation of neither consonants nor vowels was significantly different for a group of nine children with DS who had received palatal plate therapy for 4 years compared with a control group of 11 children with DS. Kumin (2003) suggested exercises to strengthen palatal muscles to decrease hypernasality and exercises to strengthen the adductor muscles to reduce breathiness. Because hypernasality and breathiness can contribute to reduced intelligibility, these exercises have the potential to improve intelligibility.

Phonological approaches to speech intelligibility treatment have been widely recommended (Cholmain, 1994; Dodd et al., 1994; Dodd & Thompson, 2001; Kumin, 2003; Rosin & Swift, 1999). Only two treatment studies have been reported in the literature, and both have indicated that a phonological approach positively affects intelligibility. In the first study (Cholmain, 1994), parents of six 4- and 5-year-olds with DS implemented therapy focused on phonological processes with their children for 6–14 weeks. Parents read selected word lists using amplification, and children practiced producing target words and sounds. All children demonstrated growth in phonological skills, as well as in grammatical skills. The percentage of consonants correctly produced ranged from 19% to 88% posttreatment, compared with 3%–38% prior to intervention. In the second study (Dodd et al., 1994), nine children with DS ranging in age from 2 to 6 years old, whose language levels ranged from nonverbal to multiword utterances, participated in a 12-week parent-directed treatment program focused on reducing variability in word productions. Parents were trained to accept as correct only one pronunciation of each word in a set of core vocabulary words selected for each child. Children's productions could contain developmental but not deviant errors. In general, the children demonstrated improved intelligibility posttreatment; they produced fewer developmental and deviant errors and fewer inconsistent productions.

Speech Intelligibility Treatment in Fragile X Syndrome

The speech of males with FXS has been reported as being difficult to understand, particularly in conversation (Lachiewicz & Mirrett, 2000; Madison et al., 1986;

Paul et al., 1984; Scharfenaker, O'Connor, Stackhouse, Braden, & Gray, 2002; Spinelli et al., 1995). This decreased speech intelligibility may be associated with a variety of factors. Common phonological difficulties include consonant substitutions, omissions, and distortions, though phonological errors are similar to those of younger mental age matches (Abbeduto & Hagerman, 1997; Hanson, Jackson, & Hagerman, 1986; Newell, Sanborn, & Hagerman, 1983; Roberts et al., 2005). The speech rate of males with FXS has been described as variable, shifting from rapid to slower rates, and may contribute to difficulties with intelligibility (Borghgraef, Frons, Dielkens, Pyck, & Van Den Berghe, 1987; Hanson et al., 1986; Lachiewicz & Mirrett, 2000; Spinelli et al., 1995). Belser and Sudhalter (2001) suggested that the pattern of accelerated speech is often accompanied by increased repetitive dysfluencies. Hypotonia of the oral mechanism has also been documented in males with FXS and may contribute to decreased intelligibility (Hagerman, 2002; Lachiewicz & Mirrett, 2000). Finally, it has been hypothesized that verbal dyspraxia may underlie the speech difficulties of some children with FXS (Lachiewicz & Mirrett, 2000; Paul et al., 1984; Spinelli et al., 1995).

As noted earlier in this chapter, intelligibility is jointly determined by speaker, transmission channel, and listener. When listening to atypical speech, the listener may compensate or adapt in various ways. For instance, variations in speaking rate have an effect on the way a listener categorizes phonetic and lexical stimuli (Miller & Volaitis, 1989; Sommers, Nygaard, & Pisoni, 1994). Therefore, changes in speaking rate, as are thought to occur in FXS, may cause listeners to alter their phonetic interpretation of acoustic cues. Particularly if the changes in speaking rate occur in a larger context of phonological errors, listeners may find it difficult to establish stable perceptual criteria for processing of the speech signal.

To our knowledge, no intervention studies for improving speech intelligibility in children with FXS have been conducted. Scharfenaker and colleagues (2002), however, suggested that therapy to reduce rate, normalize the rhythm of speech, and improve oral-motor functioning may increase intelligibility.

Other Approaches to Increase Speech Intelligibility

Hodson (1989) recommended a modified cycles approach to increase speech intelligibility in children with intellectual disability. In the cycles approach (Hodson & Paden, 1991), phonological patterns are targeted in cycles lasting from 6 to 18 hours. Error patterns are selected according to a developmental sequence, targeting primary patterns (e.g., syllableness, anterior/posterior contrasts, /s/ clusters) first, then secondary patterns (e.g., voicing contrasts, vowel contrasts, palatal sibilants), and finally advanced patterns (e.g., complex consonant sequences, multisyllabic words). The cycles approach also includes auditory bombardment, in which the child listens to words containing the target pattern slightly amplified. For children with intellectual disability, Hodson (1989) recommended modifying the cycles approach by doubling the duration of each cycle. She also cautioned that 3 or more years of treatment may be needed in order to increase intelligibility, though no efficacy data are provided. In addition, Shriberg and Widder (1990) suggested that intervention focus on improving articulatory precision and normalizing prosody to improve intelligibility in individuals with intellectual disability.

Because many children with FXS demonstrate characteristics of autism (Hagerman 2002), techniques used to increase intelligibility in children with autism may also be useful for children with FXS. In a study of five children with autism ages 3–7 years who had poor speech intelligibility, Koegel, Camarata, Koegel, Ben-Tall, and Smith (1998) compared the outcomes of a drill-based "analog" phonological intervention with a play-based "naturalistic" phonological intervention that incorporated social and natural reinforcers. Only the naturalistic intervention resulted in increased correct production of target phonemes in conversation and increased intelligibility levels, as rated by blind listeners. Such play-based, naturalistic phonological interventions may also be appropriate for children with FXS.

Some literature suggests that many children with FXS (Lachiewicz & Mirrett, 2000; Paul et al., 1984; Spinelli et al., 1995) or DS (Kumin, 2006; Kumin & Adams, 2000) have characteristics of developmental apraxia of speech or difficulty with oral-motor skills. Techniques used to increase intelligibility in developmental apraxia of speech may prove beneficial for these populations; there are, however, almost no efficacy data for this type of treatment for any population. Strand and Debertine (2000) reported on the use of integral stimulation for a child diagnosed with developmental apraxia of speech. Description of the intervention included information on treatment frequency, number and type of stimuli, a response hierarchy, and feedback. Scaled scoring was used to rate the child's intelligibility, which improved with intervention. The investigators believed that motor-learning principles—such as therapy sessions scheduled four times weekly, multiple opportunities for repetitive drill within sessions, and practice with highly functional phrases—contributed to the treatment effects.

Though treatment techniques for developmental apraxia of speech vary widely, some of the most commonly recommended approaches include 1) building memory for motor sequences by gradually increasing movement sequences, starting with meaningful, phonetically simple, single-syllable words such as "hi" and "bye"; 2) starting therapy at low linguistic levels (i.e., single-syllable words), progressing to multiple-syllable words, carrier phrases (e.g., "I see a _____"), and conversation; 3) incorporating many repetitions with a limited number of stimuli during each therapy session; 4) targeting prosodic features such as rate, rhythm, stress, and intonation; 5) incorporating a multimodal approach using visual, motor, and tactile cues during treatment; and 6) varying the social and linguistic context of treatment to promote flexibility (Hall, Jordan, & Robin, 1993; Velleman, 2003; Velleman & Strand, 1994). (For further discussion of intervention techniques used for developmental apraxia of speech, see Chapter 6.)

Finally, for children at early stages of language development with unintelligible speech, teaching signs for frequently used vocabulary words may increase communication effectiveness. This technique has been recommended for children with DS (Camarata & Nelson, 2006; Miller & Leddy, 1999) and may also be effective for children with FXS. In addition, systems for augmentative and alternative communication for children with limited or highly unintelligible speech are recommended, as discussed in Chapter 11.

CONCLUSION

Although published reports on DS and FXS clearly point to reduced speech intelligibility as a major communication problem, progress in understanding the intelligibility impairment and minimizing it through interventions has been quite limited. It is likely that in both DS and FXS, reduced intelligibility is the result of a combination of factors. Intelligibility is a relatively global aspect of speech that combines syntax, lexical choice, phonological patterns, and execution of the motor plan for speech. Difficulty in any combination of these can reduce a speaker's intelligibility.

REFERENCES

Abbeduto, L., & Chapman, R. (2005). Language development in Down syndrome and fragile X syndrome: Current research and implications for theory and practice. In P. Fletcher & J. F. Miller (Eds.), *Developmental theory and language disorders* (pp. 53–72). Amsterdam, Netherlands: John Benjamins.

Abbeduto, L., & Hagerman, R. (1997). Language and communication in fragile X syndrome. *Mental Retardation and Developmental Disabilities Research Reviews, 3*, 313–322.

Abbeduto, L., & Murphy, M.M. (2004). Language, social cognition, maladaptive behavior, and communication in Down syndrome and fragile X syndrome. In M.L. Rice & S.F. Warren (Eds.), *Developmental language disorders: From phenotypes to etiologies* (pp. 77–97). Mahwah, NJ: Lawrence Erlbaum Associates.

Balkany, T.J. (1980). Otologic aspects of Down's syndrome. *Seminars in Speech, Language, and Hearing, 1*, 39–48.

Barefoot, S.M., Bochner, J.H., Johnson, B.A., & vom Eigen, B.A. (1993). Rating deaf speakers' comprehensibility: An exploratory investigation. *American Journal of Speech-Language Pathology, 2*, 31–35.

Belser, R.C., & Sudhalter, V. (2001). Conversational characteristics of children with Fragile X syndrome: Repetitive speech. *American Journal of Mental Retardation, 106*, 28–38.

Borghgraef, M., Frons, J.P., Dielkens, A., Pyck, K., & Van Den Berghe, H. (1987). Fragile X syndrome: A study of the psychological profile in 23 prepubertal patients. *Clinical Genetics, 32*, 179–186.

Bradlow, A.R., Torretta, G.M., & Pisoni, D.B. (1996). Intelligibility of normal speech: I. Global and fine-grained acoustic-phonetic talker characteristics. *Speech Communication, 20*, 255–272.

Camarata, S.M., & Nelson, K. (2006). Conversational recast intervention with preschool and older children. In R.J. McCauley & M.E. Fey (Vol. Eds.) & S.F. Warren & M.E. Fey (Series Eds.), *Communication and language intervention series: Treatment of language disorders in children* (pp. 237–264). Baltimore: Paul H. Brookes Publishing Co.

Carlstedt, K., Henningsson, G., & Dahllof, G. (2003). A four-year longitudinal study of palatal plate therapy in children with Down syndrome: Effects on oral motor function, articulation, and communication preferences. *Acta Odontologica Scandinavica, 62*, 39–46.

Chapman, R.S., Seung, H., Schwartz, S.E., & Kay-Raining Bird, E. (2000). Predicting language production in children and adolescents with Down syndrome: The role of comprehension. *Journal of Speech, Language, and Hearing Research, 43*, 340–350.

Cholmain, C.N. (1994). Working on phonology with young children with Down syndrome. *Journal of Clinical Speech and Language Studies, 1*, 14–35.

Dodd, B., McCormack, P., & Woodyatt, G. (1994). Evaluation of an intervention program: Relation between children's phonology and parents' communicative behavior. *American Journal on Mental Retardation, 98*(5), 632–645.

Dodd, B., & Thompson, L. (2001). Speech disorder in children with Down's syndrome. *Journal of Intellectual Disabilities Research, 45*, 308–316.

Downs, M.P. (1980). The hearing of Down's individuals. *Seminars in Speech, Language, and Hearing, 1*(1), 25–38.

Flanagan, J.L. (1972). *Speech analysis, synthesis and perception.* New York: Springer-Verlag.

Grant, K.W., & Seitz, P.F. (2000). The recognition of isolated words and words in sentences: Individual variability in the use of sentence context. *Journal of the Acoustical Society of America, 107*, 1000–1011.

Hagerman, R.J. (2002). The physical and behavioral phenotype. In R.J. Hagerman & P.J. Hagerman (Eds.), *Fragile X syndrome: Diagnosis, treatment, and research* (3rd ed., pp. 3–109). Baltimore: The Johns Hopkins University Press.

Hall, P.K., Jordan, L.S., & Robin, D.A. (1993). *Developmental apraxia of speech: Theory and clinical practice.* Austin, TX: PRO-ED.

Hanson, D.M., Jackson, A.W., & Hagerman, R.J. (1986). Speech disturbances (cluttering) in mildly impaired males with the Martin-Bell/fragile X syndrome. *American Journal of Medical Genetics, 23,* 195–206.

Hazan, V., & Markham, D. (2004). Acoustic-phonetic correlates of talker intelligibility for adults and children. *Journal of the Acoustical Society of America, 116,* 3108–3118.

Hodge, M., & Daniels, J. (2005). Test of Children's Speech and Spelling–TOCS+ (Version 4.1) [Computer software]. Edmonton, Alberta: University of Alberta.

Hodson, B.W. (1989). Phonological remediation: A cycles approach. In N.A. Creaghead, P.W. Newman, & W.A. Secord (Eds.), *Assessment and remediation of articulatory and phonological disorders* (2nd ed., pp. 323–333). New York: Macmillan.

Hodson, B.W., & Paden, E.P. (1991). *Targeting intelligible speech: A phonological approach to remediation* (2nd ed.). Austin, TX: PRO-ED.

Kent, R.D., Miolo, G., & Bloedel, S. (1994). The intelligibility of children's speech: A review of evaluation procedures. *American Journal of Speech-Language Pathology, 3,* 81–93.

Kent, R.D., Weismer, G., Kent, J.F., & Rosenbek, J.C. (1989). Toward phonetic intelligibility testing in dysarthria. *Journal of Speech and Hearing Disorders, 54,* 482–499.

Klaiman, P., Witzel, M.A., Margar-Bacal, F., & Munro, I.R. (1988). Changes in aesthetic appearance and intelligibility of speech after partial glossectomy in patients with Down syndrome. *Plastic and Reconstructive Surgery, 82*(3), 403–408.

Koegel, R.L., Camarata, S., Koegel, L.K., Ben-Tall, A., & Smith, A.E. (1998). Increasing speech intelligibility in children with autism. *Journal of Autism and Developmental Disorders, 28*(3), 241–251.

Kumin, L. (1994). Intelligibility of speech in children with Down syndrome in naturalistic settings: Parents' perspective. *Perceptual and Motor Skills, 78,* 307–313.

Kumin, L. (2003). *Early communication skills for children with Down syndrome: A guide for parents and professionals* (2nd ed.). Bethesda, MD: Woodbine House.

Kumin, L. (2006). Speech intelligibility and childhood verbal apraxia in children with Down syndrome. *Down Syndrome, Research and Practice, 10,* 10–22.

Kumin, L., & Adams, J. (2000). Developmental apraxia of speech and intelligibility in children with Down syndrome. *Down Syndrome Quarterly, 5*(3), 1–7.

Kumin, L., Councill, C., & Goodman, M. (1994). A longitudinal study of the emergence of phonemes in children with Down syndrome. *Journal of Communication Disorders, 27*(4), 293–303.

Lachiewicz, A.M., & Mirrett, P.L. (2000). The development of children with fragile X syndrome. In J.D. Weber (Ed.), *Children with fragile X syndrome: A parents' guide* (pp. 199–242). Bethesda, MD: Woodbine House.

Leddy, M. (1999). The biological bases of speech in people with Down syndrome. In J.F. Miller, M. Leddy, & L.A. Leavitt (Eds.), *Improving the communication of people with Down syndrome* (pp. 61–80). Baltimore: Paul H. Brookes Publishing Co.

Madison, L.S., George, C., & Moeschler, J.B. (1986). Cognitive functioning in the fragile X syndrome: A study of intellectual, memory, and communication skills. *Journal of Mental Deficiency Research, 30,* 129–148.

Margar-Bacal, F., Witzel, M.A., & Munro, I.R. (1987). Speech intelligibility after partial glossectomy in children with Down's syndrome. *Plastic & Reconstructive Surgery, 79,* 44–49.

Miller, J.F. (1988). The developmental asynchrony of language development in children with Down syndrome. In L. Nadel (Ed.), *The psychobiology of Down syndrome* (pp. 167–198). Cambridge, MA: MIT Press.

Miller, J.F., & Leddy, M. (1999). Verbal fluency, speech intelligibility, and communicative effectiveness. In J.F. Miller, M. Leddy, & L.A. Leavitt (Eds.), *Improving the communication of people with Down syndrome* (pp. 81–92). Baltimore: Paul H. Brookes Publishing Co.

Miller, J.L., & Volaitis, L.E. (1989). Effect of speaking rate on the perceptual structure of a phonetic category. *Perception & Psychophysics, 46,* 505–512.

Morris, S.R., Wilcox, K.A., & Schooling, T.L. (1995). The Preschool Speech Intelligibility Measure. *American Journal of Speech-Language Pathology, 4,* 22–28.

Newell, K., Sanborn, B., & Hagerman, R. (1983). Speech and language dysfunction in the fragile X syndrome. In R.J. Hagerman & P.M. McBogg (Eds.), *The fragile X syndrome: Diagnosis, biochemistry, and intervention* (pp. 175–184). Dillon, CO: Spectra.

Parsons, C.L., Iacono, T.A., & Rozner, L. (1987). Effects of tongue reduction and articulation in children with Down syndrome. *American Journal of Mental Deficiency, 91,* 328–332.

Paul, R., Cohen, D.J., Breg, W.R., Watson, M., & Herman, S. (1984). Fragile X syndrome: Its relations to speech and language disorders. *Journal of Speech and Hearing Disorders, 49,* 326–336.

Rice, M.L., Warren, S.F., & Betz, S.K. (2005). Language symptoms of developmental language disorders: An overview of autism, Down syndrome, fragile X, specific language impairment, and Williams syndrome. *Applied Psycholinguistics, 26,* 7–27.

Roberts, J.E., Long, S., Malkin, C., Barnes, E.F., Skinner, M., Hennon, E.A., et al. (2005). A comparison of phonological skills of boys with fragile X syndrome and Down syndrome. *Journal of Speech, Language, and Hearing Research, 48*(5), 980–995.

Roizen, N.J. (2001). Down syndrome: Progress in research. *Mental Retardation and Developmental Disabilities Research Reviews, 7,* 38–44.

Rosin, M., & Swift, E. (1999). Communication interventions: Improving the speech intelligibility of children with Down syndrome. In J.F. Miller, M. Leddy, & L.A. Leavitt (Eds.), *Improving the communication of people with Down syndrome* (pp. 133–160). Baltimore: Paul H. Brookes Publishing Co.

Rosin, M., Swift, E., Bless, D., & Vetter, D. (1988). Communication profiles of adolescents with Down syndrome. *Journal of Childhood Communication Disorders, 12,* 49–64.

Scharfenaker, S., O'Connor, R., Stackhouse, T., Braden, M.L., & Gray, K. (2002). An integrated approach to intervention. In R.J. Hagerman & P.J. Hagerman (Eds.), *Fragile X syndrome: Diagnosis, treatment, and research* (3rd ed., pp. 363–427). Baltimore: The Johns Hopkins University Press.

Schiavetti, N. (1992). Scaling procedures for the measurement of speech intelligibility. In R.D. Kent (Ed.), *Intelligibility in speech disorders: Theory, measurement and management* (pp. 11–34). Amsterdam, Netherlands: John Benjamins.

Shriberg, L.D., Aram, D.M., & Kwiatkowski, J. (1997). Developmental apraxia of speech: II. Toward a diagnostic marker. *Journal of Speech, Language, and Hearing Research, 40,* 286–312.

Shriberg, L.D., & Widder, C.J. (1990). Speech and prosody characteristics of adults with mental retardation. *Journal of Speech and Hearing Research, 33,* 627–653.

Sommers, M.S., Nygaard, L.C., & Pisoni, D.B. (1994). Stimulus variability and spoken word recognition, I. Effects of variability in speaking rate and overall amplitude. *Journal of the Acoustical Society of America, 96,* 1314–1324.

Spinelli, M., Rocha, A., Giacheti, C., & Richieri-Costa, A. (1995). Word finding difficulties, verbal paraphasias, and verbal dyspraxia in ten individuals with fragile X syndrome. *American Journal of Medical Genetics, 60,* 39–43.

Stoel-Gammon, C. (2003). Speech acquisition and approaches to intervention. In J.A. Rondal & S. Buckley (Eds.), *Speech and language intervention in Down syndrome* (pp. 49–62). London: Whurr.

Strand, E., & Debertine, P. (2000). The efficacy of integral stimulation with developmental apraxia of speech. *Journal of Medical Speech-Language Pathology, 8*(4), 295–300.

Subtenly, J. (1977). Assessment of speech with implications for training. In F. Bess (Ed.), *Childhood deafness* (pp. 183–194). New York: Grune and Stratton.

Swift, E., & Rosin, P. (1990). A remediation sequence to improve speech intelligibility for students with Down syndrome. *Language, Speech, and Hearing Services in Schools, 21,* 140–146.

Turner G.S., Tjaden, K., & Weismer, G. (1995). The influence of speaking rate on vowel space and speech intelligibility for individuals with amyotrophic lateral sclerosis. *Journal of Speech and Hearing Research, 38,* 1001–1013.

Velleman, S. (2003). *Childhood apraxia of speech resource guide.* Clifton Park, NY: Thomson.

Velleman, S.L., & Strand, K. (1994). Developmental verbal dyspraxia. In J.E. Bernthal & N.W. Bankson (Eds.), *Child phonology: Characteristics, assessment, and intervention with special populations* (pp. 110–139). New York: Thieme.

Weismer, G., Jeng, J.-Y., Laures, J.S., Kent, R.D., & Kent, J.F. (2001). Acoustic and intelligibility characteristics of sentence production in neurogenic speech disorders. *Folia Phoniatrica et Logopaedica, 53,* 1–18.

Weismer, G., & Martin, R.E. (1992). Acoustic and perceptual approaches to the study of intelligibility. In R.D. Kent (Ed.), *Intelligibility in speech disorders: Theory, measurement and management* (pp. 68–118). Amsterdam, Netherlands: John Benjamins.

Weiss, C.E., Gordon, M.E., & Lillywhite, H.S. (1987). *Clinical management of articulatory and phonologic disorders* (2nd ed.). Philadelphia: Lippincott Williams & Wilkins.

Yarter, B.H. (1980). Speech and language programs for the Down's population. *Seminars in Speech, Language, and Hearing, 1,* 49–61.

Yorkston, K.M., & Beukelman, D.R. (1981). Communication efficiency of dysarthric speakers as measured by sentence intelligibility and speaking rate. *Journal of Speech and Hearing Disorders, 46,* 296–301.

Yorkston, K.M., Strand, E.A., & Kennedy, M.R.T. (1996). Comprehensibility of dysarthric speech: Implications for assessment and treatment planning. *American Journal of Speech-Language Pathology, 5,* 55–66.

CHAPTER 10

Increasing Literacy Learning for Individuals with Down Syndrome and Fragile X Syndrome

SUE BUCKLEY AND MINA C. JOHNSON-GLENBERG

Very little published information exists on the development of reading in individuals with fragile X syndrome (FXS). Thus, this chapter draws mainly on the literature on literacy in children and adults with Down syndrome (DS). The very small amount of information available on literacy in individuals with FXS is included in full. This data indicate that there are some similar patterns in these individuals' literacy progress and that similar intervention advice might be relevant at this time.

THE IMPORTANCE OF LITERACY INSTRUCTION

Few would argue with the view that learning to read and developing literacy skills that can be useful in everyday life are worthwhile goals for individuals with DS or FXS. There may, however, be additional benefits, as some studies suggest that progress in literacy can lead to progress in spoken language and verbal short-term memory for children with DS, children with autism, and individuals with specific language impairment (SLI). Research into the reading development of children with DS also indicates that these children are often able to read better than might be expected in relation to their other language and cognitive abilities. They may also demonstrate the ability to read from a very early age, which opens up the possibility that reading activities can be used to develop better spoken language and verbal short-term memory skills from the preschool years. The evidence reported here indicates that individuals with FXS may also read better than expected for their cognitive abilities. Research is also beginning to explore the strategies that children with DS and FXS may be using as they begin to read, and this work suggests that they may use a different pattern of strategies when compared with comparison groups matched for reading abilities. The research findings on each of these issues are briefly reviewed in this chapter and used to suggest possible intervention strategies.

LITERACY DEVELOPMENT FOR INDIVIDUALS WITH DOWN SYNDROME

The literature is reviewed to identify the range of reading skills that may be achieved by children and adults with DS, the relationships between reading and other abilities that may explain individual differences in progress, the evidence that reading instruction may improve other language and cognitive skills, and the strategies that these individuals use when they begin learning to read. This information is intended to demonstrate the value of literacy instruction for individuals with DS and set the scene to identify the principles that should guide effective literacy teaching.

What Literacy Skills Do Individuals with Down Syndrome Achieve?

An increasing number of studies report on the reading abilities of children and adults with DS. During elementary school years (ages 7–14 years), the reading ages of children with DS are reported to range between 5 years and 5 months and 10 years (Byrne, 1997; Byrne, Buckley, MacDonald, & Bird 1995; Byrne, Mac-Donald, & Buckley, 2002; Hulme, Goetz, Snowling, Brigstocke, & Nash, 2005; Irwin, 1989; Kay-Raining Bird, Cleave, & McConnell, 2000; Pieterse, 1988; Pieterse & Center, 1984; Snowling, Hulme, & Mercer, 2002). Studies that include children through elementary and high school years (5–17 years) report reading ages ranging from 4 years and 11 months to 14 years and 3 months (Hulme et al., 2005; Snowling et al., 2002).

There are considerable individual differences, with some children reading at levels that are commensurate with their chronological age. For example, in a study of 49 children with DS in mainstream schools who were receiving daily literacy instruction in the United Kingdom, four were nonreaders. The reading ages of the rest ranged from 4 years and 11 months to 14 years and 3 months, and four children read at their chronological age level (Hulme et al., 2005). Case studies have also reported individual children with DS reading at or ahead of levels expected for their chronological age (Buckley, 1985, 2003; Buckley & Bird, 1993; Buckley, Bird, & Byrne, 1996a, 1996b; Groen, Laws, Nation, & Bishop, 2006). Case studies, parent reports, and a small group study have also reported early reading skills, with children with DS beginning to read at 2–3 years of age (Appleton, 2000; Appleton, Buckley, & MacDonald, 2002; Buckley, 2003; Dickinson, 2002; Groen et al., 2006, Kotlinski & Kotlinski, 2002; Oke, 2002; Rozen, 2002). Two studies report on the reading abilities of groups of adults ranging in age from 17 to 36 years with reading abilities ranging from 6 years 7 months to 12 years 7 months (Bochner, Outhred, & Pieterse, 2001; Fowler, Doherty, & Boynton,1995).

The majority of studies report only the word reading abilities of the individuals, with very few studies reporting on spelling or reading comprehension. Spelling abilities appear to be close to word reading abilities (Byrne et al., 2002), whereas reading comprehension tends to be at least a year behind word reading abilities (Byrne et al., 2002; Fletcher & Buckley, 2002; Fowler et al., 1995; Groen et al., 2006). The only information on the writing abilities of children or adults is based on case studies (see Bird, Beadman, & Buckley, 2001; Bird & Buckley, 2001,

2002; and Buckley, 2001, 2003, for examples). Here again, wide variability is seen, with some children with DS writing and composing stories at age-appropriate levels but with most progressing more slowly. The best writers seem to be those who were introduced to reading in their preschool years.

A number of other issues are raised in the papers cited, including the fact that children with DS may read better than would be expected from their cognitive and/or language levels (Bochner et al., 2001; Byrne et al., 2002; Fowler et al., 1995; Groen et al., 2006; Hulme et al., 2005; Irwin, 1989; Laws & Gunn, 2002; Snowling et al., 2002); that the better readers have better language (Bochner et al., 2001); that those educated in inclusive classrooms are better readers and talkers (Bochner et al., 2001); and that word reading skills are often, but not always, better than decoding skills (Buckley, 2001; Byrne, 1997; Byrne et al., 2002; Cupples & Iacono, 2000; Kay-Raining Bird et al., 2000; Verucci, Menghini, & Vicari, 2006).

Current research studies are small, and access to good literacy teaching is still not available to all children; therefore, these data should not be taken to indicate the full reading potential of children with DS. Accurate estimates of what might be expected must be documented by studying larger samples of children known to be receiving quality literacy teaching adapted to their needs.

Can We Explain the Wide Range of Individual Differences Reported?

Individual differences in reading progress for typically developing children have been reported to be influenced by general cognitive ability (Boudreau, 2002; Ellis & Large, 1988); visual and verbal short-term memory skills (Brady, Mann, & Schmidt, 1987; Brady, Shankweiler, & Mann, 1983; Ellis & Large, 1988); and oral language skills, particularly receptive grammar skills (Muter & Snowling, 1998). Some studies have begun to explore factors contributing to the individual differences in literacy achievements reported for children and adults with DS, and these same factors seem to be important, but the type or intensity of reading instruction received is not documented in any of these studies, and it may play a role that is not accounted for in the analyses. Given that reading instruction may lead to improved speech, language, and verbal short-term memory function, the significance of reported correlations is difficult to interpret.

When comparing readers and nonreaders with DS, Laws and Gunn (2002) reported that readers performed better than nonreaders on measures of nonverbal ability, even after controlling for differences in hearing status. In contrast, Boudreau (2002) found that nonverbal cognitive ability was not significantly correlated with word recognition but was correlated with nonword reading (i.e., decoding skill) in a study that also included readers and nonreaders with DS.

Word recognition abilities in individuals with DS have been reported as significantly correlated with visual and verbal short-term memory spans in a number of studies (Fidler, Most, & Guiberson, 2005; Fowler et al., 1995; Kay-Raining Bird et al., 2000; Laws, 1998; Laws, Buckley, Bird, MacDonald, & Broadley, 1995; Laws & Gunn, 2002). In their longitudinal study, Kay-Raining Bird et al. (2000) reported that progress in decoding ability was predicted by verbal short-term memory span at the start of the study after controlling for chronological age, mental age, and phoneme segmentation. Similarly, in a 5-year study of 30 children and young adults with DS, Laws and Gunn (2002) reported that verbal short-term memory at the start of the study was a significant predictor of reading progress 5 years later. These findings imply that verbal short-term memory plays a causal role in reading progress, and this finding should be taken into account when designing teaching strategies.

Individuals with stronger oral language skills have been reported to show stronger word recognition and decoding skills (Fowler et al., 1995; Kay-Raining Bird et al., 2000; Laws et al., 1995; Laws & Gunn, 2002). Hulme et al. (2005) reported a significant correlation between word reading abilities and vocabulary comprehension at the start of their longitudinal study but not with phonological skills. They report the reverse pattern for typically developing children—their phonological skills but not their vocabulary comprehension scores correlate with word reading.

Does Literacy Instruction Improve Speech, Language, and Memory Skills?

The possible benefits of reading instruction for the speech and language development of children with DS was brought to the attention of the first chapter author in 1979 by Leslie Duffen, the father of Sarah, a young girl with DS. Leslie described how he had introduced Sarah to reading at the age of 3 years, specifically teaching her to read words and sentences that were developmentally appropriate and that she could use in her speech. When he started, Sarah spoke very few words, and Leslie observed that the words that they were reading appeared in her spoken language much more quickly than words she had only heard. He felt that her advanced progress by the age of 11 years (Sarah was speaking well, reading at almost an age-appropriate level, and being educated in a general education classroom) had been due to discovering reading as a key to Sarah's learning (Duffen, 1976). Sarah could learn language more effectively by seeing and processing it visually rather than by merely hearing it, suggesting that the language learning of children with DS was being held back by difficulties of accessing language in the auditory mode.

More than 20 years later, the research evidence confirms that this is the case. It is now agreed that children with DS have specific speech and language impairment—that is, their speech and language skills are significantly delayed relative to their nonverbal mental abilities (Chapman, 1999; Chapman & Hesketh, 2001; Miller, 1999). In addition, children with SLI in the general population and children with DS matched for nonverbal mental age have been shown to have very similar profiles of speech, language, and verbal short-term memory deficits (Eadie, Fey, Douglas, & Parsons, 2002; Laws & Bishop, 2003). This evidence indicates that it is not simply cognitive delay that is holding back speech and language development in children with DS. Hearing, auditory processing, and verbal short-term memory difficulties are also major factors. Children with DS are at high risk for mild to moderate hearing loss, with some 80% of preschoolers suffering from conductive losses, some of whom will also have sensorineural losses (Shott, 2001). During their teenage and early adult years, some 50% of individuals with DS still have mild to moderate losses (Marcell, 1995).

In addition to hearing loss, there has been growing evidence for the presence of verbal short-term memory difficulties, which would compromise language processing in the auditory mode (Conners, 2002). Reviews of the working memory research in DS highlight the evidence for a degree of phonological loop impairment (Jarrold & Baddeley, 2001; Jarrold, Baddeley, & Phillips, 1999). Visual short-term memory spans tend to be as expected for nonverbal mental age for individuals with DS, although verbal short-term memory spans are specifically impaired. Any impairment in phonological loop function is likely to significantly affect one's ability to understand and say single words from infancy to adult life (Dodd & Thompson, 2001; Gathercole & Baddeley, 1993a, 1993b).

Research has also identified that growth in the processing capacity of the working memory system as measured by word or digit spans is significantly impaired relative to the nonverbal abilities of children with DS, which will make processing sentences and learning grammar more difficult (Hulme & Mackenzie, 1992). A number of studies have produced evidence to link expressive language skills and verbal short-term memory skills in children and teenagers with DS (see Chapman & Hesketh, 2001, for a review). Hence, there is evidence to support the view that learning a language solely from listening will be difficult for children with DS and thus the hypothesis that reading may be a particularly important "way in" to spoken language for children with DS because it makes language visual. Still, researchers ask if there is any evidence demonstrating that reading actually does improve the spoken language of children with DS.

The author and colleagues have reported case studies of early readers since 1983. One paper provides a very detailed single case study of K.S., an 8-year-old girl with DS, who was considered by educators to be an exceptional reader (Groen et al., 2006). Case studies indicated that children who were introduced to reading activities designed to teach spoken language as early as 2–3 years of age showed significantly advanced speech, language, literacy, and verbal short-term memory skills in childhood and teenage years (Buckley, 2003; Groen et al., 2006). These children showed more advanced speech, language, and literacy skills as teenagers than did children introduced to reading after 5 or 6 years of age. Children introduced to reading at any age after 5 years significantly benefited from reading activities; however, as is demonstrated in the deaf literature (Mayberry, Lock, & Kazmi, 2002), language progress in sign or speech before 5 years is very important. Those starting later progress extensively, but they do not catch up with the early starters.

The first author of this chapter (Buckley, 2000), drawing on the work of Locke (1994, 1997) and others, has argued that the brain is optimally ready to learn a first language from 12 months to 5–6 years. When print is used to support first language learning from 2 to 3 years of age, it seems to have a qualitatively different and much greater effect, possibly as a result of brain plasticity at this age. The link between reading and improved phonology and grammar could be explained by Locke's view that as a child begins to express inflectional morphology (e.g., -ing, -ed, and -s endings), more sophisticated control is promoted in phonology (Locke, 1994, 1997). The child not attempting to express grammar may be missing a phase that is important for the development of phonology and morphosyntax. Reading activities enable children to practice production of sentence grammar not yet fully used in their spontaneous talking. In addition, a child with DS, especially with any degree of hearing loss, may benefit from the visual representation of brief speech events.

An experimental training study with teenagers with DS (Buckley, 1993, 1995) demonstrated that language teaching activities could significantly improve the teenagers' comprehension and production of grammar. The teaching method that used print was more effective than spoken language practice only, and the least able teenagers in this special school group, nonreaders at the start, showed the greatest benefit of using print. They were also found to be the students with the poorest verbal short-term memories. The methods used are described in full in Buckley (2000).

The first small piece of evidence of the benefits of ordinary literacy instruction in school is based on group data from a longitudinal study of short-term memory development collected by the first author's research team (Laws et al., 1995). In this study, two groups of children with DS matched for language, short-term memory, and nonverbal mental age were compared over a 4-year period. One group was receiving more intensive reading instruction than the other. At the end of the period, the readers were significantly ahead of the nonreaders in spoken language comprehension and verbal short-term memory measures. The gains were approximately equivalent to 2 years of typical developmental progress, meaning that the readers were 2 years ahead of the nonreaders on the measures, although the two groups had scored at the same level on all of the measures 4 years earlier and were still matched on nonverbal cognitive ability at the end of the study. This effect of reading progress on language and memory development has been demonstrated for typically developing children (Ellis & Large, 1988; Gathercole & Baddeley, 1993a, 1993b), for children with SLI (Conti-Ramsden & Durkin, 2007; Stothard, Snowling, Bishop, Chipchase, & Kaplan, 1998) and for a child with autism (Craig & Telfer, 2005).

Some of the recent studies of the effects of reading progress for children with DS are, however, confounded by school placement effects. In the Laws et al. (1995) study, all but one of the readers had been in mainstream schools, and all of the nonreaders were in special schools in the United Kingdom. This study took place at a time when full inclusion for children with DS was developing for all in the United Kingdom, regardless of an individual's level of ability. In some areas, education authorities were quicker to offer inclusion than in other areas, and thus children of a similar wide range of abilities were in inclusive schools in one area or in special schools in the neighboring area.

The children in the mainstream schools were fully included in age-appropriate classes and therefore in a much richer spoken language environment than the children in the special schools or classrooms, where most of their peers had significant speech, language, and cognitive delays. Therefore, the speech and language gains may be in part due to the language environment and in part due to literacy experience and progress. In a further study of mainstream and special school outcomes, Laws, Byrne, and Buckley (2000) reported significantly advanced language comprehension and short-term memory skills for the children in the mainstream schools. Significant differences in favor of the children in the mainstream schools were reported for vocabulary comprehension, grammar comprehension, sentence memory, and both auditory and visual digit span. However, although 22 of the 24 children in the mainstream schools could score on a standardized reading test, only 3 of the 24 children in the special schools could achieve a raw score. Therefore, the advantage for the mainstream children may have been linked to reading progress, but this could not be systematically explored in this study.

In a follow-up study of 30 children attending special schools for children with severe learning difficulties in the United Kingdom, Laws and Gunn (2002) reported an increase in reading ability over a 5-year period. The number of readers had risen from 10 to 16 children. The readers had significantly better scores on nonverbal ability, language, and short-term memory measures, but these could not be demonstrated to be the result of reading progress. However, there was some evidence that early reading skills did predict mean length of utterance 5 years later. The average age of this group was 11 years at the first assessment point and 16 years (range 10–24 years) at the second assessment. The actual reading achievements were limited, and there is no information on the methods used or the time spent on reading activities. It is possible that greater gains for spoken language will be seen when teachers are planning to use reading to teach language, and reading activities are engaged on a daily basis. It is also possible that optimal gains for language will be seen when reading is a consistent activity from at least 5 years of age, preferably from 2 to 3 years of age.

In the Byrne (1997) study, all of the children were in mainstream placements, and there was no significant association between independent reading performance on standardized tests at one phase and language progress at the next phase to provide specific evidence of reading ability influencing spoken language progress. However, all of the children in the Byrne study, regardless of their independent reading ability, received daily reading instruction and inclusion in literacy activities as they recorded their work across the curriculum with the support of classroom assistants. This group had significantly better language and short-term memory abilities (Laws et al., 2000) and expressive language (Buckley, Bird, Sacks, & Archer, 2006) than comparable special school groups. This may suggest that it is the daily involvement in reading experience rather than the child's independent reading skills that leads to gains in spoken language. In the mainstream versus special education studies, comparisons were being made between children who received a high level of daily reading instruction and literacy experience and those who received very limited, if any, literacy instruction or experience of print. More longitudinal research studies are needed to clarify the links between reading and spoken language, but at the present time, the evidence does suggest that reading experience and reading attainments do benefit speech, language, and working memory development.

What Strategies Are Children with Down Syndrome Using to Read?

Research with typically developing children indicates that there is a strong relationship between both phonological awareness skills and phonemic awareness skills and learning to read. Studies also show that phonological awareness skills are similarly associated with word-recognition and decoding ability in children with DS (Cardoso-Martins & Frith, 2001; Cupples & Iacono, 2000; Fletcher & Buckley, 2002; Fowler et al., 1995; Gombert, 2002; Kay-Raining Bird et al., 2000; Kennedy & Flynn, 2003a; Laws & Gunn, 2002; Snowling et al., 2002; for contrary evidence, see Hulme et al., 2005).

Some researchers suggest that phonological awareness and skills may develop differently in children with DS. They are reported to perform more poorly on rhyme tasks than controls matched for nonverbal mental age and/or reading ability (Boudreau, 2002; Gombert, 2002; Snowling et al., 2002). In one study, children with DS also found a rhyme matching task more difficult than a middle phoneme matching task, whereas the reverse was true for typically developing children (Cardoso-Martins, Michalick, & Pollo, 2002). One research group suggested that children with DS may be selectively more sensitive to sounds at the beginnings than at the ends of words (Snowling et al., 2002), which could perhaps be linked to teaching experience.

When considering phonemic awareness skills, children with DS seem to fare better at phoneme identity than at phoneme manipulation tasks. Their performance on phoneme-matching tasks that required judgments as to whether a target word began with same sound as one of the test words was not significantly different from the performance of typically developing children matched on nonverbal mental age or on reading ability (Cardoso-Martins & Frith, 2001; Snowling et al., 2002). However, children with DS performed significantly worse than the control group in two studies in which the phoneme matching tasks employed an odd-one-out procedure (Boudreau, 2002; Gombert, 2002). They also performed significantly worse on phoneme manipulation tasks involving tapping and segmentation (Gombert, 2002). They did, however, perform as well as nonverbal mental age matched controls on phoneme blending in the Boudreau (2002) study but worse than the reading age matched controls in the Gombert (2002) study.

Intervention studies are beginning to indicate that children with DS can be taught phonological skills (Kennedy & Flynn, 2003b; van Bysterveldt, Gillon, & Moran, 2006) and that phonological instruction improves their ability to read unfamiliar words (Cupples & Iacono, 2002). Four studies that reported scores on a nonword reading test (the Word Attack subtest of the Woodcock Reading Mastery Tests–Revised; Woodcock, 1998) suggested that some decoding skills are present but that they are reduced compared with word recognition skills (Boudreau, 2002; Cupples & Iacono, 2000; Fowler, et al., 1995; Hulme et al., 2005; Kay-Raining Bird et al., 2000).

Individual differences must be noted as the five most able readers in the Fowler et al. (1995) study had word attack skills that were more advanced than their word reading skills, as is also the case for K.S., the previously mentioned exceptional reader (Groen et al., 2006). Mean scores and group trends may be very misleading and may not actually represent the patterns seen in all or even a majority of individuals within the group. It is especially important to bear this in mind when considering the progress and needs of atypical groups. It is also important to remember that children with DS have significant speech and language difficulties; thus, their experience of the language is different. In addition, they may not have received the same teaching and learning opportunities. There is a need for training studies to systematically explore the levels of competence that can be achieved by children with DS across all of these skills and the ways in which they are linked to reading progress.

A number of authors agree that children with DS may rely on a logographic (i.e., whole-word) strategy for a longer time (Byrne, 1997; Hulme et al., 2005; Kay-Raining Bird et al., 2000; Verucci et al., 2006) than other children, and each stage may need to be supported for longer to ensure success. All children initially use a logographic strategy to read (i.e., they memorize the whole word pattern and recognize the word by matching it with their stored word pattern) (Frith, 1985; Gathercole & Baddeley, 1993a; Oakhill & Beard, 1999; Seymour, 1993; Seymour & Elder, 1986).

There is some evidence that as some children with DS learn the letter–sound links and increase their experience of reading, they do reach a stage at which they can use alphabetic strategies (i.e., they can decode by sounding out the letters in words for reading and for spelling) (Byrne, 1997; Cupples & Iacono, 2000; Kay-Raining Bird et al., 2000). Given that most children with DS have some degree of hearing difficulty and that the phonological loop impairment may mean that they are not storing accurately specified sound patterns for words, it can be predicted that they will have more difficulty with phonics and the use of an alphabetic strategy. Most children and teenagers with DS cannot say all of the sounds (i.e., phonemes) in the language, clearly adding a further level of difficulty for them.

The data collected by Byrne (1997) and Fletcher and Buckley (2002) indicate that children with DS with mean word reading and spelling ages of about 7 years and older can use an alphabetic strategy to decode words and that some are using phonic spelling strategies (Buckley, 2001). Interestingly, these children showed very good skills in the phonological awareness tasks that required them to detect rhyme and alliteration or to blend, but they found segmenting tasks much more difficult. The alphabetic children in this study (i.e., those who could read words they had never seen before because they were nonsense words made up as an alphabetic test) had good phonological awareness skills. However, other children with equally good phonological awareness skills were unable to apply them to decoding new words or spelling, highlighting the need to explicitly teach these strategies (Hatcher, Hulme, & Ellis, 1994; Torgesen, 2005).

For the English language, it usually takes typically developing children 2 years to progress from learning the letter–sound links from a phonics teaching program to becoming an alphabetic reader and speller (Gathercole & Baddeley, 1993b), suggesting that extensive experience with the printed language is necessary to develop alphabetic skills. Many languages have more regular correspondence between the written and spoken forms of the language than English, and these written languages may be easier for children with DS to master, although this does not seem to be the case for Italian (Verucci et al., 2006)

Reading Comprehension

Most children with DS have word reading and spelling ages ahead of reading comprehension ages (Byrne, 1997; Byrne et al. 2002; Fowler et al., 1995; Groen et al., 2006). The reasons for this have not been systematically explored. In the studies reported, reading comprehension was usually as good as or better than grammar comprehension. It might be expected that both vocabulary and grammar comprehension levels would predict reading comprehension (Nation & Norbury, 2005; Roberts & Scott, 2006; Snowling & Hayiou-Thomas, 2006). Some of the differences reported for children with DS (in which reading comprehension is ahead of language comprehension) may be artifacts of the different test norms, or they may actually demonstrate that some children comprehend written language better than spoken language. More research is needed to explore reading comprehension in children with DS, drawing on the growing literature on reading comprehension difficulties in other groups of children (Nation, 2005; Nation & Norbury, 2005).

Another factor that can be expected to influence reading comprehension for children with DS is their limited working memory capacity. This will influence their ability to decode new text while retaining the meaning of what has already been read (Gathercole & Pickering, 2000, 2001). Practitioners and parents report that most children with DS show better comprehension skills when they are reading about activities or characters that are familiar to them (e.g., reading from their news book, diary, or school books in which they have recorded information about activities in which they have participated in; reading about familiar television or cartoon characters). The case report of K.S., the exceptional reader, indicates that she had age-appropriate reading comprehension for literal text but more difficulty with text requiring inferencing from linguistic clues or from her existing knowledge.

Writing

Many children with DS who can read quite well with good comprehension still find writing (i.e., putting their own thoughts on paper) very difficult, and they need support to write sentences or short stories or to record their work. Working memory difficulties will again be part of the explanation, as those influence the ability to think about what to write next while still recording the previous sentence (Gathercole & Pickering, 2001). Writing difficulties resulting from motor skill delays are a separate issue. Computer software packages may help considerably with both composition and writing, including those that combine symbols (i.e., icons) with print. The first author and colleagues encourage reading instruction using print from the outset rather than symbols, but each child should be assessed on an individual basis, and symbol systems will help some children to get started, especially if they have experienced reading failure.

READING PROCESSES AND MALES WITH FRAGILE X SYNDROME

Several experiments by Johnson-Glenberg (2007a, 2007b) probe the differences between the reading skills of males with FXS and typically developing children. The Word Identification (Word ID) and Word Attack subtests of the Woodcock Reading Mastery Tests–Revised (Woodcock, 1998) were administered to these two different groups. The males with FXS (age range 11.42–38.08 years) and the typically developing children (age range 3.92–8.25 years) were originally recruited for a memory experiment (Johnson-Glenberg, 2007). Later in the study, the following reading measures were added to address hypotheses regarding reading and the performance of a neural network model (Johnson-Glenberg, 2007b). The typically developing children were matched for nonverbal mental age using two Stanford-Binet subtests—Bead Memory and Pattern Analysis (Thorndike, Hagen, & Sattler, 1986). These subtests have been used extensively with individuals with developmental disabilities (Abbeduto et al., 2003), and they scale properly for populations with delays. The Word ID subtest of the Woodcock Reading Mastery Tests–Revised (Woodcock, 1998) contains a list of real words that individuals read until six consecutive errors are made.

The males with FXS were on average 20 years old, and the typically developing mental age match children were $5^{1}/_{2}$ years old. The group with FXS performed significantly better on the Word ID task, with an age equivalent score of 8.00 (1.34) compared with the typically developing match's average score of 5.97 (1.51). The interpretation of these data suggest that when matched for nonverbal mental age, the males with FXS named real words significantly better than the typically developing children did. This makes sense, as the males with FXS have more world experience and have been exposed to written words more often. Their mean age is almost four times that of the typically developing children. This result is a stepping stone to the next question of interest—are the males with FXS using the same processes as the typically developing children to decode words? To answer this, several nonword and phonological awareness measures were administered. In an effort to control for effects that might be due to word-level memorization skills associated with the matching on mental age, a new typically developing match group was created. The Word ID subtest became the matching variable, and nonverbal mental age was allowed to vary.

Creating the Reading Match Group

Seven of the original typically developing participants were retained, and six new older typically developing (TD) participants were recruited (TD $n = 13$; FXS $n = 15$). The groups were matched on word ID skills. The Word Attack subtest of the Woodcock Reading Mastery Tests–Revised (Woodcock, 1998), a nonword task, was then administered. The new typically developing reading match group was more than 2 years older (7 years and 6 months) than the previous typically developing nonverbal mental age match group (5 years and 5 months). After word reading skills were matched, the nonverbal mental age scores were significantly discrepant (TD = 8.71; FXS = 5.19). In addition, the typically developing children were decoding nonwords significantly better than the males with FXS, TD age equivalent = 8.67 (SD = 3.43); FXS 6.45 (SD = 1.57), $t(16.83) = 2.14$, $p = .04$). Although the groups could name real words similarly, TD = 8.08 (2.63) and FXS = 7.99 (1.30), they varied in the underlying skills used to decode non-words. Somewhere between 5 and 7 years of age, the average typically developing children surpassed the males with FXS in these skills.

Phonological Subprocesses

There are many processes that feed into the naming of nonwords. These principally include phonemic awareness and sequencing. Not much is known about phonological subprocesses in males with FXS. In the expressive arena, Roberts, Hennon, and Anderson (2003) reported that males with FXS had expressive difficulty with consonant substitutions, omissions, and distortions, which are characteristic of developmentally younger children. In addition, Roberts et al. (2003) reported oral motor difficulties for males with FXS when repeating multisyllablic sequences and problems with motor planning. More recently, Roberts et al. (2005) found that young males with FXS did not differ from nonverbal mental age–matched typically developing children in the percentage of correct early, middle, and late developing consonants; phonological processes; or whole-word proximity scores when tested at the isolated single-word level.

Phonological processing is a key component in reading. Reviewing the reading literature reveals that for *all* types of readers, even after ruling out IQ, later reading ability is predicted by phonological processing (Siegel, 1993; Stanovich, Cunningham, & Feeman, 1984). Conners, Atwell, Rosenquist, and Sligh (2001) gave several language and phonological measures to a mixed etiology group of individuals with intellectual disability. The participants were either relatively stronger or weaker decoders with IQs that ranged from 40 to 70. When age was covaried out, Conners et al. (2001) found that the most reliable difference between the two groups was the ability to refresh phonological codes in working memory. The refresh score was a composite measure comprised of the mean Z score of 1) the difference between repeating three or four syllable words, and 2) the Z score for individual articulation speed. The Conners et al. (2001) result has implications both for working memory processing and for assembly (i.e., the sequencing of phonemes for speech). Although assembly is important, it is also the case that the internal phonemic representations themselves must be "crisp" and well represented. To assess the strength of the phonemic representations, Johnson-Glenberg (2003) administered several phonemic measures from the Phonological Awareness Test (PAT; Robertson & Salter, 1997) to a subset of FXS participants.

Four relevant subtests from PAT—rhyming, segmentation, deletion, and isolation—were administered. Only two of the three levels of isolation were examined: 1) the *initial* sound in a consonant–vowel–consonant word and 2) the *final* sound, as medial sound was too difficult for these individuals. The PAT percentile scores for the males with FXS were gathered using the Woodcock Reading Mastery Tests–Revised Word ID age-equivalent score as a base. Chronological age was not used because the males were so much older than the typically developing participants, and this would have resulted in a meaningless "less than 1 percentile" score across the board. By matching on the ability to read real words, a dissociation between the FXS and the typically developing Word ID–matched reading skills could be examined and differences amongst the subtests had the potential to be detected.

The PAT test was only given to the final six participants in the FXS study. Typically developing Word ID matches were expected to score at the 50th percentile on average. The males with FXS performed at the 7th percentile on rhyme, the 8th percentile on segmentation, the 2nd percentile in isolation, and the 8th percentile on phoneme deletion.

These preliminary data suggest that males with FXS have compromised phonological subprocesses. On average, they can read real words similar to 8-year-old typically developing children, but they sounded out nonwords equivalent to $6\frac{1}{2}$-year-olds. This may be because phonemic awareness is relatively underdeveloped in males with FXS. Perhaps they rely on memory skills to name the real words on the Word ID test, but when they must rely on phonological recoding resources to pronounce and sequence novel combinations (i.e., nonwords in the Word Attack test), they do not adequately possess the needed subskills. This may be due to memory limitations, as sequencing is a problem for males with FXS (Johnson-Glenberg, 2007a, 2007b). It may also be an outcome of a certain type of teaching. As with individuals with DS, little is known about most prevalent teaching methods utilized in the schools. It is probable that the students with FXS were taught using the whole-word method, or logographic method, only.

Reading and phonological awareness are considered to be reciprocal. The FXS participants were readers and had been exposed to print for many more years than the typically developing children, yet their phonological skills were all below the 10th percentile based on their real word reading skills. This suggests a divergence in the type of processing that the two groups use to read. Nothing is known about the genetics of reading and individuals with FXS. There is, however, information from the substantive dyslexia research literature stating that individuals with phonological processing deficits who are taught only with whole-word methods may be able to add to a sight word vocabulary but that they do poorly when expected to decode novel print sequences. These individuals generally remain poor readers as they age (Byrne, 1998).

A review of the reading programs available for those with intellectual disability revealed that the majority of the programs were based on syllable or whole-word drill and practice sets. Individuals with developmental delays did not appear to be receiving the in-depth phonological awareness training that has been so helpful for many individuals with dyslexia.

Byrne, Fielding-Barnsley, and Ashley (2000) found that children who participated in a highly structured preschool training program for phoneme awareness performed better than untrained controls 6 years later on several tests of irregular word, real word, and nonword reading. The best preschool predictor of their later reading development was the number of training sessions needed to reach a criterion level for phoneme awareness. There now seems to be an emphasis on the early assessment of children's response to intervention (RTI).

Recommendations are strongly made for more phonological awareness training for individuals with FXS. The instruction should be sensitive to RTI and will be more intense for individuals with intellectual disability. It is important that individuals with FXS become more independent readers and that they have access to research-supported interventions. Giving individuals with FXS the opportunity to acquire the phonological tools that will allow them to sound out new words may greatly expand their reading skills and affect quality of life.

SIMILARITIES BETWEEN INDIVIDUALS WITH FRAGILE X SYNDROME AND THOSE WITH DOWN SYNDROME

The reading studies indicate that both individuals with DS and those with FXS tend to read better than might be expected from their mental age levels and that both groups find decoding more difficult than sight word reading. This suggests that reading can be viewed as a potential strength to be developed; that initially, sight word strengths should be used to teach reading; and that extra attention must be paid to developing the understanding and use of letter–sound rules and decoding skills.

EFFECTIVE TEACHING METHODS THAT LINK LITERACY AND SPEECH-LANGUAGE GOALS

Most authors consider the principles for teaching children with DS to be largely the same as for all children (Farrell, 1996; Farrell & Gunn, 2000; Oelwein, 1995, 1999). In addition, teachers should recognize that reading instruction is a very powerful way to teach spoken language. Teaching methods should also take account of some of the evidence of this, particularly the data showing that children with DS are using their good visual skills and may depend on sight word, or logographic, strategies to higher reading ages than typically developing children. Males with FXS are typically not advanced in phonological processes and also overly rely on logographic methods to read.

Reading is a complex activity, and for children with significant cognitive difficulties, it is also important to consider how they understand what they are learning to do. The aim of reading is to obtain meaning from text, and therefore, the first author of this chapter and her colleagues suggest that a child or adult with DS should learn 30–40 sight words that can be made into meaningful sentences so that they can enjoy reading for meaning from the outset. The vocabulary and sentences should be chosen to be appropriate for the language comprehension level and the interests of the individual. Once the individual is successfully reading in this way, he or she can begin learning about the ways in which the letters represent sounds and the ways the letters and sounds make up words (see Table 10.1). The process of understanding this is helped by using the words the individual can already competently read to illustrate how the letters and sounds work in those words. Phonics (i.e., decoding and blending) are not introduced before success is achieved with some sight words. In the experience of the first author of this chapter and her colleagues, if teaching phonic strategies begins before successful sight word reading is achieved, the child may think every word has to be sounded out as letter sounds and may fail to see and read the whole word. Many of the children with DS with whom they have worked steadily master phonics and can decode new words and can spell, but doing so takes time and consistent instruction through the elementary years.

Previously reviewed research findings highlight the influence of verbal short-term memory skills on phonemic awareness; phoneme manipulation; and word attack skills, or decoding skills. Most children and adults with DS have relatively poor verbal short-term memory skills; therefore, the memory demands of tasks should always be considered. Teaching methods that use visual materials to support learning are likely to be the most successful.

Reading intervention studies are needed to identify the most effective teaching methods. There are none published at present, but some small intervention studies in the United Kingdom are beginning to report their findings (Baylis & Snowling, 2005; Goetz, Carroll, Nasir, Snowling, & Hulme, in press). The Goetz

Table 10.1.   Ten tips for increasing early literacy outcomes

1. Teach a small sight vocabulary first. Choose vocabulary that the student understands.
2. Use these sight words in sentences.
3. Ensure that the sentences can be read and understood.
4. Teach letter names and letter sounds.
5. Begin to teach decoding and blending only when Step 3 has been achieved.
6. Always make the activities fun, model correct responses, and prompt success.
7. Make personal books together about the student's life and interests to support the school curriculum. Get out the digital camera for this.
8. Make use of computer software for creating text.
9. Teach text comprehension strategies (e.g., visualizing, retelling, predicting, question generating).
10. Look for good software to support all aspects of literacy learning.

For more advice on successful strategies and practical ideas for literacy teaching, see Bird, Beadman, and Buckley (2001) and Bird and Buckley (2001, 2003).

et al. (in press) study reported the results of a controlled short-term intervention study providing individually planned one-to-one teaching for 40-minute daily sessions over an 8-week period. The intervention program taught children phoneme segmentation and blending skills in the context of learning letter–sound correspondences and working with words in books. The children in the intervention group improved significantly on measures of early literacy skills compared with a waiting control group. The waiting group then joined the intervention, and both groups made progress that was maintained 5 months after the intervention project finished. The Baylis and Snowling (2005) study also reported gains in reading outcomes for 10 children, each receiving two 1-hour individual reading instruction sessions per week for 11 weeks. The program focused on improving the children's sight vocabulary and their alphabetic/decoding skills. There is still much to learn about effective interventions that take account of the particular language and cognitive profiles of individuals, but those engaged in this work will also benefit from being familiar with the research into reading development and reading instruction for typically developing children (Roberts & Scott, 2006; Snowling & Hulme, 2005).

When to Start?

These previously outlined principles can be applied with beginning readers of any age, although evidence of early reading abilities previously reviewed in the chapter supports the view that reading activities should begin early. The first author of this chapter and her colleagues introduce reading as soon as children can match and select pictures and have a comprehension vocabulary of some 50–100 words. They then choose words for two and three key-word sentences and teach these as sight words by playing a matching and selecting game with the words without pictures (Bird & Buckley, 2001; Didden, de Graff, Nelemans, Vooren, & Lancioni, 2006). At the same time, they make books illustrating the words and sentences that are personalized for each child and his or her family. Reading activities are embedded in a speech and language program for each child. The emphasis is on fun and supported learning. The words and sentences are read together, and the child is prompted to succeed. Even if the child does not learn to read the words, the materials support language learning.

Older Learners

Although the importance and particular benefits of introducing reading before 5 years of age has been emphasized, children with DS or FXS may make progress at any age. Teenagers may be motivated to learn to read as they see the practical benefits of learning, and some authors (Farrell, 1996; Farrell & Elkins, 1991; Fowler et al., 1995) have emphasized that the cognitive skills of teenagers may mean that they are better able to make progress than in earlier years and that schools therefore should not give up formal literacy teaching in teenage years. An adult literacy program in Australia is reporting reading progress for young adults with DS, making use of a variety of whole language approaches, as well as traditional teaching methods, to support students in experiencing successful literacy (Gallaher, van Kraayenoord, Jobling, & Moni, 2002; Moni & Jobling, 2001; Morgan, Moni, & Jobling, 2004; van Kraayenoord, Moni, Jobling, & Ziebarth, 2001).

This project is also making full use of computer-assisted learning, and there is now a wide variety of excellent software to support literacy teaching. The benefits of computer-assisted learning for language and literacy for children with DS have been demonstrated by Meyers (1988, 1990).

Role of the Family in Supporting Literacy Teaching

For all children, the experience of being read to and then encouraged to read in the family home is an important factor in their progress. Family involvement in literacy teaching may be even more important for children with DS or FXS, as they need more support and more practice to progress. In the first chapter author's experience, all of the skilled readers with DS whom she has worked with or assessed have received more literacy teaching at home than at school. With higher expectations in schools, however, this may be changing. All of the readers who have started to read by 3 years of age have been taught by their families, including K.S. (Groen et al., 2006). Some families have had good support in planning reading programs from home-visiting teachers or speech and language therapists, but other parents have successfully worked alone, taking their guidance from written information.

There is little published work on the role of families in the literacy achievements of children with DS. A survey of 224 parents or guardians in Canada (Trenholm & Mirenda, 2006) indicated that families provided many opportunities for their children to observe reading activities and a wide range of literacy materials. Although most families read to their children and discussed the pictures, fewer than one third reported that they asked their child to retell a story or answer comprehension questions. Families had the highest expectations for literacy goals during elementary school years, and Trenholm and Mirenda commented on the need to inform families about the effective ways that they can support literacy development in an ongoing manner. There is clearly a need for more guidance to be developed for both families and teachers to enable them to teach literacy skills effectively.

Role of the Speech-Language Pathologist in Supporting Literacy Teaching

The speech-language pathologist (SLP) can play an important role in supporting literacy teaching in the classroom and in the preschool years. Most importantly, the SLP can ensure that reading is at an appropriate language level for the child, with vocabulary and sentence structures within the child's comprehension. The SLP can help the teacher or parent construct reading activities to specifically teach new vocabulary and grammar to a child, from preschool and throughout later school years. In addition, all speech and language targets can be incorporated into reading, spelling, and phonics activities.

CONCLUSION

This chapter has reviewed the available literature on reading outcomes and processes for individuals with DS and FXS. It has also emphasized the potential benefits of being involved in reading activities and instruction for speech, language, and working memory development. Although many individuals with these conditions can achieve useful levels of literacy skills, the authors would draw attention to the benefits for those who do not become independent readers. They may still gain in language and world knowledge. Others have also stressed the benefits of valuing all literacy achievements, regardless of how small (Kliewer, 1998), and of being involved in the world of literacy and storytelling (Grove, 1998). Many individuals with developmental disabilities do not receive quality (or any) reading instruction during their education. It is hoped that teachers, parents, and SLPs will be encouraged to have higher expectations for reading achievements and to further develop quality instruction and literacy experiences for all.

REFERENCES

Abbeduto, L., Murphy, M.M., Cawthon, S.W., Richmond, E., Weissman, M.D., Karadottir, S., et al. (2003). Receptive language skills of adolescents and young adults with Down or FXS syndrome. *American Journal on Mental Retardation, 108*(3), 149–160.

Appleton, M. (2000). *Reading and its relationship to language development: A comparison of preschool children with Down syndrome, hearing impairment, or typical development.* Unpublished master's thesis, University of Portsmouth, United Kingdom.

Appleton, M., Buckley, S., & MacDonald, J. (2002). The early reading skills of preschoolers with Down syndrome and their typically developing peers: Findings from recent research. *Down Syndrome News and Update, 2,* 9–10.

Baylis, P., & Snowling, M. (2005, September). *A reading training study for children with Down syndrome.* Paper presented at the 4th International Conference on Developmental Issues in Down Syndrome, Portsmouth, United Kingdom.

Bird, G., Beadman, J., & Buckley, S. (2001). *Reading and writing for children with Down syndrome (5–11 years).* Portsmouth, United Kingdom: The Down Syndrome Educational Trust.

Bird, G., & Buckley, S. (2001). *Reading and writing for infants with Down syndrome (0–5 years).* Portsmouth, United Kingdom: The Down Syndrome Educational Trust.

Bird, G., & Buckley, S. (2002). *Reading and writing development for teenagers with Down syndrome (11–16 years).* Portsmouth, United Kingdom: The Down Syndrome Educational Trust.

Bochner, S., Outhred, L., & Pieterse, M. (2001). A study of functional literacy skills in young adults with Down syndrome. *International Journal of Disability, Development and Education, 48*(1), 67–90.

Boudreau, D. (2002). Literacy skills in children and adolescents with Down syndrome. *Reading and Writing: An Interdisciplinary Journal, 15,* 497–525.

Brady, S., Mann, V., & Schmidt, R. (1987). Errors in short-term memory for good and poor readers. *Memory and Cognition, 15,* 444–453.

Brady, S., Shankweiler, D., & Mann, V. (1983). Speech perception and memory coding in relation to reading ability. *Journal of Experimental Child Psychology, 35,* 345–367.

Buckley, S.J. (1985). Attaining basic educational skills: Reading, writing and number. In D. Lane & B. Stratford (Eds.), *Current approaches to Down syndrome* (pp. 315–343). London: Holt Saunders.

Buckley, S.J. (1993). Developing the speech and language skills of teenagers with Down syndrome. *Down Syndrome Research and Practice, 1*(2), 63–71.

Buckley, S.J. (1995). Improving the expressive language skills of teenagers with Down syndrome. *Down Syndrome Research and Practice, 3*(3), 110–115.

Buckley, S.J. (2001). *Reading and writing for individuals with Down syndrome: An overview.* Portsmouth, United Kingdom: The Down Syndrome Educational Trust.

Buckley, S.J. (2000). *Speech and language development for individuals with Down syndrome: An overview.* Portsmouth, United Kingdom: The Down Syndrome Educational Trust.

Buckley, S.J. (2002). Literacy and language. In J.A. Rondal & S. Buckley (Eds.), *Speech and language intervention in Down syndrome* (pp. 132–153). London: Whurr.

Buckley, S.J., & Bird, G. (1993). Teaching children with Down syndrome to read. *Down Syndrome Research and Practice, 1*(1), 34–41.

Buckley, S.J., Bird, G., & Byrne, A. (1996a). The practical and theoretical significance of teaching literacy skills to children with Down syndrome. In J. Rondal & J. Perera (Eds.), *Down syndrome: Psychological, psychobiological, and socio-educational perspectives* (pp. 119–128). London: Whurr Publishers.

Buckley, S.J., Bird, G., & Byrne, A. (1996b). Reading acquisition by young children. In B. Stratford & P. Gunn (Eds.), *New approaches to Down syndrome* (pp. 268–279). London: Cassell.

Buckley, S., Bird, G., Sacks, B., & Archer, T. (2006). A comparison of mainstream and special education for teenagers with Down syndrome: Implications for parents and teachers. *Down Syndrome Research and Practice, 9*(3), 54–67.

Byrne, A. (1997). *Teaching reading to children with Down syndrome.* Unpublished doctoral dissertation, University of Portsmouth.

Byrne, A., Buckley, S.J., MacDonald, J., & Bird, G. (1995). Investigating the literacy, language, and memory skills of children with Down syndrome and their mainstream peers. *Down Syndrome Research and Practice, 3*(2), 53–58.

Byrne, A., MacDonald, J., & Buckley, S.J. (2002). Reading, language and memory skills: A comparative longitudinal study of children with Down syndrome and their mainstream peers. *British Journal of Educational Psychology, 72,* 513–529.

Byrne, B. (1998). *The foundation of literacy: The child's acquisition of the alphabetic principle.* Hove, England: Psychology Press.

Byrne, B., Fielding-Barnsley, R., & Ashley, L. (2000). Effects of phoneme identity training after six years: Outcome level distinguished from rate of response. *Journal of Educational Psychology, 92,* 659–667.

Cardoso-Martins, C., & Frith, U. (2001). Can individuals with Down syndrome acquire alphabetic literacy skills in the absence of phoneme awareness? *Reading and Writing: An Interdisciplinary Journal, 14,* 361–375.

Cardoso-Martins, C., Michalick, M.F., & Pollo, T.C. (2002). Is sensitivity to rhyme a developmental precursor to sensitivity to phoneme? Evidence from individuals with Down syndrome. *Reading and Writing: An Interdisciplinary Journal, 15,* 439–454.

Chapman, R.S. (1999). Language development in children and adolescents with Down syndrome. In J.F. Miller, M. Leddy, & L.A. Leavitt. (Eds.), *Improving the communication of people with Down syndrome* (pp. 41–60). Baltimore: Paul H Brookes Publishing Co.

Chapman, R.S., & Hesketh, L.J. (2001). Language, cognition, and short-term memory in individuals with Down syndrome. *Down Syndrome Research and Practice, 79,* 1–8.

Conners, F.A. (2002). Phonological working memory difficulty and related interventions. In J.A. Rondal & S. Buckley (Eds.), *Speech and language intervention in Down syndrome* (pp. 31–48). London: Whurr.

Conners, F.A., Atwell, J.A., Rosenquist, C.J., & Sligh, A.C. (2001). Abilities underlying decoding differences in children with intellectual disability. *Journal of Intellectual Disability Research, 45,* 292–299.

Conti-Ramsden, G., & Durkin, F. (2007). Phonological short-term memory, language, and literacy: Developmental relationships in early adolescence in young people with SLI. *Journal of Child Psychology and Psychiatry, 48*(2), 147–156.

Craig, H.K., & Telfer, A.S. (2005). Hyperlexia and autism spectrum disorder: A case study of scaffolding language growth over time. *Topics in Language Disorders, 25*(4), 364–375.

Cupples, L., & Iacono, T. (2000). Phonological awareness is related to reading skill in children with Down syndrome. *Journal of Speech, Language, and Hearing Research, 43,* 595–608.

Cupples, L., & Iacono, T. (2002). The efficacy of 'whole word' versus 'analytic' reading instruction for children with Down syndrome. *Reading and Writing: An Interdisciplinary Journal, 15,* 549–574.

Dickinson, L.L. (2002). The use of a reading programme and signing to develop language and communication skills in a toddler with Down syndrome. *Down Syndrome News and Update, 2*(1), 2–4.

Didden, R., de Graff, S., Nelemans, M., Vooren, M., & Lancioni, G. (2006). Teaching sight words to children with moderate to mild mental retardation: Comparison between instructional procedures. *American Journal on Mental Retardation, 111*(5), 366–377.

Dodd, B., & Thompson, L. (2001). Speech disorder in children with Down's syndrome. *Journal of Intellectual Disability Research, 45*(4), 308–316.

Duffen, L. (1976). Teaching reading to children with little or no language. *Remedial Education, 11*(3), 139–142.

Eadie, P.A., Fey, M.E., Douglas, J.M., & Parsons, C.L. (2002). Profiles of grammatical morphology and sentence imitation in children with specific language impairment and Down syndrome. *Journal of Speech, Language and Hearing Research, 45*, 720–732.

Ellis, N., & Large, B. (1988). The early stages of reading: A longitudinal study. *Applied Cognitive Psychology, 2*(1), 47–76.

Farrell, M. (1996). Continuing literacy development. In B. Stratford & P. Gunn (Eds.), *New approaches to Down syndrome* (pp. 280–299). London: Cassell.

Farrell, M., & Elkins, J. (1991). Literacy and the adolescent with Down syndrome. In C.J. Denholm & J. Ward (Eds.), *Adolescents with Down syndrome: International perspectives on research and programme development. Implications for parents, researchers, and practitioners* (pp. 15–26). British Columbia, Canada: University of Victoria.

Farrell, M., & Gunn, P. (2000). *Literacy for children with Down syndrome: Early days.* Queensland, Australia: Post Pressed.

Fidler, D.J., Most, D.E., & Guiberson, M.M. (2005). Neuropsychological correlates of word identification in Down syndrome. *Research in Developmental Disabilities, 26*, 487–501.

Fletcher, H., & Buckley, S.J. (2002). Phonological awareness in children with Down syndrome. *Down Syndrome Research and Practice, 8*(1), 11–18.

Fowler, A.E., Doherty, B.J., & Boynton, L. (1995). The basis of reading skill in young adults with Down Syndrome. In L. Nadel & D. Rosenthal (Eds.), *Down syndrome: Living and learning in the community* (pp. 182–196). New York: Wiley Liss.

Frith, U. (1985). Beneath the surface of developmental dyslexia. In K.E. Patterson, J.C. Marshall, & M. Coltheart (Eds.), *Surface dyslexia* (pp. 361–397). London: Routledge and Kegan Paul.

Gallaher, K.M., van Kraayenoord, C.E., Jobling, A., & Moni, K.B. (2002). Reading with Abby: A case study of individual tutoring with a young adult with Down syndrome. *Down Syndrome Research and Practice, 8*(2), 59–66.

Gathercole, S.E., & Baddeley, A.D. (1993a). Phonological working memory: A critical building block for reading development and vocabulary acquisition? *European Journal of Psychology of Education, 8*(3), 259–272.

Gathercole, S., & Baddeley, A. (1993b). *Working memory and language.* Hove, United Kingdom: Lawrence Erlbaum Associates.

Gathercole, S.E., & Pickering, S.J. (2000). Working memory deficits in children with low achievements in the national curriculum at 7 years of age. *British Journal of Educational Psychology, 70*(2), 177–194.

Gathercole, S.E., & Pickering, S.J. (2001). Working memory deficits in children with special educational needs. *British Journal of Special Education, 28*(2), 89–97.

Goetz, K., Carroll, J., Nasir, L., Snowling, M., & Hulme, C. (in press). Training reading and phonological awareness skills in children with Down syndrome. *Reading and Writing.*

Gombert, J.-E. (2002). Children with Down syndrome use phonological knowledge in reading. *Reading and Writing: An Interdisciplinary Journal, 15*, 455–469.

Groen, M., Laws, G., Nation, K., & Bishop, D.V.M. (2006). A case of exceptional reading accuracy in a child with Down syndrome: Underlying skills and the relation to reading comprehension. *Cognitive Neuropsychology, 23*(8), 1190–1214.

Grove, N. (1998). *Literature for All: Developing.* London: David Fulton.

Hatcher, P., Hulme, C., & Ellis, A.W. (1994). Ameliorating early reading failure by integrating the teaching of reading and phonological skills: The phonological link hypothesis. *Child Development, 65*, 41–57.

Hulme, C., Goetz, K., Snowling, M., Brigstocke, S., & Nash, H. (2005, September). *Reading development in children with Down syndrome: relationships with oral language and phonological skills.* Paper presented at the 4th International Conference on Developmental Issues in Down Syndrome, Portsmouth, United Kingdom.

Hulme, C., & Mackenzie, S. (1992). *Working memory and severe learning difficulties.* Mahwah, NJ: Lawrence Erlbaum Associates.

Irwin, K.C. (1989). The school achievement of children with Down's syndrome. *New Zealand Medical Journal, 102*(860), 11–13.

Jarrold, C., & Baddeley, A.D. (2001). Short-term memory in Down syndrome: Applying the working memory model. *Down Syndrome Research and Practice, 7*(1), 17–23.

Jarrold, C., Baddeley, A.D., & Phillips, C. (1999). Down syndrome and the phonological loop: Evidence for, and importance of, a specific verbal short term memory deficit. *Down Syndrome Research and Practice, 6*(2), 61–75.

Johnson-Glenberg, M.C. (2003). Literacy and working memory in those with FXS syndrome. Poster session presented at Symposium on Research on Children's Language Disorders, Madison, WI.

Johnson-Glenberg, M.C. (2007a). FXS syndrome: Memory skills and the emergence of reading in males. In R. Paul (Ed.), *Language disorders from a developmental perspective: Essays in honor of Robin Chapman.* Mahwah, NJ: Lawrence Erlbaum Associates.

Johnson-Glenberg, M.C. (2007b). *FXS syndrome: A neural network model of sequential memory in males.* Manuscript submitted for publication.

Kay-Raining Bird, E., Cleave, P.L., & McConnell, L.M. (2000). Reading and phonological awareness in children with Down syndrome: A longitudinal study. *American Journal of Speech-Language Pathology, 9,* 319–330.

Kennedy, E.J., & Flynn, M.C. (2003a). Early phonological awareness and reading skills in children with Down syndrome. *Down Syndrome Research and Practice, 8,* 100–109.

Kennedy, E.J., & Flynn, M.C. (2003b). Training phonological awareness skills in children with Down syndrome. *Research in Developmental Disabilities, 24,* 44–57.

Kliewer, C. (1998). Citizenship in the literate community: An ethnography of children with Down syndrome and the written word. *Exceptional Children, 64*(2), 167–180.

Kotlinski, J., & Kotlinski, S. (2002). Teaching reading to develop language. *Down Syndrome News and Update, 2*(1), 5–6.

Laws, G. (1998). The use of nonword repetition as a test of phonological memory in children with Down syndrome. *Journal of Child Psychology and Psychiatry, 29,* 1119–1130.

Laws, G., & Bishop, D.V.M. (2003). A comparison of language impairment in adolescents with Down syndrome and children with specific language impairment. *Journal of Speech, Language and Hearing Research, 46,* 1324–1339.

Laws, G., Buckley, S.J., Bird, G., MacDonald, J., & Broadley, I. (1995). The influence of reading instruction on language and memory development in children with Down syndrome. *Down Syndrome Research and Practice, 3*(2), 59–64.

Laws, G., Byrne, A., & Buckley, S.J. (2000). Language and memory development in children with DS at mainstream and special schools: A comparison. *Educational Psychology, 20*(4), 447–457.

Laws, G., & Gunn, D. (2002). Relationships between reading, phonological skills, and language development in individuals with Down syndrome: A five-year follow up study. *Reading and Writing: An Interdisciplinary Journal, 15,* 527–548.

Locke, J.L. (1994). Gradual emergence of developmental language disorders. *Journal of Speech and Hearing Research, 37*(3), 608–616.

Locke, J.L. (1997). A theory of neurolinguistic development. *Brain and Language, 58,* 265–326.

Marcell, M.M. (1995). Relationships between hearing and auditory cognition in Down syndrome youth. *Down Syndrome Research and Practice, 3*(3), 373–398.

Mayberry, R.I., Lock, E., & Kazmi, H. (2002). Linguistic ability and early language exposure. *Nature, 417,* 38.

Meyers, L.F. (1988). Using computers to teach children with Down syndrome spoken and written language skills. In L. Nadel (Ed.), *The psychobiology of Down syndrome* (pp. 247–265). Cambridge, MA: MIT Press.

Meyers, L.F. (1990). Language development and intervention. In D.C. Van Dyke, D. Lang, F. Heide, S. Van Duyne, & M.J. Soucek (Eds.), *Clinical perspectives in the management of Down syndrome* (pp. 153–164). New York: Springer-Verlag.

Miller, J.F. (1999). Profiles of language development in children with Down syndrome. In J.F. Miller, M. Leddy, & L.A. Leavitt. (Eds.), *Improving the communication of people with Down syndrome.* (pp. 41–60). Baltimore: Paul H. Brookes Publishing Co.

Moni, K.B., & Jobling, A. (2001). Reading-related literacy learning of young adults with Down syndrome: Findings from a three year teaching and research program. *International Journal of Disability, Development, and Education, 48,* 377–394.

Morgan, M., Moni, K.B., & Jobling, A. (2004). What's it all about? Investigating reading comprehension strategies in young adults with Down syndrome. *Down Syndrome Research and Practice, 9*(2), 37–44.

Muter, V., & Snowling, M. (1998). Concurrent and longitudinal predictors of reading: The role of meta-linguistic and short-term memory skills. *Reading Research Quarterly, 33,* 320–337.

Nation, K. (2005). Children's reading comprehension difficulties. In M.J. Snowling & C. Hulme (Eds.), *The science of reading: A handbook* (pp. 521–537). Oxford, United Kingdom: Blackwell.

Nation, K., & Norbury, C.F. (2005). Why reading comprehension fails: Insights from developmental disorders. *Topics in Language Disorders, 25*(1), 21–32.

Oakhill, J., & Beard, R. (Eds.). (1999). *Reading development and the teaching of reading: A psychological perspective.* Oxford, United Kingdom: Blackwell Science.

Oelwein, P.L. (1995). *Teaching reading to children with Down syndrome: A guide for parents and teachers.* Bethesda, MD: Woodbine House.

Oelwein, P.L. (1999). Individualizing reading for each child's ability and needs. In T.J. Hassold & D. Patterson (Eds.), *Down syndrome: A promising future together* (pp. 155–164). New York: Wiley Liss.

Oke, M.K., (2002). Teaching Nazli in Turkish and English. *Down Syndrome News and Update, 2*(1), 8.

Pieterse, M. (1988). The Down syndrome program at Macquarie University: A model early intervention program. In M. Pieterse, S. Bochner, & S. Bettison (Eds.), *Early intervention for children with disabilities: The Australian experience* (pp. 81–96). Sydney: Macquarie University.

Pieterse, M., & Center, Y. (1984). The integration of eight Down's Syndrome children into regular schools. *Australia and New Zealand Journal of Developmental Disabilities, 10*(1), 20.

Roberts, J., Hennon, E.A., & Anderson, K. (2003). FXS syndrome and speech and language. *The ASHA Leader, 8*(19), 6–10.

Roberts, J.A., & Scott, K.A. (2006).The simple view of reading: Assessment and intervention. *Topics in Language Disorders, 26*(2), 127–143.

Roberts, J.E., Long, S.H., Malkin, C., Barnes, E., Skinner, M., Hennon, E.A., et al. (2005). A comparison of phonological skills of young males with fragile X syndrome and Down syndrome. *Journal of Speech, Language, and Hearing Research, 48,* 980–995.

Robertson, C., & Salter, W. (1997). *The Phonological Awareness Test.* East Moline, IL: LinguiSystems.

Rozen, G. (2002). Teaching Charlotte spoken language through reading. *Down Syndrome News and Update, 2*(1), 7.

Seymour, P.H.K. (1993, January). *A "dual foundation" model of orthographic development.* Presented at Acquisition de la lecture-écriture et psychologie cognitive, Paris.

Seymour, P.H., & Elder, L. (1986). Beginning reading without phonology. *Cognitive Neuropsychology, 3*(1), 1–36.

Shott, S.R. (2001). Hearing loss in children with Down syndrome. *International Journal of Pediatric Otorhinolaryngology, 61*(3), 199–205.

Siegel, L.S. (1993). Phonological processing deficits as the basis of a reading disability. *Developmental Review, 13,* 246–257.

Snowling, M.J., & Hayiou-Thomas, M.E. (2006). The dyslexia spectrum: Continuities between reading, speech, and language impairments. *Topics in Language Disorders, 26*(2), 110–126.

Snowling, M.J., & Hulme, C. (Eds.). (2005). *The science of reading: A handbook.* Oxford, United Kingdom: Blackwell.

Snowling, M.J., Hulme, C., & Mercer, R.C. (2002). A deficit in rime awareness in children with Down syndrome. *Reading and Writing: An Interdisciplinary Journal, 15,* 471–495.

Stanovich, K.E., Cunningham, A.E., & Feeman, D.J. (1984). Intelligence, cognitive skills, and early reading progress. *Reading Research Quarterly, 19,* 278–303.

Stothard, S.E., Snowling, M.J., Bishop, D.V., Chipchase, B.B., & Kaplan, C.A. (1998). Language impaired preschoolers: A follow up into adolescence. *Journal of Speech Language Hearing Research, 41*(2), 407–418.

Thorndike, R.L., Hagen, E.P., & Sattler, J.M. (1986). *Stanford-Binet Intelligence Scale* (4th ed.). Itasca, IL: Riverside.

Torgesen, J.K. (2005). Recent discoveries on remedial interventions for children with dyslexia. In M.J. Snowling & C. Hulme (Eds.), *The science of reading: A handbook.* (pp. 521–537). Oxford, United Kingdom: Blackwell.

Trenholm, B., & Mirenda, P. (2006). Home and community literacy experiences of individuals with Down syndrome. *Down Syndrome Research and Practice, 10*(1), 30–40.

van Bysterveldt, A., Gillon, G., & Moran, C. (2006). Enhancing phonological awareness and letter knowledge in preschool children with Down syndrome. *International Journal of Disability, Development and Education, 53*(3), 301–329.

van Kraayenoord, C.E., Moni, K.B., Jobling, A., & Ziebarth, K. (2001). Broadening approaches to literacy education for young adults with Down syndrome. In M. Cuskelly, A. Jobling, & S. Buckley (Eds.), *Down syndrome across the life span.* London: Whurr.

Verucci, L., Menghini, D., & Vicari, S. (2006). Reading skills and phonological awareness acquisition in Down syndrome. *Journal of Intellectual Disability Research, 50,* 477–491.

Woodcock, R.W. (1998). *Woodcock Reading Mastery Test–Revised–Normative Update* (WMRT-R/NU). Circle Pines, MN: American Guidance Service.

CHAPTER 11

Augmentative and Alternative Communication for Children with Down Syndrome or Fragile X Syndrome

NANCY C. BRADY

C hildren with developmental disabilities, including Down syndrome (DS) and fragile X syndrome (FXS), are typically delayed in learning to talk. Before talking, they communicate prelinguistically using vocalizations, gestures, and other behaviors. (For more information on prelinguistic communication intervention, please see Chapter 7.) Even after they begin to speak, children with DS or FXS may be difficult to understand (Roberts et al., 2005). One strategy that has been developed to improve communication during the period of time in which children cannot rely on speech is to use augmentative and alternative communication (AAC). This chapter discusses the use of AAC with children with developmental disabilities, with a special emphasis on children with DS or FXS.

Although few empirical studies specifically address AAC in DS, and, to the author's knowledge, none address AAC in FXS, there is a larger body of literature concerning children with other disabilities to draw on. Information from this literature, along with increasing information about the phenotypic language characteristics in children with DS or FXS (cf. Abbeduto & Hagerman, 1997; Chapman, Seung, Schwartz, & Kay-Raining Bird, 2000; Mundy, Kasari, Sigman, & Ruskin, 1995; Roberts, Mirrett, Anderson, Burchinal, & Neebe, 2002; Roberts, Mirrett, & Burchinal, 2001; Yoder & Warren, 2004), provides the foundation for this discussion. A brief description of various forms of AAC is presented first, followed by a discussion of specific applications relevant for children with DS or FXS.

WHAT IS AUGMENTATIVE AND ALTERNATIVE COMMUNICATION?

AAC is a set of strategies used by individuals with limited or no speech abilities to aid in their communication. Some individuals rely on AAC for a period of time in which speech is temporarily unavailable, whereas others use AAC as their primary mode of communication for their entire life. Most systems that describe

255

AAC break it into two categories based on symbol type: aided and unaided (Beukelman & Mirenda, 2005; Lloyd, Fuller, & Arvidson, 1997; Siegel & Cress, 2002). Aided symbols include some external aid, such as a picture board, or a speech-generating device called a voice output communication aid (VOCA). Unaided symbols include natural gestures and sign language systems.

Children with developmental disabilities can learn to use both aided and unaided symbols, often in combination, to communicate (Iacono, Mirenda, & Beukelman, 1993; Reichle & Ward, 1985). In addition, it is important to remember that children with developmental disabilities frequently continue to rely on vocal communication as they learn to communicate with AAC. For example, children often vocalize while communicating with pictures or VOCA devices. Sometimes these vocalizations help convey pragmatic aspects of communication, such as stress, and other times the vocalizations may be word approximations that are more intelligible when combined with AAC.

A common concern for parents and intervention teams considering AAC is that it will discourage speech development. They may worry that children will continue to use an "easier" alternative such as manual signs or pictures instead of speech (Beukelman & Mirenda, 2005). Fortunately there is growing evidence that AAC does not inhibit speech. Participants have been reported to increase speech production following implementation of both aided and unaided AAC (Charlop-Christy, Carpenter, LeBlanc, & Kellet, 2002; Millar, Light, & Schlosser, 2006; Romski & Sevcik, 1993; Schaeffer, 1980). For both children with DS and children with FXS, it has been observed that AAC use diminishes as their use of speech increases and improves (Brady, Skinner, Roberts, & Hennon, 2006; Kumin, 2003). Speech is more efficient than any form of AAC because it is faster and is more likely to be understood by more partners. Therefore, once children can convey their messages through speech, AAC use often decreases.

WHY USE AUGMENTATIVE AND ALTERNATIVE COMMUNICATION WITH CHILDREN WITH DOWN SYNDROME OR FRAGILE X SYNDROME?

AAC has been developed for and has been used with individuals with severely delayed language onset associated with a number of disabilities. The following sections discuss potential benefits for using AAC specifically with individuals with DS or FXS, based on characteristics associated with these two developmental disabilities.

Down Syndrome

Significantly delayed onset of speech and poor intelligibility are two primary reasons for introducing AAC to children with DS. Children with DS often begin speaking much later than typically developing children. Kumin (2003) reported that most children with DS do not use speech until they are between 3 and 5 years of age. In addition to the cognitive delays associated with DS, anatomical and physiological factors also are associated with these speech delays (Miller, 1999; Miller & Leddy, 1998). Most children with DS have anomalies of the skeletal system resulting in a smaller oral cavity. In addition, facial musculature is often poorly developed. A large percentage of children with DS also have hearing losses associated with frequent episodes of otitis media (Rice, Warren, & Betz, 2005). Combined, these factors are likely to contribute to the observation that most children with DS demonstrate particular difficulty acquiring productive language. In a longitudinal analysis of 43 children with DS, Miller (1999) reported that most children showed poorer language production scores relative to either comprehension or general cognitive status. These gaps became more pronounced with age, but the author suggested this may have been due to lack of adequate measures during early development. That is, it is difficult to measure early language comprehension and production or cognitive development, and hence it is difficult to determine whether gaps in skills become greater or if the sensitivity in measuring differences improves over time.

The relative strength in comprehension by children with DS during early stages of language development has been used as one of the rationales in favor of implementing AAC. The rationale is that if children with DS are able to understand more than they are able to produce and if there is a way to bypass the production problem, they should become more effective communicators (Kay-Raining Bird, Gaskell, Dallaire Babineau, & Macdonald, 2000; Kumin, 2003; Miller, 1999). As literature reviewed in later sections will illustrate, AAC may be a key transitional means of communication during this period of delayed speech onset.

Once children with DS do begin to speak, they are often difficult to understand. Decreased intelligibility has been reported in spontaneous speech (Abbeduto & Murphy, 2004) and during single-word productions (Roberts et al., 2005). Roberts and colleagues reported that children with DS had significantly more incorrect consonant productions during single-word productions than either children with FXS or younger, typically developing children. Thus, children with DS may continue to use AAC as they begin to speak because it may increase intelligibility. For example, a child may use a picture or letter representing an initial sound to help disambiguate an unintelligible utterance (Brady & Halle, 2002).

Fragile X Syndrome

Like children with DS, children with FXS, particularly males, are usually delayed in learning to speak. Children with FXS often say their first words 1 year or more later than typically developing children (Roberts et al., 2001), and some children with FXS remain nonverbal for life. Children with FXS also have some of the same anatomical and physiologic factors as those described for children with DS. For example, increased ear infections and oral-motor sensitivity and weakness have been described as characteristics of young children with FXS (Rice et al., 2005). Mothers have reported using AAC with a majority of young children with FXS during this period of prolonged prelinguistic communication (Brady et al., 2006).

Children with FXS may also be difficult to understand once they begin to speak. Conversational speech may be particularly unintelligible (Abbeduto & Hagerman, 1997). Intelligibility may be affected by harshness in vocal tone and speaking in a rapid and variable rate (Rice et al., 2005). In single-word production, however, speech was similar between children with FXS and younger, typically developing children who were matched to children with FXS according to nonverbal mental age (Roberts et al., 2005). Thus, although speech intelligibility in children with FXS may not be as compromised as it is in children with DS, it is still an issue and may contribute to a decision to use AAC with children with FXS during the initial stages of learning to speak.

A relatively large proportion of children with FXS (25%–30%) also meet the diagnostic criteria for autism (Bailey et al., 2004). Children who have both FXS and autism may share many of the same characteristics, including hand flapping, poor verbal development, increased stereotypic behaviors, and sometimes challenging behaviors. Challenging behaviors may include aggression toward self or others. AAC may have additional benefits for children with challenging behaviors. A body of research has demonstrated that AAC can be a functional alternative for these challenging behaviors (Brady & Halle, 1997; Durand, 1999; Reichle & Wacker, 1993). As AAC use increases, concomitant decreases in challenging behaviors may be observed (Mirenda, 1997; Mirenda, 2003).

AUGMENTATIVE AND ALTERNATIVE COMMUNICATION APPROACHES USED WITH CHILDREN WITH DISABILITIES

The following sections present examples of AAC approaches that are used with children with disabilities, including children with DS or FXS. Examples of systems that are used alone are presented first, followed by a discussion of multimodal systems. Examples of use with children with DS are highlighted when possible, and implications for children with FXS are discussed. The literature on using AAC with children with autism is particularly relevant because many children with FXS also meet diagnostic criteria for autism (Bailey et al., 2004). Therefore, examples of use with children with autism also are presented.

Natural Gestures

Natural gestures (e.g., pointing, giving objects, leading by the hand, open palm requests) are important early communication forms. Typically developing children use gestures in conjunction with vocalizations as their primary means of communication during their first year of life (Crais, Day Douglas, & Cox Campbell, 2004; Volterra, Caselli, Capirci, & Pizzuto, 2005). Natural gestures may also be considered as unaided forms of AAC (Beukelman & Mirenda, 2005). In their eagerness to find the most word-like form of communication, parents and intervention teams may not always recognize natural gestures as potential intervention targets. Several studies, however, have found that children with a variety of disabilities show improved communication after participating in interventions aimed at increasing use of natural gestures (Calculator, 2003; Fey et al., 2006; Yoder & Warren, 2002).

Descriptive studies have documented that children with DS, like typically developing children, communicate with gestures during mother–child interactions. In a longitudinal study of three children with DS, Chan and Iacono (2001) reported that all three children communicated with a variety of gestures and used these gestures to communicate a variety of functions (e.g., to request and comment). Iverson, Longobardi, and Caselli (2003) compared five children with DS with five typically developing children matched according to language ages and found that the children with DS produced fewer gestures than the typically developing children but that the children with DS still frequently communicated with gestures.

The advantages of natural gestures include their portability and comprehensibility. Children who are able to move their upper extremities are physically able to make most gestures whenever they want to communicate, without additional materials. When a child points to an object, most adult communication partners will follow the direction of the point and will often name the object to which the child has pointed. Similarly, when a child unsuccessfully tries to open an object and then gives the object to a communication partner, the child's meaning is readily apparent. In a recent longitudinal study, Brady, Marquis, Fleming, and McLean (2004) found that children with developmental disabilities who used more advanced forms of gestures, such as pointing, had better language outcomes than children who did not use pointing gestures. These early forms of communication can help set the stage for later communication by promoting caregiver interactions and input. It is often necessary, however, to teach parents and teachers to recognize the communicative value of these gestures (Coulter & Gallagher, 2001; Girolametto, Greenberg, & Manolson, 1986; Keen, Sigafoos, & Woodyatt, 2005).

The disadvantage of natural gestures is that they can only be used to refer to objects and events present in the child's immediate environment. Because they are nonsymbolic, natural gestures can only refer to concrete referents. If a child wants to communicate about something that happened yesterday or wants to ask for something that is not present, natural gestures will be inadequate. Symbolic forms of communication such as those discussed in the following sections allow individuals to communicate about objects and events outside of the immediate context and to communicate abstract ideas and feelings.

Manual Sign Systems

Many examples of efforts to teach signs derived from formal sign language systems to individuals with developmental disabilities can be found in the literature (Bonvillian & Nelson, 1976; Carr, Binkoff, Kologinsky, & Eddy, 1978; Schepis et al., 1982). These studies showed acquisition of signs by children with a variety of disabilities and across different contexts. As Mirenda (2003) pointed out, however, the majority of these studies demonstrated only acquisition of labels. That is, children learned to respond to questions such as "What is this?" but were rarely observed to generalize production to requests, comments, or other functional communication contexts.

A concern often voiced about sign language is that it may limit children's communication success because of the need for communication partners familiar with sign language (Mirenda & Bopp, 2003). In addition, the motor configurations of some signs can result in very similar-looking gestures. For example, the signs for "eat" and "drink" share similar hand shapes, movement patterns, and locations (Reichle, Cooley Hidecker, Brady, & Terry, 2003). Such similarities among signs may lead to ambiguous interpretations (communication breakdowns), particularly with unfamiliar partners.

An advantage associated with sign language is portability. Like natural gestures, no extra equipment is needed to produce signs. In addition, children learning to sign do not have to make discriminations between graphic stimuli, as is needed with certain types of AAC, which may be difficult for some children with severe disabilities (Brady & Saunders, 1991; Michael, 1985; Sundberg & Sundberg, 1990). Several studies have documented speech development in children after learning to communicate with sign language (Barrera, Lobato-Barrera, & Sulzer-Azaroff, 1980; Kay-Raining Bird et al., 2000; Kouri, 1989; Layton & Savino, 1990). Some research suggests that teaching sign language early on may offer an advantage to young children, even if they do not need AAC (Abrahemsen, Cavallo, & McCluer, 1985; Goodwyn & Acredolo, 1993). A recent review of results from many studies of sign language effects for typically developing infants, however, concluded that there is insufficient evidence to support claims that signing facilitates spoken language development (Johnston, Durieux-Smith, & Bloom, 2005).

The following sections review sign language studies specifically applicable to children with DS and children with autism. As mentioned previously, no studies specifically deal with AAC with children with FXS, but studies from children with autism may be instructive.

Down Syndrome

Sign language has remained a popular form of AAC for children with DS. Kumin (2003) reported that sign language is the most commonly used transitional language system for children with DS. Kay-Raining Bird and Chapman (1994) reported that one estimate of the frequency of sign language intervention for young children with DS was 85%. Perhaps the particular popularity for children with DS (relative to other types of developmental disability) stems from identification of these children at or before birth. Parents and professionals are often eager to start intervention early in infancy, and signing to their children is one way to intervene. It has also been suggested that sign language may be easier to learn because the symbols rely on a visual mode, and children with DS have been found to have better visual than auditory memories (Kay-Raining Bird & Chapman, 1994). In addition, signs may be easier for children to form and for teachers to physically prompt than spoken words.

Total communication refers to the use of signs in combination with word production. Teachers or parents implementing a total communication approach often sign some or all of the words as they are speaking to their children. This total approach is thought by some to provide additional linguistic input that may facilitate word learning (Beukelman & Mirenda, 2005; Layton & Savino, 1990). In a study directly comparing word learning through sign presentation alone, sign combined with spoken presentation, and speech presentation alone, Kay-Raining Bird and colleagues (2000) found no significant differences in production and comprehension probes. They did, however, find differences in imitation—children imitated more often following the simultaneously presented models. This study included 10 children with DS and a group of typically developing children matched according to mental age. The authors speculated that the children might have attended more when signs were combined with speech and that this increased attention facilitated imitation.

Although signed input through total communication is often considered facilitative, little attention has been devoted to details about how to sign to children with DS. Clibbens, Powell, and Atkinson (2002) compared strategies used by mothers signing to their children with DS with strategies used by deaf mothers signing to their deaf infants. The authors pointed out that mothers of deaf children often use a number of strategies to increase joint attention between referent and sign. For example, mothers of deaf children frequently displace their signs to be within the child's visual field or signing space. Clibbens and colleagues found that mothers of children with DS rarely used displaced signs. They used different strategies, including molding of their children's hands. The authors observed, however, that during the initial stages of sign learning, molding their children's hands often disrupted the child's joint engagement with the referent and mother. The authors suggested that some of the strategies used by deaf mothers may facilitate sign learning by children with DS.

Autism and Fragile X Syndrome

According to Beukelman and Mirenda (2005), prior to 1990, manual signing was the form of AAC used most often with people diagnosed as having autism or cognitive disabilities. A number of studies showed that children with autism could acquire a vocabulary of productive signs (Barrera et al., 1980; Bonvillian & Nelson, 1976; Carr, Kologinsky, & Leff-Simon, 1987; Fulwiler & Fouts, 1976; Remington & Clarke, 1993; Schepis et al., 1982). Manual sign instruction or total communication combining sign with speech is still often recommended for children with autism and appears popular for nonverbal children with FXS as well. A recent study reported the results of 55 interviews with mothers of young children with FXS, in which many of the children were nonspeaking (Brady et al., 2006). Twenty-seven of these mothers reported using signs with their children to help them communicate.

The rationale for teaching manual signs to children with autism and/or FXS are similar to those given for children with DS. Namely, sign language is a visual system, and many children with autism also show relative strengths in processing visual versus auditory information (Mirenda, 2003). In addition, signs are easier to prompt than are vocalizations. Several studies have demonstrated increased speech production after using a total communication approach with children with autism (Carr & Kologinsky, 1983; Layton, 1988; Schepis et al., 1982).

Some additional characteristics of autism and FXS may impede sign language use, however. Some research suggests that sequencing the fine motor movements required for many signs may be difficult for children with autism (Seal & Bonvillian, 1997). Issues of motor control have been described in children with FXS as well (Baranek et al., 2005). In addition, Roberts and colleagues (2002) found that young children with FXS showed relative weaknesses in gesture use compared with vocal and verbal communication. In response to these potential limitations and the problem of limited audience (i.e., children who learn signs as their primary form of communication are only able to communicate with others who can understand signs), more recent studies of AAC use by children with autism spectrum disorders and other developmental disabilities have tended to favor other types of visual systems (see Mirenda, 2003, for a review).

Picture Exchange Communication System

An AAC mode that has been frequently used in recent years with children with autism and/or severe intellectual disability is the Picture Exchange Communication System (PECS; Charlop-Christy et al., 2002; Frost & Bondy, 1994; Schwartz, Garfinkle, & Bauer, 1998). In PECS, children are initially taught to select pictures and exchange them to request items depicted in the pictures. Later phases of instruction include teaching children to combine pictures to form basic sentences and exchange them to make requests and comments, such as "I see a dog."

Like all aided systems, PECS requires access to a communication aid, in this case symbols and the display. PECS symbols are typically housed in a large binder, and children locate and extract symbols from this binder and affix them to a strip of cardboard with Velcro—this is known as the "sentence strip." Thus, successful communication in some environments, such as the playground, can be difficult with PECS because the symbol set and sentence strip may not be available. Although symbols used in PECS may represent all of the parts of speech (e.g., determiner, nouns, verbs), the PECS communicator is limited to the symbol set available at any one time. In other words, children cannot communicate about a referent unless they have the symbol for that referent. This increases the dependency on a teacher or caregiver to provide adequate vocabulary selection.

An advantage to PECS is that it systematically teaches persistence. Early on in the program, children are taught to persist in attempting to exchange symbols with a communication partner who is not attending to them. Communication partners will purposefully turn their backs away from a child and fail to respond until the child has given the symbol to them. In a sense, this phase of training directly teaches children to repair communication breakdowns by repeating their communication attempts. Another advantage of PECS is that many of the pictures used to symbolize referents may be more readily understood by inexperienced communication partners than signs.

In addition to increasing communication, PECS has also been associated with increased speech production (Bondy & Frost, 1993; Charlop-Christy et al., 2002; Schwartz et al., 1998). Schwartz and colleagues reported results from implementing PECS with 31 preschool children who had a variety of developmental disabilities, including DS and autism. The authors reported that the average length of time to acquire and use PECS was 11 months. Forty-four percent of the children were reported to also begin speaking after learning to communicate with PECS. The authors acknowledged, however, that many variables other than PECS could have contributed to speech development.

Although no studies have been found that have specifically focused on using PECS with children with DS, the study by Schwartz and colleagues (1998) included several students with DS. Children with DS in this study appeared to show patterns similar to those of the other participants.

Autism and Fragile X Syndrome

Several studies investigating PECS acquisition by children with autism have been reported. In one of the original reports on PECS, Bondy and Frost (1993) reported that 67 children with autism learned to use PECS in a school setting where it was incorporated throughout classroom activities. For example, children chose play activities and lunch items with PECS. The authors also reported that 59% of the children developed speech as their primary communication mode after using PECS. Although this report is merely descriptive, it has led to more rigorously controlled studies of PECS with children with autism.

A study by Charlop-Christy and colleagues (2002) demonstrated increased spoken communication following PECS instruction for three individuals with autism using a multiple-baseline-across-participants design. All three participants, however, were able to at least imitate a few words at the outset of PECS instruction, and imitation has been identified as a predictor of later speech (McCathren, Yoder, & Warren, 1999). Kamps, Kemmerer, and Potucek (2002) also showed increased spontaneous speech and PECS use by a school-age child with autism following PECS instruction.

PECS and manual sign training were directly compared in two studies. Adkins and Axelrod (2001) taught a boy with autism spectrum disorder to use both manual signs and PECS to request preferred objects, and they evaluated relative performance using an alternating-treatments design. The results favored PECS—the boy learned PECS faster and showed greater generalization with PECS. Tincani (2004) reported slightly different results, however. Two school-age children with autism spectrum disorders were each taught to request one set of items with manual signs and another set of items with PECS using an alternating-treatments design. The results showed that one child learned signs quicker, whereas the other child learned PECS quicker. Both children produced more spoken words in the sign condition. Once again, however, both children were able to produce at least some speech at the outset of the study. The authors concluded that interventionists should evaluate individual children's skills in areas such as motor and vocal imitation in order to determine whether one modality is likely to be more beneficial than another.

Although no research studies with children with FXS have been reported, PECS appears to be frequently implemented for children with FXS. In the interview study described previously (Brady et al., 2006), mothers of young children with FXS frequently reported using PECS with their children. Fifteen of the 55 participating mothers reported using PECS or picture selection systems. The popularity of PECS appears related to two factors. First, PECS is an approach grounded in behavior analytic teaching strategies and is compatible with popular behavioral education approaches. Second, PECS workshops are widely available, and teachers and clinicians can readily obtain training in how to implement PECS. It is a prepackaged program that contains information about teaching each step of PECS, which may also appeal to some education teams who are relatively unfamiliar with AAC.

Other Graphic Augmentative and Alternative Communication Systems

Long before PECS was available, other graphic (picture-based) communication systems were developed and used with individuals with developmental disabilities, including DS and autism (Calculator & Dollaghan, 1982; Glennen & Calculator, 1985; Reichle & Brown, 1986; Reichle & Yoder, 1985). The primary distinction between PECS and other graphic AAC approaches is the means of message transmittal. In PECS, the picture-symbol is physically exchanged with the communication partner. In other graphic AAC approaches, the learner selects the symbol by either touching the symbol directly or by selecting the symbol through the use of a switch interface (as in scanning approaches used with individuals with limited motor abilities). Graphic selection may have some advantages over manual sign systems because it takes advantage of recognition instead of recall memory (Iacono & Duncum, 1995; Mirenda, 2003; Reichle et al., 2003). That is, producing a graphic symbol response requires selecting from among a fixed array of possible symbols, but producing a sign requires recall without such an array.

Individuals with developmental disabilities have learned to select symbols to request items or activities (Kozleski, 1991; Reichle & Sigafoos, 1991; Sigafoos & Reichle, 1992), to reject nonpreferred items (Martin, Drasgow, Halle, & Brucker, 2005; Sigafoos, Drasgow, Reichle, et al., 2004) and to label objects (Reichle, Barrett, Tetlie, & McQuarter, 1987; Sigafoos, Doss, & Reichle, 1989). The symbols may be photographs, line drawings, or more abstract images that represent referents. It is recommended that consideration be given to individual learners' abilities to associate various symbol types with referent objects before deciding on a specific symbol type (Mineo Mollica, 2003).

As with the other types of AAC discussed thus far, graphic selection communication input has also been described as facilitative of word learning. It has been suggested that for children learning AAC, partners' use of AAC in addressing the child (*augmented input*) will have positive effects on the child's acquisition and use of AAC and receptive language development (Harris & Reichle, 2004; Romski & Sevcik, 1993; Schlosser, Belfiore, Nigam, Blischak, & Hetzroni, 1995). Although very few studies focus solely on augmented input's effects, Harris and Reichle (2004) found that three children with moderate disabilities increased their comprehension and use of picture symbols after an intervention that focused on augmented input.

Down Syndrome

Several studies on ACC used by individuals with developmental disabilities included children with DS (e.g., Sigafoos, 1992; Sigafoos & Reichle, 1989). Use of graphic AAC has been described as an appropriate strategy for children with DS because it is visual in nature and may capitalize on the visual strengths of children with DS (Clibbens et al., 2002; Kumin, 2003; Miller, 1999). Hunt, Alwell, and Goetz (1991) demonstrated how use of graphic symbols could promote peer interactions, in addition to augmenting basic communication functions such as requesting. Three students, including one student with DS, were taught to initiate conversations through the use of a notebook containing pictures and drawings that represented favorite activities. Each of the children increased their conversational turns through the use of the notebooks.

Autism and Fragile X Syndrome

There have been many demonstrations of teaching children with autism to use graphic forms of AAC to communicate across a variety of contexts. As discussed by Mirenda (2003), participants in most of these studies were taught to request desired objects or activities. A recent article also described procedures for teaching a 10-year-old student with autism to reject nonpreferred activities by selecting a symbol (Martin et al., 2005). As pointed out by the authors, teaching an explicit rejecting response may result in a decrease in less desirable behaviors such as tantrums or aggression. Picture selection may also be a way for children with autism to increase social interactions. For example, Johnston, Nelson, Evans, and Palazolo (2003) taught three preschool-age children to initiate play interactions by selecting a graphic symbol indicating play. All three children also showed decreases in off-task behaviors, and teachers reported satisfaction with the teaching procedures.

As was the case for children with DS, graphic forms of AAC have been proposed for children with autism because they are a good match with their relative strengths in processing visual information (Mirenda & Erickson, 2000). Some evidence suggests that children with FXS may also show relative strengths with visual processing (Goldson & Hagerman, 1992). There is no research available supporting the use of graphic AAC with children with FXS, however. One variable that is likely to affect outcomes for children with FXS is severity of cognitive impairment in general and severity of autism. A number of outcomes have been linked to the degree of autism in children with FXS. For example, Roberts and colleagues (2001) found that children with FXS and autism with higher scores on the Childhood Autism Rating Scale (CARS; Schopler, Reichler, & Rochen Renner, 1988) had poorer language scores compared with children with lower CARS scores.

Voice Output Communication Aids

The use of VOCAs with children with a variety of disabilities is also increasing (DiCarlo & Banajee, 2000; Durand, 1999; Schepis, Reid, Behrmann, & Sutton, 1998). This mode of AAC requires the child to select a symbol that then produces a corresponding spoken word. For example, when a child selects a picture of a ball, he or she may hear the word "ball" (or whatever word or words are programmed to correspond to the picture of the ball). VOCA communication may be more successful than other forms of AAC because the production of an auditory signal may alert communication partners that the child is communicating and may recruit partner attention while not requiring that the partner be knowledgeable of anything beyond spoken speech.

Like PECS and sign language, use of VOCAs by children with developmental disabilities has also been associated with speech development (Sevcik & Romski, 2003; Sigafoos, Didden, & O'Reilly, 2003). These authors have suggested that hearing a spoken word consistently paired with the symbol and referent may facilitate speech development in some children, particularly those with relatively advanced receptive language (Romski & Sevcik, 1996). Brady (2000) presented two case studies that further supported the role of language comprehension in VOCA production. Brady found that children learned to select symbols on a VOCA in fewer trials if they comprehended the spoken names prior to VOCA intervention. Hence, there appears to be a strong link among spoken word comprehension, VOCA production, and speech production.

Jones Bock, Stoner, Beck, Hanley, and Prochnow (2005) compared learning to use a VOCA with learning to use PECS among six 4-year-old children who were reportedly nonspeaking and had developmental delays. The researchers employed an alternating-treatments design and used the prescribed teaching strategy that is recommended for PECS to teach both PECS and VOCA use. For example, when children were taught to use the VOCA, they were taught to pick up the device and move toward their communication partners. The results showed that three of the six children progressed through the first two stages of learning faster in the PECS condition than the VOCA condition. On generalization probes conducted in the classroom, three children produced more responses using the VOCA, and the other three children produced more responses using PECS. Interestingly, the generalization probes did not always correspond to the acquisition data—some children used VOCAs more during generalization, even if they learned PECS faster, and other children used PECS more during generalization, even if they learned VOCA use faster. The authors concluded that it is important to evaluate individual preference for one mode over another. Furthermore, they suggested that children should not be taught to use only one mode; rather, they should be taught and encouraged to use multiple modes of communication.

Down Syndrome

No studies were found that specifically addressed teaching children with DS to use VOCAs, although research studies on VOCAs have included children with DS (e.g., Romski & Sevcik, 1996). In general, most children with DS appear to have the physical and cognitive abilities to operate a VOCA, and the apparent advantages in using VOCAs would be expected to apply equally to children with and without DS.

Autism

A number of studies have shown that children with autism can learn to use VOCAs (Brady, 2000; Schepis et al., 1998; Sigafoos et al., 2003). Most of the studies on VOCA use by children with autism have focused on teaching initiated requests (Mirenda, 2003). A study by Sigafoos, Drasgow, Halle, and colleagues (2004), however, taught two students with autism spectrum disorders to repair communication breakdowns by using a VOCA. Interventionists purposefully ignored initial communication attempts, which included prelinguistic behaviors such as reaching or guiding a partner's hand to a desired object. The students learned to select the VOCA to repair these communication breakdowns, and the investigators noted that the students also began to use the VOCA to initiate requests when there had been no breakdown in communication. Halle, Brady, and Drasgow (2004) explained such outcomes in terms of response efficiency: Participants will learn to communicate using a mode that is more efficient over time.

As mentioned previously, use of AAC may also lead to decreases in challenging behaviors. Durand (1999) demonstrated that individuals could learn to use VOCAs instead of challenging behaviors to communicate. Following a functional analysis to determine the motivations for their challenging behaviors, five individuals, including two with autism spectrum disorders, were taught to use VOCAs to request objects and assistance in their classrooms. Data from all five participants showed decreases in challenging behaviors that mirrored increases in VOCA usage.

Multimodal Augmentative and Alternative Communication

It may seem counterintuitive for children in the beginning stages of learning AAC to learn more than one mode (e.g., PECS and sign; VOCA and PECS), but some authors have suggested that multimodal instruction may be beneficial (Iacono & Duncum, 1995; Iacono et al., 1993; Jones Bock et al., 2005). In a study with a young girl with DS, Iacono and Duncum reported more frequent responding when her instructor modeled both sign and VOCA productions than when the instructor modeled only sign. The study did not compare learning in a VOCA-alone condition, however. The child who participated in this study had a history of learning to produce signs, so the combined approach may have reinforced previous word learning while taking advantage of the benefits of the VOCA that were described previously.

One potential benefit to a multimodal approach is the availability of different modes with different partners (Iacono et al., 1993; Reichle & Ward, 1985). For example, Reichle and Ward taught an adolescent with severe disabilities who used manual signs to use a communication board when communicating with someone who didn't understand manual signs. *Mode switching* indicates this switch from one mode, such as sign language or picture selection, to another mode, such as natural gestures or vocalizations. Mirenda and Bopp (2003) reported a case in which a young man was taught to approach new communication partners and begin a conversation by presenting a written question, "Do you use sign language?" If the person answered "Yes," the young man would sign. If the person answered "No," the young man would use a typing device.

It has been proposed that increases in the number of modes available in one's repertoire may also facilitate repairs of communication breakdowns (Brady, 2003). Communication breakdowns that result from environmental constraints, such as noise or poor lighting, or from partner unfamiliarity with a particular mode of AAC, may best be repaired through mode switching (Mirenda & Bopp, 2003). Thus, the availability of multiple modes of communication may facilitate successful communication across multiple contexts.

A number of investigators have also demonstrated that multimodal *inputs* can be beneficial for acquiring AAC and/or speech (American Speech-Language-Hearing Association, 2004; Barrera et al., 1980; Harris & Reichle, 2004). When sign and speech are presented together, the term *simultaneous communication* has been used, whereas pointing to graphic stimuli while speaking is known as *augmented input*. Augmented input has been linked to both receptive and expressive vocabulary gains (Harris & Reichle, 2004; Romski, Sevcik, Robinson, Mervis, & Bertrand, 1996).

CONCLUSION

This chapter has presented an overview of issues related to use of AAC with children with DS and children with FXS. Relative advantages and disadvantages are associated with each mode. Although different individuals or different intervention programs may favor the use of one mode over another, at present, no widely accepted decision rules exist regarding the selection of the mode or modes of AAC instruction for an individual child or population of children who have similar characteristics or etiologies (American Speech-Language-Hearing Association, 2004). As a number of the studies reviewed within this chapter indicate, determining an optimum mode for an individual child requires careful documentation of learning rate and use across communication contexts.

In general, characteristics that have been attributed to children with DS or FXS favor use of some kind of AAC system but not necessarily one mode of AAC over another. Both groups reportedly process and respond better to visual as opposed to auditory information, and all of the modes described take advantage of visual channels. In addition, all of the modes have been reported to facilitate speech production, although the evidence for the benefit is often only suggestive. The speech effects are important, and more research is needed in this area because AAC is most often viewed as a transitional rather than permanent strategy for children with DS or FXS.

A number of factors are likely to contribute to successful AAC learning for all individuals with developmental disabilities, including children with DS or FXS. These variables include the child's extant skills in communication at the outset of intervention. For example, a child who communicates prelinguistically at a high rate, with multiple partners, and for a variety of communication functions may have a very different prognosis compared with a child with much less developed extant skills (Brady et al., 2004; Brady, Steeples, & Fleming, 2005). Similarly, a child with better speech comprehension may have better outcomes, particularly speech outcomes, than a child with poorer comprehension.

In addition to these child variables, a number of environmental variables are likely to affect outcomes. One of the most obvious sets of environmental variables is the instructional strategies employed. The studies reviewed in this chapter incorporated different strategies such as functional communication training (Durand, 1999), using scripted naturalistic routines (Iacono & Duncum, 1995; Johnston et al., 2003), and strategies that emphasized augmented input as well as output (Romski & Sevcik, 1996). Unfortunately, the number of research studies using these different approaches is small, and it is typically impossible to evaluate the relative contributions of the teaching strategies, child characteristics, AAC mode, or other environmental variables such as partner responsivity. Much more research is needed to enable practitioners to determine an optimal teaching strategy for a child based on individual learning characteristics.

Several strategies have been suggested for promoting AAC in both school and home settings. Von Tetzchner, Merete Brekke, Sjothun, and Grindheim (2005) emphasized the importance of teaching children to communicate a range of communicative functions so that children can better communicate with peers about a variety of topics. In addition, these authors point out that teacher competence with using the AAC system is also likely to affect child competence with AAC. For example, if a teacher only signs a few words or is not comfortable using a picture-based system, it is unlikely that other children in the classroom will learn to use the child's AAC. In such situations, the child often falls into a passive role, answering yes/no questions spoken by peers and teachers, rather than initiating and responding about a variety of topics.

Parents and family members are also key participants in children's AAC learning programs. For children younger than 3 years of age, the home is often the primary intervention site, and for older children, carryover to home environments is often targeted by in-school interventions. An article by Stiebel (1999) presented the results of teaching parents of children with autism not only how to use their children's AAC systems (a graphic selection system) but also how to problem solve when children were not communicating with AAC at home. The problem-solving strategy involved identifying possible reasons why their children did not use picture cards during home routines and then brainstorming solutions aimed at increasing card use. The results showed that parents learned to provide more opportunities for AAC after the problem-solving intervention.

The emphasis of this chapter has been on teaching beginning or transitional AAC to children with DS and children with FXS. This has also been the emphasis of most of the research conducted thus far. It has been observed that children with developmental disabilities who learn to use AAC rarely develop expressive language beyond a basic (single symbol/sign) level (Powell & Clibbens, 2003). For children who make the transition to speech in a relatively short period of time, this is not a huge issue. But for the reportedly smaller number of children who rely on AAC for extended periods of time or for their entire life, more research is needed on ways to increase semantic, syntactic, and pragmatic aspects of language through AAC.

A number of resources are available for those interested in learning more about how to teach the various AAC systems discussed in this chapter. One method used to teach natural gestures, Prelinguistic Milieu Teaching, is described by Warren and colleagues (2006). Web sites, such as the one produced at the University of Washington (http://depts.washington.edu/augcomm), contain current resources about teaching AAC that are helpful for a variety of populations. The Rehabilitation Engineering Research Center (RERC) web site (http://www.aac-rerc.com/) contains links to AAC resources at Duke University; Augmentative Communication, Inc.; Children's Hospital Boston; Pennsylvania State University; State University of New York at Buffalo; Temple University; and the University of Nebraska–Lincoln. In addition, information about PECS, including educational opportunities, can be found at the PECS web site (http://www.pecs.com).

REFERENCES

Abbeduto, L., & Hagerman, R. (1997). Language and communication in fragile X syndrome. *Mental Retardation and Developmental Disabilities Research Reviews, 3*(4), 313–322.

Abbeduto, L., & Murphy, M. (2004). Language, social cognition, maladaptive behavior, and communication in Down syndrome and fragile X syndrome. In M.L. Rice & S.F. Warren (Eds.), *Developmental language disorders: From phenotypes to etiologies* (pp. 77–97). Mahwah, NJ: Lawrence Erlbaum Associates.

Abrahemsen, A., Cavallo, M., & McCluer, J. (1985). Is the sign advantage a robust phenomenon? From gesture to language in two modalities. *Merrill-Palmer Quarterly, 31*(2), 177–209.

Adkins, T., & Axelrod, S. (2001). Topography-based versus selection-based responding: Comparison of mand acquisitions in each modality. *The Behavior Analyst Today, 2*(3), 259–266.

American Speech-Language-Hearing Association. (2004). Roles and responsibilities of speech-language pathologists with respect to augmentative and alternative communication: Technical report. *ASHA Supplement 24, 9*(8), 93–95.

Bailey, D.B., Roberts, J.E., Hooper, S.R., Hatton, D.D., Mirrett, P.L., Roberts, J.E., et al. (2004). Research on fragile X syndrome and autism: Implications for the study of genes, environments, and developmental language disorders. In M.L. Rice & S.F. Warren (Eds.), *Developmental language disorders: From phenotypes to etiologies* (pp. 121–150). Mahwah, NJ: Lawrence Erlbaum Associates.

Baranek, G., Danko, C., Skinner, M., Hatton, D., Roberts, J., & Mirrett, P. (2005). Video analysis of sensory-motor features in infants with fragile X syndrome at 9–12 months of age. *Journal of Autism and Developmental Disorders, 35*, 645–656.

Barrera, R.D., Lobato-Barrera, D., & Sulzer-Azaroff, B. (1980). A simultaneous treatment comparison of three expressive language training programs with a mute autistic child. *Journal of Autism and Developmental Disorders, 10*, 21–37.

Beukelman, D., & Mirenda, P. (2005). *Augmentative and alternative communication: Supporting children and adults with complex communication needs* (3rd ed.). Baltimore: Paul H. Brookes Publishing Co.

Bondy, A.S., & Frost, L.A. (1993). Mands across the water: A report on the application of the picture-exchange communication system in Peru. *The Behavior Analyst, 16*(1), 123–128.

Bonvillian, J., & Nelson, K.E. (1976). Sign language acquisition in a mute autistic boy. *Journal of Speech and Hearing Disorders, 41*, 339–347.

Brady, N. (2000). Improved comprehension of object names following voice output communication aid use: Two case studies. *Augmentative and Alternative Communication, 16,* 197–204.

Brady, N. (2003). *Communication repair strategies by young children with developmental disabilities.* Paper presented at the Thirty-Sixth Annual Gatlinburg Conference on Research and Theory in Intellectual and Developmental Disabilities, Annapolis, MD.

Brady, N., & Halle, J. (1997). Functional analysis of communicative behaviors. *Focus on Autism and Other Developmental Disabilities, 12,* 95–104.

Brady, N.C., & Halle, J.W. (2002). Breakdowns and repairs in conversations between beginning AAC users and their partners. In D.R. Beukelman & J. Reichle (Series Eds.) & J. Reichle, D., Beukelman, & J. Light (Vol. Eds.), *Augmentative and alternative communication series: Exemplary practices for beginning communicators. Implications for AAC* (pp. 323–351). Baltimore: Paul H. Brookes Publishing Co.

Brady, N., Marquis, J., Fleming, K., & McLean, L. (2004). Prelinguistic predictors of language growth in children with developmental disabilities. *Journal of Speech, Language and Hearing Research, 47*(3), 663–667.

Brady, N., & Saunders, K. (1991). Considerations in the effective teaching of object-to-symbol matching. *Augmentative and Alternative Communication, 7,* 112–116.

Brady, N., Skinner, M., Roberts, J., & Hennon, E. (2006). Communication in young children with fragile X syndrome: A qualitative study of mothers' perspectives. *American Journal of Speech-Language Pathology, 15,* 353–364.

Brady, N., Steeples, T., & Fleming, K. (2005). Effects of prelinguistic communication levels on initiation and repair of communication in children with disabilities. *Journal of Speech, Language and Hearing Research, 48*(5), 1098–1113.

Calculator, S. (2003). Use of enhanced natural gestures to foster interactions between children with Angelman syndrome and their parents. *American Journal of Speech-Language Pathology, 11*(4), 340–355.

Calculator, S., & Dollaghan, C. (1982). The use of communication boards in a residential setting: An evaluation. *Journal of Speech and Hearing Disorders, 47,* 281–287.

Carr, E., & Kologinsky, E. (1983). Acquisition of sign language by autistic children, II: Spontaneity and generalization effects. *Journal of Applied Behavior Analysis, 16,* 297–314.

Carr, E.G., Binkoff, J.A., Kologinsky, E., & Eddy, M. (1978). Acquisition of sign language by autistic children, 1: Expressive labelling. *Journal of Applied Behavior Analysis, 11,* 489–501.

Carr, E.G., Kologinsky, E., & Leff-Simon, S. (1987). Acquisition of sign language by autistic children, III: Generalized descriptive phrases. *Journal of Autism and Developmental Disorders, 17,* 217–229.

Chan, J., & Iacono, T. (2001). Gesture and word production in children with Down syndrome. *Augmentative and Alternative Communication, 17,* 73–87.

Chapman, R., Seung, H., Schwartz, S., & Kay-Raining Bird, E. (2000). Predicting language production in children and adolescents with Down syndrome: The role of comprehension. *Journal of Speech and Hearing Research, 43*(2), 340–350.

Charlop-Christy, M., Carpenter, M., LeBlanc, L., & Kellet, K. (2002). Using the Picture Exchange Communication System (PECS) with children with autism: Assessment of PECS acquisition, speech, social-communicative behavior and problem behavior. *Journal of Applied Behavior Analysis, 35*(3), 213–231.

Clibbens, J., Powell, G., & Atkinson, E. (2002). Strategies for achieving joint attention when signing to children with Down's syndrome. *International Journal of Language and Communication Disorders, 37*(3), 309–323.

Coulter, L., & Gallagher, C. (2001). Evaluation of the Hanen Early Childhood Educators Programme. *International Journal of Language and Communication Disorders, 36,* 264–269.

Crais, E., Day Douglas, D., & Cox Campbell, C. (2004). The intersection of the development of gestures and intentionality. *Journal of Speech, Language and Hearing Research, 47,* 678–694.

DiCarlo, C., & Banajee, M. (2000). Using voice output devices to increase initiations of young children with disabilities. *Journal of Early Intervention, 23*(3), 191–199.

Durand, M. (1999). Functional communication training using assistive devices: Recruiting natural communities of reinforcement. *Journal of Applied Behavior Analysis, 32*(3), 247–267.

Fey, M., Warren, S., Brady, N., Finestack, L., Bredin-Oja, S., & Fairchild, M. (2006). Early effects of prelinguistic milieu teaching and responsivity education for children with developmental delays and their parents. *Journal of Speech, Language and Hearing Research, 49*(3), 526–547.

Frost, L., & Bondy, A. (1994). *The picture exchange communication system: Training manual.* Cherry Hill, NJ: Pyramid Educational Consultants.

Fulwiler, R.L., & Fouts, R.S. (1976). Acquisition of American Sign Language by a non-communicating autistic child. *Journal of Autism and Childhood Schizophrenia, 4,* 43–51.

Girolametto, L.E., Greenberg, J., & Manolson, H.A. (1986). Developing dialogue skills: The Hanen Early Language Parent Program. *Seminars in Speech and Language, 7,* 367–382.

Glennen, S.L., & Calculator, S.N. (1985). Training functional communication board use: A pragmatic approach. *Augmentative and Alternative Communication, 1,* 134–142.

Goldson, E., & Hagerman, R. (1992). The fragile X syndrome. *Developmental Medicine and Child Neurology, 34*(9), 826–832.

Goodwyn, S.W., & Acredolo, L.P. (1993). Symbolic gesture versus word: Is there a modality advantage for onset of symbol use? *Child Development, 64,* 688–701.

Halle, J., Brady, N., & Drasgow, E. (2004). Enhancing socially adaptive communicative repairs of beginning communicators with disabilities. *American Journal of Speech-Language Pathology, 13*(1), 43–55.

Harris, M., & Reichle, J. (2004). The impact of aided language stimulation on symbol comprehension and production in learners with moderate cognitive disabilities. *American Journal of Speech-Language Pathology, 13*(2), 155–167.

Hunt, P., Alwell, M., & Goetz, L. (1991). Interacting with peers through conversation turn-taking with a communication book adaptation. *Augmentative and Alternative Communication, 7,* 117–126.

Iacono, T., & Duncum, J. (1995). Comparison of sign alone and in combination with an electronic communication device in early language intervention: Case study. *Augmentative and Alternative Communication, 11*(4), 249–254.

Iacono, T., Mirenda, P., & Beukelman, D. (1993). Comparison of unimodal and multimodal AAC techniques for children with intellectual disabilities. *Augmentative and Alternative Communication, 9,* 83–93.

Iverson, J., Longobardi, E., & Caselli, M.C. (2003). Relationship between gestures and words in children with Down's syndrome and typically developing children in the early stages of communicative development. *International Journal of Language and Communication Disorders, 38*(2), 179–197.

Johnston, J.C., Durieux-Smith, A., & Bloom, K. (2005). Teaching gestural signs to infants to advance child development: A review of the evidence. *First Language, 25*(2), 235–251.

Johnston, S., Nelson, C., Evans, J., & Palazolo, K. (2003). The use of visual supports in teaching young children with autism spectrum disorder to initiate interactions. *Augmentative and Alternative Communication, 19*(2), 86–103.

Jones Bock, S., Stoner, J., Beck, A., Hanley, L., & Prochnow, J. (2005). Increasing functional communication in non-speaking preschool children: Comparison of PECS and VOCA. *Education and Training in Developmental Disabilities, 40*(3), 264–278.

Kamps, D., Kemmerer, K., & Potucek, J. (2002). Brief report: Increasing communication skills for an elementary-aged student with autism using the picture exchange communications system. *Journal of Autism and Developmental Disorders, 32*(3), 225–230.

Kay-Raining Bird, E., & Chapman, R. (1994). Sequential recall in individuals with Down syndrome. *Journal of Speech and Hearing Research, 37,* 1369–1380.

Kay-Raining Bird, E., Gaskell, A., Dallaire Babineau, M., & Macdonald, S. (2000). Novel word acquisition in children with Down syndrome: Does modality make a difference? *Journal of Communication Disorders, 33,* 241–266.

Keen, D., Sigafoos, J., & Woodyatt, G. (2005). Teacher responses to the communicative attempts of children with autism. *Journal of Developmental and Physical Disabilities, 17*(1), 19–33.

Kouri, T. (1989). How manual sign acquisition relates to the development of spoken language: A case study. *Language, Speech, and Hearing Services in the Schools, 20*(1), 50–62.

Kozleski, E.B. (1991). Expectant delay procedure for teaching requests. *Augmentative and Alternative Communication, 7,* 11–19.

Kumin, L. (2003). *Early communication skills for children with Down syndrome*. Bethesda, MD: Woodbine House.

Layton, T.L. (1988). Language training with autistic children using four different modes of presentation. *Journal of Communication Disorders, 21,* 333–350.

Layton, T.L., & Savino, M.A. (1990). Acquiring a communication system by sign and speech in a child with Down syndrome: A longitudinal investigation. *Child Language Teaching and Therapy, 6,* 59–76.

Lloyd, L., Fuller, D., & Arvidson, H. (1997). *Augmentative and alternative communication: A handbook of principles and practices.* Boston: Allyn & Bacon.

Martin, C., Drasgow, E., Halle, J., & Brucker, J. (2005). Teaching a child with autism and severe language delays to reject: Direct and indirect effects of functional communication training. *Educational Psychology, 25*(2–3), 287–304.

McCathren, R., Yoder, P., & Warren, S. (1999). The relationship between prelinguistic vocalization and later expressive vocabulary in young children with developmental delay. *Journal of Speech, Language and Hearing Research, 42,* 915–924.

Michael, J. (1985). Two kinds of verbal behavior plus a possible third. *The Analysis of Verbal Behavior, 3,* 2–5.

Millar, D., Light, J., & Schlosser, R. (2006). The impact of augmentative and alternative communication intervention on the speech production of individuals with developmental disabilities: A research review. *Journal of Speech, Language and Hearing Research, 49*(2), 248–265.

Miller, J.F. (1999). Profiles of language development in children with Down syndrome. In J.F. Miller, M. Leddy, & L.A. Leavitt (Eds.), *Improving the communication of people with Down syndrome* (pp. 11–39). Baltimore: Paul H. Brookes Publishing Co.

Miller, J.F., & Leddy, M. (1998). Down syndrome: The impact of speech production on language development. In S.F. Warren & J. Reichle (Series Eds.) & R. Paul (Vol. Ed.), *Communication and language intervention series: Vol.8. Exploring the speech–language connection* (pp. 163–177). Baltimore: Paul H. Brookes Publishing Co.

Mineo Mollica, B. (2003). Representational competence. In D.R. Beukelman & J. Reichle (Series Eds.) & J. Light, D. Beukelman, & J. Reichle (Vol. Eds.), *Augmentative and alternative communication series: Communicative competence for individuals who use AAC. From research to effective practice* (pp. 107–145). Baltimore: Paul H. Brookes Publishing Co.

Mirenda, P. (1997). Supporting individuals with challenging behavior through functional communication training and AAC: Research review. *Augmentative and Alternative Communication, 13,* 207–224.

Mirenda, P. (2003). Toward functional augmentative and alternative communication for students with autism: Manual signs, graphic symbols, and voice output communication aids. *Language, Speech, and Hearing Services in Schools, 34,* 203–216.

Mirenda, P., & Bopp, K.D. (2003). "Playing the game": Strategic competence in AAC. In D.R. Beukelman & J. Reichle (Series Eds.) & J. Light, D. Beukelman, & J. Reichle (Vol. Eds.), *Augmentative and alternative communication series: Communicative competence for individuals who use AAC. From research to effective practice* (pp. 401–437). Baltimore: Paul H. Brookes Publishing Co.

Mirenda, P., & Erickson, K. (2000). Augmentative communication and literacy. In S.F. Warren & J. Reichle (Series Eds.) & A.M. Wetherby & B.M. Prizant (Vol. Eds.), *Communication and language intervention series: Vol. 9. Autism spectrum disorders: A transactional developmental perspective* (pp. 333–367). Baltimore: Paul H. Brookes Publishing Co.

Mundy, P., Kasari, C., Sigman, M., & Ruskin, E. (1995). Nonverbal communication and early language acquisition in children with Down syndrome and in normally developing children. *Journal of Speech and Hearing Research, 38,* 157–167.

Powell, G., & Clibbens, J. (2003). Augmentative communication. In J. Rondal & S. Buckley (Eds.), *Speech and language intervention in Down syndrome* (pp. 116–131). London: Whurr publishers.

Reichle, J., Barrett, C., Tetlie, R.R., & McQuarter, R.J. (1987). The effect of prior intervention to establish generalized requesting on the acquisition of object labels. *Augmentative and Alternative Communication, 3,* 3–11.

Reichle, J., & Brown, L. (1986). Teaching the use of a multipage direct selection communication board to an adult with autism. *The Journal of the Association for Persons with Severe Handicaps, 11,* 68–73.

Reichle, J., Cooley Hidecker, M., Brady, N., & Terry, N. (2003). Intervention strategies for communication: Using aided augmentative communication systems. In D.R. Beukelman & J. Reichle (Series Eds.) & J. Light, D. Beukelman, & J. Reichle (Vol. Eds.), *Augmentative and alternative communication series: Communicative competence for individuals who use AAC. From research to effective practice* (pp. 441–479). Baltimore: Paul H. Brookes Publishing Co.

Reichle, J., & Sigafoos, J. (1991). Establishing an initial repertoire of requesting. In J. Reichle, J. York, & J. Sigafoos (Eds.), *Implementing augmentative and alternative communication: Strategies for learners with severe disabilities* (pp. 89–114). Baltimore: Paul H. Brookes Publishing Co.

Reichle, J., & Wacker, D.P. (Vol. Eds.) & S.F. Warren & J. Reichle (Series Eds.). (1993). *Communication and language intervention series: Vol. 3. Communicative alternatives to challenging behavior: Integrating functional assessment and intervention strategies.* Baltimore: Paul H. Brookes Publishing Co.

Reichle, J., & Ward, M. (1985). Teaching discriminative use of an encoding electronic communication device and Signing Exact English to a moderately handicapped child. *Language, Speech, and Hearing Services in the Schools, 16,* 58–63.

Reichle, J., & Yoder, D. (1985). Communication board use in severely handicapped learners. *Language, Speech, and Hearing Services in Schools, 16,* 146–157.

Remington, B., & Clarke, S. (1993). Simultaneous communication and speech comprehension, Part II: Comparison of two methods of overcoming selective attention during expressive sign training. *Augmentative and Alternative Communication, 9,* 49–60.

Rice, M.L., Warren, S., & Betz, S. (2005). Language symptoms of developmental language disorders: An overview of autism, Down syndrome, fragile X, specific language impairment, and Williams syndrome. *Applied Psycholinguistics, 26,* 7–27.

Roberts, J., Long, S., Malkin, C., Barnes, E., Skinner, M., Hennon, E., et al. (2005). A comparison of phonological skills of boys with fragile X syndrome and Down syndrome. *Journal of Speech, Language and Hearing Research, 48*(5), 980–996.

Roberts, J., Mirrett, P., Anderson, K., Burchinal, M., & Neebe, E. (2002). Early communication, symbolic behavior, and social profiles of young males with fragile X syndrome. *American Journal of Speech-Language Pathology, 11,* 295–304.

Roberts, J.E., Mirrett, P., & Burchinal, M. (2001). Receptive and expressive communication development of young males with fragile X syndrome. *American Journal on Mental Retardation, 106*(3), 216–231.

Romski, M.A., & Sevcik, R.A. (1993). Language learning through augmented means: The process and its products. In S.F. Warren & J. Reichle (Series Eds.) & A.P. Kaiser & D.B. Gray (Vol. Eds.), *Communication and language intervention series: Vol. 2. Enhancing children's communication: Research foundations for intervention* (pp. 85–104). Baltimore: Paul H. Brookes Publishing Co.

Romski, M.A., & Sevcik, R.A. (1996). *Breaking the speech barrier: Language development through augmented means.* Baltimore: Paul H. Brookes Publishing Co.

Romski, M.A., Sevcik, R.A., Robinson, B.F., Mervis, C.B., & Bertrand, J. (1996). Mapping the meanings of novel visual symbols by youth with moderate or severe mental retardation. *American Journal of Mental Retardation, 100,* 391–402.

Schaeffer, B. (1980). Spontaneous language through signed speech. In R.L. Schiefelbusch (Ed.), *Nonspeech language and communication: Analysis and intervention* (pp. 421–447). Baltimore: University Park Press.

Schepis, M.M., Reid, D.H., Behrmann, M.M., & Sutton, K.A. (1998). Increasing communicative interactions of young children with autism using a voice output communication aid and naturalistic teaching. *Journal of Applied Behavior Analysis, 31,* 561–579.

Schepis, M., Reid, D., Fitzgerald, J., Faw, G., van den Pol, R., & Welty, P. (1982). A program for increasing manual signing by autistic and profoundly retarded youth within the daily environment. *Journal of Applied Behavior Analysis, 15,* 363–379.

Schlosser, R., Belfiore, P., Nigam, R., Blischak, D., & Hetzroni, O. (1995). The effects of speech output technology in the learning of graphic symbols. *Journal of Applied Behavior Analysis, 23,* 537–549.

Schopler, E., Reichler, R., & Rochen Renner, B. (1988). *Childhood Autism Rating Scale (CARS).* Los Angeles: Western Psychology Services.

Schwartz, I., Garfinkle, A., & Bauer, J. (1998). The Picture Exchange Communication System: Communicative outcomes for young children with disabilities. *Topics in Early Childhood Special Education, 18*(3), 144–159.

Seal, B., & Bonvillian, J. (1997). Sign language and motor functioning in students with autistic disorder. *Journal of Autism and Developmental Disorders, 27*(4), 437–466.

Sevcik, R., & Romski, M. (2003). Longitudinal designs. In R. Schlosser (Ed.), *The efficacy of augmentative and alternative communication: Toward evidence-based practice* (pp. 163–181). San Diego: Academic Press.

Siegel, E.B., & Cress, C.J. (2002). Overview of the emergence of early AAC behaviors: Progression from communicative to symbolic skills. In D.R. Beukelman & J. Reichle (Series Eds.) & J. Reichle, D.R. Beukelman, & J.C. Light (Vol. Eds.), *Augmentative and alternative communication series: Exemplary practices for beginning communicators. Implications for AAC* (pp. 25–57). Baltimore: Paul H. Brookes Publishing Co.

Sigafoos, J. (1992). Assessing choice making among children with multiple disabilities. *Journal of Applied Behavior Analysis, 3,* 747–756.

Sigafoos, J., Didden, R., & O'Reilly, M. (2003). Effects of speech output on maintenance of requesting and frequency of vocalizations in three children with developmental disabilities. *Augmentative and Alternative Communication, 19,* 37–47.

Sigafoos, J., Doss, S., & Reichle, J. (1989). Developing mand and tact repertoires in persons with severe developmental disabilities using graphic symbols. *Research in Developmental Disabilities, 10,* 183–200.

Sigafoos, J., Drasgow, E., Halle, J., O'Reilly, M., Seely-York, S., Edrisinha, C., et al. (2004). Teaching VOCA use as a communicative repair strategy. *Journal of Autism and Developmental Disorders, 34*(4), 411–422.

Sigafoos, J., Drasgow, E., Reichle, J., O'Reilly, M., Green, V., & Tait, K. (2004). Tutorial: Teaching communicative rejecting to children with severe disabilities. *American Journal of Speech-Language Pathology, 13*(1), 31–42.

Sigafoos, J., & Reichle, J. (1992). Comparing explicit to generalized requesting in an augmentative communication mode. *Journal of Developmental and Physical Disabilities, 4*(2), 167–188.

Stiebel, D. (1999). Promoting augmentative communication during daily routines: A parent problem-solving intervention. *Journal of Positive Behavior Interventions, 1*(3), 159–169.

Sundberg, C.T., & Sundberg, T.L. (1990). Comparing topography-based verbal behavior with stimulus selection-based verbal behavior. *The Analysis of Verbal Behavior, 8,* 31–41.

Tincani, M. (2004). Comparing the Picture Exchange Communication system and sign language training for children with autism. *Focus on Autism and Other Disabilities, 19*(3), 152–164.

Volterra, V., Caselli, M.C., Capirci, O., & Pizzuto, E. (2005). Gesture and the emergence and development of language. In M. Tomasello & D. Slobin (Eds.), *Beyond nature–nurture: Essays in honor of Elizabeth Bates* (pp. 3–41). Mahwah, NJ: Lawrence Erlbaum Associates.

Von Tetzchner, S., Merete Brekke, K., Sjothun, B., & Grindheim, E. (2005). Constructing preschool communities of learners that afford alternative language development. *Augmentative and Alternative Communication, 21*(2), 82–100.

Warren, S.F., Bredin-Oja, S.L., Fairchild, M., Finestack, L.H., Fey, M.E., & Brady, N.C. (2006). Responsivity education/prelinguistic milieu teaching. In S.F. Warren & M.E. Fey (Series Eds.) & R.J. McCauley & M.E. Fey (Eds.), *Communication and language intervention series: Treatment of language disorders in children* (pp. 47–75). Baltimore: Paul H. Brookes Publishing Co.

Yoder, P., & Warren, S. (2002). Effects of prelinguistic milieu teaching and parent responsivity education on dyads involving children with intellectual disabilities. *Journal of Speech, Language and Hearing Research, 45*(6), 1158–1175.

Yoder, P., & Warren, S. (2004). Early predictors of language in children with and without Down syndrome. *American Journal of Mental Retardation, 109*(4), 285–300.

CHAPTER 12

Family Well-Being in Down Syndrome and Fragile X Syndrome

ANNA J. ESBENSEN, MARSHA MAILICK SELTZER, AND LEONARD ABBEDUTO

The impact on families of raising a child with a developmental disability has been a topic of interest to researchers for several decades. Some researchers have found negative effects on the mental health and self-competence of parents and siblings and disruption of relationships within the family (as reviewed in Cummings, 1976; Cummings, Bayley, & Rie, 1966; Dyson, 1991, 1993; Fisman, Wolf, & Noh, 1989; Friedrich & Friedrich, 1981; Gath & Gumley, 1984; Romans-Clarkson et al., 1986; Singhi, Goyal, Pershad, Singhi, & Walia, 1990; Smith, Innocenti, Boyce, & Smith, 1993; Stoneman, 1997; Wilton & Renaut, 1986). Other researchers, however, have not replicated these findings, instead finding comparable outcomes to those of families of children without disabilities (Dumas, Wolf, Fisman, & Culligan, 1991; Gamble & McHale, 1989; Gowen, Johnson-Martin, Goldman, & Appelbaum, 1989; Harris & McHale, 1989; Houser & Seligman, 1991; Koegel, Schreibman, O'Neill, & Burke, 1983; Krauss & Seltzer, 1999; McKinney & Peterson, 1987; Van Riper, Ryff, & Pridham, 1992).

In order to better understand the inconsistent research findings related to the impact of having a child with developmental disabilities, recent efforts have focused on investigating the variability in well-being among families having a child with a developmental disability. This effort has included examining the impact of raising children with specific disorders, such as Down syndrome (DS), fragile X syndrome (FXS), and autism. Genetic syndromes predispose a child to particular behavioral profiles (Dykens, 1995), which may lead those in the child's family to respond to the child in unique ways (Hodapp, Ly, Fidler, & Ricci, 2001). Evidence also suggests that the psychological well-being of families varies with the challenges and behavior problems associated with different disabilities (Abbeduto et al., 2004).

This chapter focuses on the well-being of families of children with DS or FXS. Although both are genetic syndromes, DS and FXS are associated with different behavioral phenotypes, different patterns of heritability, and different paths to the child's diagnosis. This chapter reviews how characteristics associated

This chapter was supported in part by grants from the National Institute on Child Health and Human Development (P30 HD03352, T32 HD07489, R01 HD024356, and R03 HD048884) and the National Institute on Aging (R01 AG08768).

with these two genetic syndromes affect family well-being and then reviews the literature examining the impact of a child with DS or FXS on the family life course. Research limitations and directions for research and practice are also reviewed.

EFFECTS OF GENETIC SYNDROMES ON FAMILIES

Genetic syndromes can affect family well-being as a result of issues related to the pattern of heritability, the certainty and timing of the diagnosis, the knowledge base that exists about the syndrome, and the behavioral characteristics associated with the syndrome. Different genetic syndromes are associated with different, albeit often overlapping, profiles of behavior, or behavioral phenotypes. As Dykens (1995) put it, there is a heightened likelihood that individuals with a given genetic syndrome "will exhibit certain behavioral and developmental sequelae relative to those without the syndrome" (p. 523). These behavioral phenotypes can influence parental well-being and have indirect effects on the child's subsequent development (Hodapp, 1997). For example, genetic syndromes associated with high rates of behavior problems or psychopathology can create stress for parents, compromising their psychological well-being as well as their capacity to interact with their child in ways that are supportive of their child's optimal development, which could strengthen or even exacerbate a child's problem behaviors, creating more stress for parents, and the cycle would continue. Patterns of temperament and sociability could also affect the interactions between the family and the child, in addition to the well-being of family members.

The genetic origin of a syndrome is also highly likely to affect family well-being. In some cases, the gene(s) that lead to a child's disability may also predispose his or her parents to less than optimal outcomes and to an increased vulnerability to the challenge of parenting a child with a specific syndrome (Franke et al., 1996). Parents who are carriers of the gene(s) leading to their child's disabilities may also suffer from self-blame and guilt, seeing themselves as the cause of their child's condition (Kay & Kingston, 2002). Choices regarding continuing a pregnancy and having additional children can also be affected when a parent knows that he or she carries a gene that can lead to a disability in a child (Kay & Kingston, 2002; McConkie-Rosell, Spiridigliozzi, Iafolla, Tarleton, & Lachiewicz, 1997). If a parent does not know that he or she is a carrier of a problematic gene, the family is at risk of conceiving multiple affected children (Bailey, Skinner, & Sparkman, 2003). A heritable syndrome can also have an impact on siblings and extended relatives. Discovering whether other family members have the syndrome or are at risk for passing on the syndrome can strain relationships among extended family members (Bailey et al., 2003).

Learning that a child's developmental disability has a genetic cause can have a positive effect on families, providing parents with a clear and coherent explanation of their child's condition and a reasonable expectation of what the future holds. The timing of the receipt of that diagnosis, however, can vary dramatically across different genetic syndromes. Practices for diagnostic screening at birth vary from state to state (Bailey, 2004). Thus, genetic syndromes without physical characteristics identifiable at birth may not be diagnosed until developmental delays are well established and recognized by parents (Bailey, Skinner, Hatton, & Roberts, 2000). Receiving a diagnosis prenatally or at birth allows parents to begin the process of adapting to their child's condition when their child is a new-born (Van Riper, 1999; Van Riper & Selder, 1989). In contrast, when a diagnosis is received after testing for causes of a developmental delay, this diagnosis may not come until the child is older than 2 or 3 years of age (Huang, Sadler, O'Rior-dan, & Robin, 2002). In the case of genetic syndromes that have become identi-fiable only through recent technological advances, many families are receiving the diagnosis for the first time when their children have reached adolescence or adulthood (Carmichael, Pembrey, Turner, & Barnicoat, 1999; Huang et al., 2002). In such an instance, parents will have experienced, at minimum, years of uncer-tainty and worry about the cause of their child's delay. Although knowing the diagnosis can be helpful to the parents, it is also likely that the uncertainty of the early years could have had a negative impact on the parents.

Receiving a diagnosis of a genetic syndrome can also bring a wealth of infor-mation to families about the syndrome and often times brings access to support and advocacy groups. Being knowledgeable about a syndrome and having access to support groups may have positive impacts on parental well-being (Erickson & Upsur, 1989).

FAMILY WELL-BEING IN DOWN SYNDROME

The research examining the well-being of families of children with DS spans more than 40 years. For families of children with DS, parents of children born in the 1970s tend to have more positive experiences compared with parents of children born earlier (Gath, 1990). Many factors are likely to contribute to these differ-ences, including improvements in diagnostic processes and training of medical professionals, the increased availability of supports, improvements based on research about family well-being, and the reduction of stigma associated with dis-abilities. The possibility of cohort effects thus requires caution in interpreting findings from any single study or studies from any single historical period.

At Diagnosis

Individuals with DS are generally diagnosed at birth. Of children brought to term, up to 87% of children with DS are identified as having DS postnatally (Skotko, 2005a). A diagnosis of DS at birth leads to a period of distress for parents. This dis-tress often results from an unexpected diagnosis, as well as parental concerns about the future of their child, their ability to parent a child with special needs, and the quality of the information received from medical professionals (Van Riper & Selder, 1989). Indeed, many parents report feeling dissatisfied with the way in which they were told of the diagnosis from their medical professional (Van Riper, Pridham, & Ryff, 1992). Mothers report feeling angry and frustrated at how they were informed of the diagnosis and feeling anxious and scared about what impli-cations the diagnosis has for the future of her child (Skotko, 2005a; Skotko & Bedia, 2005). Many mothers also report that medical professionals delayed informing them of the diagnosis, told them when their partner was not around or in inappropriate settings, did not provide enough information, or provided misinformation about the negative aspects of raising a child with DS. Mothers who report being optimistic about raising a child with DS report receiving infor-mation from their medical professional that emphasized the positive aspects of DS

(Skotko & Bedia, 2005), which suggests that the way in which the diagnosis is delivered may help to shape early parenting beliefs and, perhaps, practices. In a related topic, mothers of children with DS born in the 2000s were more likely to report that their medical professionals talked about or emphasized the positive aspects of DS than did mothers of those born prior to that time, suggesting changes in professional practice that bode well for parental well-being in current and future cohorts (Skotko, 2005a). Support from genetic counseling has also been helpful in relieving guilt and blame experienced by parents of newborn children with DS (Collins, Halliday, Kahler, & Williamson, 2001).

Advances in prenatal screening for fetuses at increased risk for developmental disorders (e.g., screening for maternal serum alpha-fetoprotein) have resulted in some parents being given a diagnosis of DS in the first trimester of pregnancy. In one study of 304 cases of DS in Hawaii that spanned 10 years, 43% were identified prenatally (Forrester & Merz, 1999). In a survey of more than 1,000 mothers of children with DS, 12.5% reported receiving the diagnosis prenatally (Skotko, 2005b). The factors that affect parental well-being when being given a diagnosis of DS at birth are the same factors that affect the parents at a prenatal diagnosis. In particular, mothers receiving the diagnosis prenatally report feeling shocked, scared, and anxious. In addition, these parents also report feeling pressure to make a decision regarding whether to continue or terminate their pregnancy (Skotko, 2005b). Approximately 84%–88% of fetuses with DS identified prenatally are electively terminated (Forrester & Merz, 1999; Glover & Glover, 1996; Williamson, Harris, Church, Fiddler, & Rhind, 1996). In the study conducted in Hawaii (Forrester & Merz, 1999), the decision to electively terminate the pregnancy was found to vary by ethnicity, with East Asians (93%), Caucasians (84%), and Filipinos (82%) being more likely to do so than Pacific Islanders (56%). Although there have been no published reports of studies that examined the well-being of couples who elected to terminate the pregnancy following a diagnosis of DS, there are suggestions in the literature about how to support parents who have decided to terminate a pregnancy (Thayer, Ciarleglio, & Rucquoi, 1991).

For parents who choose to continue the pregnancy after a prenatal diagnosis of DS, the months before the birth become a time for adjusting future expectations and obtaining information. Investigators have retrospectively interviewed mothers who received a prenatal diagnosis of DS and elected to continue with their pregnancy (Helm, Miranda, & Chedd, 1998). These mothers reported needing printed material; up-to-date information; and medical professionals who delivered the news in a positive, nonjudgmental, and understanding manner. Some preferred talking to DS parent groups after receiving the diagnosis, whereas other parents preferred to delay talking to parent support groups until after they had made their decision as to whether to continue with the pregnancy. Most mothers reported needing but not having access to information about the nature of DS during what they viewed as a particularly stressful time in their lives (Helm et al., 1998). Many also report feeling that they were pressured into making a decision in line with the medical professionals' point of view, that they were not supported in arriving at their own informed decision, and that seeking information on their own caused additional anxiety and uncertainty. These mothers, however, also report being able to overcome the initial shock of the diagnosis of DS and being able to celebrate the birth of their child (Van Riper, 1999).

During Childhood

Raising a child with DS can have a profound impact on the lives of parents. Many parents, however, report that the positive consequences associated with raising a child with DS far outweigh the negative ones (Van Riper & Selder, 1989). The positive consequences reported by parents include bringing the family closer together, understanding unconditional love, putting things in perspective, and appreciating diversity (Van Riper & Selder, 1989).

In fact, previous research on the impact of a child's disability on parental psychological well-being has demonstrated that mothers of children with DS often fare better than mothers of children with other forms of intellectual disability. Compared with mothers of children who, as a group, are heterogeneous with respect to etiology, mothers of children with DS report lower levels of stress (Kasari & Sigman, 1997; Marcovitch, Goldberg, MacGregor, & Lojkasek, 1986) and more extensive and satisfying networks of support (Hauser-Cram, Warfield, Shonkoff, & Krauss, 2001; Shonkoff, Hauser-Cram, Krauss, & Upshur, 1992), and they perceive their children to have less difficult temperaments (Kasari & Sigman, 1997). Parents of children with DS also report being less pessimistic about their children's future compared with parents of children with either Williams syndrome or Smith-Magenis syndrome (Fidler, Hodapp, & Dykens, 2000). Like DS, Williams syndrome and Smith-Magenis syndrome are characterized by a range of physical and medical anomalies (Dykens, Hodapp, & Finucane, 2000); however, compared with DS, children with Williams syndrome are at a heightened risk for internalizing disorders, and children with Smith-Magenis syndrome exhibit elevated rates of maladaptive behaviors and sleep problems. Parents of children with DS also report fewer family problems than do parents of children with Smith-Magenis syndrome (Fidler et al., 2000), and the former are less likely to interpret child noncompliance negatively compared with mothers of children who, as a group, are heterogeneous with respect to etiology (Ly & Hodapp, 2002). Parents of children with DS are also reported to have lower divorce rates and a comparable level of marital quality compared with parents of children with a similar degree of intellectual disability of other origin (Gath & Gumley, 1986). The level of family functioning for those families with a child with DS has also been reported to be more cohesive and harmonious than other families of children with intellectual disability (Mink, Nihira, & Meyers, 1983).

Families raising a child with DS also tend to fare better when compared with families raising a child with autism. Diagnoses of autism are typically made when a child is 2 or 3 years of age and are based on a pattern of impairments in social interaction and communication along with restricted interests and repetitive behaviors. In comparison to mothers of children with autism, mothers of children with DS have reported experiencing lower levels of stress (Fisman et al., 1989; Holroyd & McArthur, 1976), lower levels of anxiety (Piven et al., 1991; Rodrigue, Morgan, & Geffken, 1990; Ryde-Brandt, 1991), and lower levels of depression (Dumas et al., 1991), while reporting more positive views of their child's characteristics (Kasari & Sigman, 1997). Both fathers and mothers of children with DS report greater marital satisfaction and lower parenting stress than do parents of children with autism (Dumas et al., 1991; Fisman et al., 1989; Rodrigue et al., 1990). In general, however, family well-being is at greater risk in families raising a child with autism compared with virtually all other developmental disabilities (for a review, see Dunn, Burbine, Bowers, & Tantleff-Dunn, 2001).

When parents of children with DS have been compared with parents of children without intellectual disability, the two groups are often found to be more comparable than different. No differences have been obtained on experienced levels of stress when mothers of children with DS were compared with mothers of outpatient clinic children (Holroyd & McArthur, 1976). In comparison to parents of children without disabilities, parents of children with DS were not reported to differ on measures of individual, marital, or family functioning (Van Riper, Ryff, et al., 1992); on mental or physical health (Gath, 1977; Gath & Gumley, 1984); or on family harmony and warmth (Gath & Gumley, 1984). Marital satisfaction and divorce rates are also comparable to or better than those of the general population (Carr, 1988; Cunningham, 1996), although in a small sample, more families of children with DS exhibited marital separations (Gath & Gumley, 1984). Mothers of children with DS also report that they feel less concerned with trivial matters, less materialistic, and less self-centered after the birth of their child (Cunningham, 1996).

It is important to recognize these findings should not be taken to mean that parents of children with DS are immune from stress. In fact, between 25% and 35% of families do experience difficulties (Cunningham, 1996). These problems show a stable pattern from childhood through adolescence and are typically related to elevated behavior problems exhibited by the child. Also, not all researchers have found families of children with DS to be associated with better psychological well-being than families of children with other disabilities (Gath, 1990; Hanson & Hanline, 1990; Ryde-Brandt, 1991; Sanders & Morgan, 1997). For example, some mothers of young children with DS have higher levels of depressed mood (Roach, Orsmond, & Barratt, 1999) and lower levels of marital satisfaction than mothers of children with similar levels of intellectual disability (Gath, 1990). This depressed mood and marital dissatisfaction has been reported to persist into adolescence (Gath, 1990; Gath & Gumley, 1986). Mothers of children with DS also are reported to exhibit comparable levels of pessimism about their child's future to mothers of children with autism and more pessimism than mothers of typically developing children (Sanders & Morgan, 1997).

The variability in findings has led Cahill and Glidden (1996) to argue that the better psychological outcomes for families of children with DS may be a result of sampling biases. They were able to reproduce the findings for better psychological outcomes for families of children with DS in comparison to families of children with other disabilities. This finding, however, was not replicated when the two samples were matched for various demographic variables. This recognizes that other characteristics of a family, such as marital status and the child's age and level of functioning, may influence its well-being beyond having a child with DS.

It is also important to note that there is some evidence that fathers of children with DS are more likely to show poor well-being than are mothers of children with DS. Thus, fathers of children with DS have been found to report higher levels of stress compared with mothers and compared with fathers of children with other disabilities (Shonkoff et al., 1992). Moreover, some researchers have found that fathers of children with DS report similar levels of marital satisfaction, parenting competence, family functioning, and social support as do fathers of children with autism (Rodrigue, Morgan, & Geffken, 1992). This has led to the hypothesis that fathers of children with disabilities may receive less support than do mothers and thus have lower levels of psychological well-being (Cunningham, 1996). More than 40% of fathers interviewed by Hornby (1995) reported restrictions being placed on family life as a result of having a child with DS and having difficulty adjusting to the diagnosis, and only one third commented that raising a child with DS had minimal effects on family life. Such findings suggest that the child's diagnosis can interact in a complex way with parent gender or role within the family.

During Adolescence

Adolescence is a period of transition for many individuals and their families, including adolescents with special needs and typically developing adolescents (Graber & Brooks-Gunn, 1996; Hamburg & Takanishi, 1989). Among families of adolescents with DS, this period of transition is accompanied by additional changes that can affect the well-being of the family. Several medical problems occur at an increased frequency among adolescents with DS, including weight gain, sleep apnea, thyroid dysfunction, skin and skeletal disorders, cardiac conditions, and psychiatric disorders (Pueschel, 1996). It is not unusual for adolescence to be a difficult time for any family, but with the additional medical concerns arising for adolescents with DS, these families may be at an elevated risk for negative effects on their well-being. At the same time, however, adolescents with DS are also reported to display gains in social skills relative to adolescents with intellectual disability of heterogeneous etiology (Hauser-Cram et al., 2001). These improved social skills may serve as protective factors during adolescence.

In fact, there are data suggesting that families of adolescents with DS continue to fare better than families dealing with other types of developmental disabilities. In a comparative study of adolescents and young adults with DS, FXS, and autism, for example, mothers of adolescents with DS displayed better psychological well-being, on average, than the other two comparison groups (Abbeduto et al., 2004). Mothers of adolescents with DS were less pessimistic about their child's future and were more likely to perceive that their child reciprocated feelings of closeness as compared with mothers of adolescents with FXS or autism. In addition, mothers of adolescents with DS reported more closeness in the relationship with their child and fewer depressive symptoms than mothers of adolescents with autism (Abbeduto et al., 2004). Such differences between mothers of adolescents with DS and FXS, however, became negligible when controlling for contextual factors, behavioral symptoms of autism, and maternal coping, suggesting that it is these associated factors rather than DS per se that should be seen as accounting for the differences in parental well-being.

In contrast to these positive findings, mothers of adolescents with DS also report a decrease in perceived satisfaction with life, which has also been associated with a decline in perceived satisfaction with social support (Cunningham, 1996). Whether this decline in satisfaction with life is a result of changes in social support or in related changes during adolescence remains to be determined; however, a trend has also been reported that during this time period, mothers of adolescents with DS feel that their child creates greater restrictions on family life than an adolescent without disabilities (Cunningham, 1996). For some adolescents with DS, social isolation becomes a problem because of making fewer social contacts and having fewer friends without disabilities (Cunningham, 1996). As a result, parents often become "social coordinators" for their adolescent. Again, the restrictions experienced by parents and the reduced social contacts have been found to be associated with elevated behavior problems exhibited by adolescents with DS (Cunningham, 1996), which may have a negative effect on family well-being.

During Adulthood

Although the vast majority of studies on family well-being and DS have focused on young children, research from the 1990s has begun to focus on the impact over the life course (Seltzer & Krauss, 1998). The life span of individuals with DS is lengthening (Bittles & Glasson, 2004), extending the caregiving time period of adults living at home with their families. Mothers of adults with DS are adjusting to their own aging and are also responsible for the continued caregiving of their adult children, who are increasingly vulnerable to health problems, including Alzheimer's disease and the dementia that accompanies it (Pueschel, 1987; Zigman, Schupf, Lubin, & Silverman, 1987). Mothers of adults with DS are themselves at risk for health problems. One study found that these mothers have an increased risk for developing dementia as compared with mothers of adults with other types of intellectual disability (Schupf, Kapell, Lee, Ottman, & Mayeux, 1994), particularly among mothers younger than 35 years of age at the time of their child's birth. Nonetheless, evidence suggests that the "advantage" of having a son or daughter with DS continues throughout life (Seltzer, Krauss, & Tsunematsu, 1993). Mothers of adults with DS report less conflicted family environments, more satisfaction with their social supports, and less stress and burden than do mothers of adults with intellectual disability due to other causes (Seltzer et al., 1993). The mothers' social support networks are also reported to be larger for mothers of adult children with DS compared with those of mothers of adult children with other types of intellectual disability (Seltzer & Krauss, 1998). These findings are similar to that found among mothers of children with DS, suggesting that despite the high rates of health problems in DS, there is a life-course pattern of continuity in positive profiles of adaptation in mothers with a son or a daughter with DS.

Indeed, there is some evidence that there is an increase in positive well-being among mothers as their adult children with DS age. These mothers report a sense of optimism and acceptance of their child's disability (Krauss & Seltzer, 1999; Seltzer et al., 1993). Although they note that earlier in life they experienced more burden, as their child has become an adult, mothers have developed an appreciation for their child's strengths (Krauss & Seltzer, 1995). This is not to say that mothers of adults with DS do not experience frustrations and stresses; however, these aging mothers typically report more gratifications than frustrations with raising their adult child (Krauss & Seltzer, 1995).

In comparison with mothers of adults with autism, mothers of adults with DS report a closer relationship with their child and less pessimism about their child's future (Greenberg, Seltzer, Krauss, Chou, & Hong, 2004; Seltzer, Krauss, Orsmond, & Vestal, 2001). No differences have been found, however, between mothers of adults with DS and autism on measures of depressive symptoms, optimism, positive psychological well-being, and physical health (Greenberg et al., 2004). This finding contrasts to the findings comparing mothers of young children with DS and autism and could reflect improvements in the psychological well-being of mothers of adults with autism after years of caregiving, perhaps because of the abatement of autism symptoms over time (Seltzer, Shattuck, Abbeduto, & Greenberg, 2004).

Studies have found adults with DS to be more likely to have hearing impairments and speech intelligibility problems as compared with adults with intellectual disability of unknown etiology (Seltzer & Krauss, 1998). Communication problems such as these have been found to be associated with behavior problems, which are known to negatively affect parental well-being (Gath & Gumley, 1986; Greenberg et al., 2004). The indirect effect of communication difficulties on the well-being of families of individuals with DS remains to be examined. Communication is critical to any interpersonal relationship and is integral to establishing ties in the community and personal relationships. As such, there is some likelihood that families of adults with communication difficulties may experience a different pattern of well-being compared with families who have adult children with relatively strong communication skills.

Well-Being of Siblings

The impact of having a sibling with DS is complex. Some researchers have found negative affects on siblings. For example, older sisters of individuals with DS have been reported to display more behavior problems (Cuskelly & Dodds, 1992; Cuskelly & Gunn, 1993), and at school, siblings of individuals with DS have been reported to display slightly elevated behavior problems (Gath & Gumley, 1986).

Not all studies, however, have reported negative consequences to siblings. Siblings of individuals with DS are reported to exhibit lower rates of social impairments and cognitive disorders as compared with siblings of individuals with autism (August, Stewart, & Tsai, 1981; Bolton et al., 1994). During adulthood, siblings of adults with DS report feeling closer to their sibling than do siblings of adults with autism (Seltzer, Krauss, et al., 2001).

Moreover, although approximately 20% of siblings of children with DS show signs of poorer adaptation, this has not been found to be directly related to the diagnosis of DS (Cunningham, 1996). Instead, sibling problems are more likely to be a result of poor parental adaptation and coping mechanisms (Cunningham, 1996). Typically, siblings report positive relations with their sibling with DS and positive to neutral effects of having a sibling with DS. They also report positive perceptions of their own self-worth (Cunningham, 1996; Van Riper, 1999) and, based on maternal reports, are relatively socially competent with a low incidence of behavior problems (Van Riper, 1999). Again, family variables, such as communication, resources, vulnerability, and self-appraisal, are likely to be important factors in determining the well-being of the siblings. Communication limitations, behavior problems, and limitations in adaptive functioning of the child with DS have also been found to be associated with behavior problems in the siblings (Gath, 1990; Gath & Gumley, 1987).

Discussion

A common explanation offered for why families of children with DS experience relative "advantages" in their well-being is the temperament and behaviors associated with the syndrome. The personality traits of children with DS are commonly described as affectionate, sociable, and easy in temperament (Bridges & Cicchetti, 1982; Gibbs & Thorpe, 1983; Kasari & Bauminger, 1998). Individuals with DS are also reported to exhibit better functional abilities (Greenspan & Delaney, 1983; Harrison, 1987; Loveland & Kelley, 1988; Zigman et al., 1987) and fewer behavior problems (Greenspan & Delaney, 1983; Hodapp & Dykens, 1994) than are individuals with other cognitive disabilities.

Another possible explanation is that support groups are more available to families of children with DS than to families of children with other genetic disorders (Erickson & Upsur, 1989). Having support groups for a particular syndrome provides families with information pertinent to their child's particular behaviors and characteristics and with social support and can lead to more adaptive coping on the part of the family. Mothers of children with DS are also reported to receive more family support than are mothers of children with other genetic disorders (Poehlmann, Clements, Abbeduto, & Farsad, 2005).

A third possibility is that more is known about the development of children and adults with DS than those with intellectual disability due to other causes. As such, the families of individuals with DS face more "certainty" about the future and thus may experience less stress (Beavers, Hampson, Hulgus, & Beavers, 1986).

FAMILY WELL-BEING IN FRAGILE X SYNDROME

FXS has received considerable research attention for more than a decade. The leading heritable cause of intellectual disability and a frequent cause of autism (Hagerman, 1999), FXS might have multiple impacts on family well-being. The effect on families of raising a child with FXS, however, has received very little attention by researchers compared with the intense effort devoted to understanding the behavioral phenotype and genetic mechanisms involved.

At Diagnosis

Unlike DS, FXS is not identifiable at birth from observable physical characteristics. Unless families have prior knowledge of a family history of FXS, the syndrome is typically not identified until the parents become concerned because of noticeable and well-established developmental delays. Significant variability exists in the age at which a diagnosis is made, but diagnoses typically are made around the age of 3 years (Bailey et al., 2000). Parents report becoming concerned about their child's development around 9–13 months of age and have that concern validated by a medical professional on average around 22–25 months of age; however, genetic testing often does not provide a diagnosis of FXS until approximately 30–35 months of age (Bailey et al., 2000). This delay between parental concern with development and a formal diagnosis has multiple impacts on family well-being (Carmichael et al., 1999). Parents often experience frustration in trying to validate their concerns and obtaining a diagnosis for their child's developmental delays. They also often doubt their own parenting skills and observations when trying to get their concerns acknowledged by a medical professional. It is important to note, however, that with regard to having caring and sensitive treatment during the diagnostic process, a comparable number of parents report experiencing supportive as report experiencing unsupportive medical professionals (Carmichael et al., 1999).

The delay in obtaining a diagnosis of FXS can also result in families not having access to genetic information and making further reproductive decisions without knowledge of the possible reoccurrence rates of the syndrome in their family. As a result, many families have multiple children with FXS (Bailey et al., 2003; Carmichael et al., 1999). For parents not receiving the diagnosis of FXS at a genetic clinic, a sizable number report that they were not referred for genetic counseling (Carmichael et al., 1999). Parents report that if they had known they were a carrier for FXS, this knowledge would have affected their reproductive plans (McConkie-Rosell et al., 1997), and for 59%, it has affected their decision about whether to have another child (Bailey et al., 2003).

Reactions of families to their child's diagnosis of FXS have been both positive and negative (Carmichael et al., 1999). Although more than 80% of parental respondents report feelings of guilt and self-blame associated with obtaining the diagnosis, very few comment on feeling anxious about their other children or feel that they themselves will be stigmatized (Carmichael et al., 1999; Poehlmann et al., 2005). Many of these parents, however, do worry about their children experiencing stigma related to a diagnosis of FXS and worry that the diagnosis has resulted in tension between them and extended family members (Carmichael et al., 1999). The majority of parents who informed their relatives about the impact the FXS diagnosis has on these extended family members reported that doing so was at least somewhat stressful (Bailey et al., 2003). Parents are easily emotionally and intellectually overwhelmed by the complexity of the syndrome (McConkie-Rosell et al., 2005) and report that receiving the diagnosis of FXS challenged them to reframe their family life and their expectations for their child and the family (Bailey et al., 2003)

Nevertheless, more than 90% of parents report that a benefit of the diagnosis is that their child will receive appropriate intervention (Carmichael et al., 1999; Roy, Johnsen, Breese, & Hagerman, 1995), and more than 70% report that genetic counseling will be a benefit to siblings and extended family members. Parents also report that they feel they are better able to understand the needs of their child and obtain appropriate information after receiving the diagnosis (Bailey et al., 2003; Carmichael et al., 1999). Although a formal diagnosis of FXS can sometimes lead to a sense of guilt associated with having passed on an X-linked disorder, for many parents, obtaining an official diagnosis also relieves the emotional and psychological burdens that come with not knowing the cause of their child's developmental delay (Roy et al., 1995).

During Childhood

In comparison with mothers of children with disabilities of unknown etiology, there is a trend for mothers of children with FXS to report having more harmonious family environments (Perry, Harris, & Minnes, 2004). In addition, mothers of children with FXS report comparable levels of stress and fewer depressive symptoms as compared with mothers of children with Williams syndrome or Prader-Willi syndrome (Sarimski, 1997). Children with Prader-Willi syndrome exhibit an extreme preoccupation with food (hyperphagia) and symptoms consistent with disrupted hypothalamic activity, such as sleep disturbances and temperature dysregulation (Dykens et al., 2000). These symptoms can severely disrupt the family home. Mothers of children with FXS also report less marital conflict, less anger, and a need for lower levels of control than do mothers of children with Prader-Willi syndrome (Van Lieshout, de Meyer, Curfs, & Fryns, 1998). In comparison with mothers of children with DS, however, mothers of children with FXS report receiving less support from family members (Poehlmann et al., 2005).

In comparison with mothers of children with typical development, mothers of children with FXS report elevated levels of parenting stress (Johnston et al., 2003; Sarimski, 1997) and a lower sense of parenting competence (Sarimski, 1997). This elevated level of stress appears to be related to the elevated behavior problems characteristic of children with FXS and to maternal feelings of competence and acceptability, but not to the child's level of intellectual ability or age (Sarimski, 1997). This is an interesting finding given that children with FXS display a declining rate of cognitive development during late childhood and adolescence (Dykens et al., 2000). Although research findings suggest that intellectual ability is not predictive of stress in mothers of children with FXS (Johnston et al., 2003), further research is needed to explore the role, if any, that the children's declining rates of cognitive, language, and adaptive ability development have on maternal well-being.

During Adolescence

In a comparative study mentioned previously in this chapter, mothers of adolescents and young adults with FXS were compared with mothers of adolescents and young adults with DS or autism (Abbeduto et al., 2004). The mothers of the adolescents with FXS were more pessimistic about their children's future than were mothers of adolescents with DS. Mothers of adolescents with FXS also reported perceiving lower levels of reciprocated closeness from their children than did mothers of adolescents with DS but reported higher levels of reciprocated closeness than did mothers of adolescents with autism (Abbeduto et al., 2004). When contextual factors were controlled for, the difference between mothers of adolescents with FXS and mothers of adolescents with autism endured. No other differences between FXS and the comparison groups of mothers were observed on measures of depressive symptoms, maternal ratings of perceived closeness with her child, or coping style. These findings suggest that by the time their children reach adolescence, mothers of children with FXS may cope comparably to mothers of children with DS.

No studies to date have compared the family well-being of adolescents with FXS with that of families of typically developing adolescents. Nor have any studies examined the family well-being of adults with FXS or the well-being of siblings of adults or children with FXS. The well-being of fathers of children with FXS also has received little attention.

Well-Being of Carriers

Evidence suggests that women who carry the premutation of the gene that is responsible for FXS (i.e., the FMR1 gene) may be vulnerable to challenges beyond those contributed by raising a child with FXS. Several concerns have been identified among women who carry the premutation, including premature ovarian failure, an awareness of their genetic identity, and regret over not knowing that they were carriers sooner (McConkie-Rosell, Spiridigliozzi, Dawson, Sullivan, & Lachiewicz, 2001). Recent findings suggest that a subgroup of women with the premutation may even have subtle cognitive impairments (Franke et al., 1999; Steyaert, Legius, Borghgraef, & Fryns, 2003), and some studies suggest more rapid physical decline with age, including the possibility of developing the Parkinson-like fragile X–associated tremor/ataxia syndrome (FXTAS; Jacquemont et al., 2004; Steyaert et al., 2003). Females with premutations have been reported to be at heightened risk for affective problems, including anxiety disorders and depression (Franke et al., 1998; Johnston et al., 2001). Importantly, the elevated risk for affective disorders among fragile X carriers has been found to be independent of the burden of raising a child with a developmental disability and the feelings of guilt associated with being a carrier (Franke et al., 1998). Indeed, there is some evidence connecting some behavioral symptoms in carriers to the genotype. Thus, some mothers of children with FXS—by virtue of their carrier status and accompanying physical, cognitive, and affective problems—may find it difficult to cope with the challenges of raising a child with a developmental disability (Hagerman & Lampe, 1999). Lower levels of maternal well-being may negatively influence the well-being and developmental outcomes of the child with FXS. Children without intellectual disability who have mothers with depression are at risk for general difficulties in functioning, increased guilt, and interpersonal difficulties, as well as problems with attachment (Beardslee, Versage, & Gladstone, 1998). It is possible that the increased risk for affective disorders among carriers of the fragile X premutation could put their children at increased risk for similar outcomes.

Discussion

Families of individuals with FXS display levels of psychological well-being and functioning that are better, on average, than those of families of individuals with autism, although somewhat worse than families of individuals with DS (Abbeduto et al., 2004). This finding is likely a result of several factors. Children with FXS, particularly males, display elevated rates of unpredictable maladaptive behaviors, including inattention, hyperactivity, and social anxiety (Hagerman, 1999; Keysor & Mazzocco, 2002). In addition, families of children with FXS need to cope with the heritability of the syndrome. The pattern of behavior problems and issues of heritability could lead to lower levels of well-being in families of children with FXS compared with DS. Greater challenges may be faced by families raising multiple children with FXS as compared with families raising only one child with a developmental disability. And some carriers of the FXS premutation have fewer psychological resources for coping with the stress associated with raising one or more affected children.

Yet, there is reason to suspect that the outcome for families of FXS may improve. Although support groups for FXS are not as extensive as the supports available for DS or autism, these groups continue to develop for FXS, as does the knowledge base. Having available support groups and a knowledge base may serve as potential protective factors for the well-being of families of individuals with FXS.

DIRECTIONS FOR RESEARCH AND PRACTICE

Research Design

Several research design concerns are relevant to studying the well-being of families of individuals with genetic syndromes. Factors such as child, parent, and family characteristics are inherently confounded with diagnostic group differences, and thus, an important concern is the selection of appropriate comparison groups (Cahill & Glidden, 1996; Seltzer, Abbeduto, Krauss, Greenberg, & Swe, 2004). Although the comparison group chosen will depend primarily on the research question being asked, it is still important to determine how the genetic syndrome group of interest will differ from the comparison group. Is the best comparison group for DS or FXS composed of individuals with another genetic syndrome group, such as Prader-Willi syndrome or Williams syndrome? Among these other genetic syndromes, there are differences in behavioral phenotypes and health concerns that could affect research findings. For example, these genetic syndromes have accompanying health concerns, but the types of concerns and the timing of the concerns differ. Health concerns in DS are greater in the first year of life and in adolescence and relate more often to the heart and thyroid, whereas health concerns in Prader-Willi syndrome are greater in early childhood and relate to dysregulation of the hypothalamus. Associated behavioral traits also differ by syndrome; for example, FXS is associated with communication and social difficulties, whereas individuals with Williams syndrome often display strengths in the interpersonal domain (Dykens et al., 2000). Also, the timing of the diagnosis varies among genetic syndromes, as do issues related to heritability. And the low prevalence of other genetic syndromes would likely result in difficulties finding cases to match on child, parent, or family characteristics. For individuals with FXS, individuals with autism might provide a suitable comparison group as the pattern of communication and interpersonal and behavioral symptoms are similar (Seltzer, Abbeduto, et al., 2004). Perhaps the most important caution, however, is that documenting differences in well-being among groups of parents of individuals with different syndromes is simply a first step for research. The next is to understand which of the many factors inherently confounded with the child's condition are causally involved in the emergence of the parental profile of well-being observed (Seltzer, Abbeduto, et al., 2004).

Another research design concern is related to the issue of causality. Parent characteristics prior to the diagnosis of a genetic syndrome are typically unknown. As such, it is difficult to determine what role these characteristics play in the risk or resiliency of some families in coping with raising a child with a genetic syndrome. Longitudinal population-based studies, such as the Wisconsin Longitudinal Study (WLS), might be able to resolve this issue. By following a random sample of 1,957 high school graduates from Wisconsin, the WLS has gathered information about parents before they have had children. The WLS sample includes some parents who had children with intellectual disability or genetic syndromes. Analyses of this sample can help to determine if parental characteristics remain stable after having a child with special needs (Seltzer, Greenberg, Floyd, Pettee, & Hong, 2001).

A third concern of studies examining family well-being is the age range of children selected for study. Concerns related to raising a child with a genetic syndrome can change from infancy though adulthood. For example, different physical and mental health problems are more or less of a risk at certain points in time. As such, investigators should be aware when the age range selected for study spans a time period with transitions or elevated risks for health problems for a particular genetic syndrome.

Future Research and Practice

There continue to be many unstudied areas of concern regarding the well-being of families of individuals with DS and FXS. Because much of the research on well-being has focused on mothers, a stronger effort needs to be made to examine the well-being of fathers and siblings, particularly for FXS in which siblings may also have FXS or may be a carrier for fragile X. There is also a need to better understand the pattern of findings. This chapter presents several factors that could mitigate the impact of genetic syndromes on family well-being; however, these factors have yet to be examined in a systematic manner. Specifically, what is it about being a family member of an individual with DS or FXS that leads to the pattern of findings relating to well-being as compared with some other disorders? Also, other variables that could play a role in the risk or resiliency of family well-being need to be examined further, particularly the role of maladaptive behaviors and level of competence.

With regard to FXS, little is known about the well-being of families of adults with FXS. Is the pattern of family well-being stable from childhood to adulthood, or does it change as the child becomes older? What impact does FXTAS among older fragile X carriers have on the family well-being, particularly when FXTAS affects the parent of a child with FXS who is living at home as an adult? Future research can address these concerns, as well as the impact of raising multiple children with FXS.

A large impact on parental well-being relates to interactions with professionals. When medical professionals provide parents with a diagnosis of a genetic syndrome, there are certain things professionals can do to have a positive impact on parental well-being. Providing parents with up-to-date information on the genetic syndrome, referrals to parent support groups, and positive aspects of the genetic syndrome in a supportive manner are reported by parents to make them feel more optimistic about the diagnosis (Helm et al., 1998). With regard to FXS, medical professionals can be more supportive in listening to parental concerns and suggesting earlier screening for FXS. As children with genetic syndromes become older, professionals should be aware of the changing health concerns and the most appropriate interventions to help the child maximize his or her potential. Addressing health concerns and providing the most support possible to the child are two methods professionals can use to help indirectly foster the well-being of the families of children with genetic syndromes.

REFERENCES

Abbeduto, L., Seltzer, M.M., Shattuck, P., Krauss, M.W., Orsmond, G., & Murphy, M.M. (2004). Psychological well-being and coping in mothers of youths with autism, Down syndrome, or fragile X syndrome. *American Journal on Mental Retardation, 109,* 237–254.

August, G.J., Stewart, M.A., & Tsai, L. (1981). The incidence of cognitive abilities in siblings of autistic children. *British Journal of Psychiatry, 138,* 416–422.

Bailey, D.B. (2004). Newborn screening for fragile X syndrome. *Mental Retardation and Developmental Disabilities Research Reviews, 10,* 3–10.

Bailey, D.B., Skinner, D., Hatton, D., & Roberts, J. (2000). Family experiences and factors associated with the diagnosis of fragile X syndrome. *Journal of Developmental and Behavioral Pediatrics, 21,* 315–321.

Bailey, D.B., Skinner, D., & Sparkman, K. (2003). Discovering fragile X syndrome: Family experiences and perceptions. *Pediatrics, 111,* 407–416.

Beardslee, W.R., Versage, E.M., & Gladstone, T.R.G. (1998). Children of affectively ill parents: A review of the past 10 years. *Journal of the American Academy of Child and Adolescent Psychiatry, 37,* 1134–1141.

Beavers, J., Hampson, R.B., Hulgus, Y.F., & Beavers, W.R. (1986). Coping in families with a retarded child. *Family Process, 25,* 365–378.

Bittles, A.H., & Glasson, E.J. (2004). Clinical, social, and ethical implications of changing life expectancy in Down syndrome. *Developmental Medicine and Child Neurology, 46,* 282–286.

Bolton, P., MacDonald, H., Pickles, A., Rios, P., Goode, S., Crowson, M., et al. (1994). A case-control family study of autism. *Journal of Child Psychology and Psychiatry, 35,* 877–900.

Bridges, F., & Cicchetti, D. (1982). Mothers' ratings of the temperament characteristics of Down syndrome infants. *Developmental Psychology, 18,* 238–244.

Cahill, B.M., & Glidden, L.M. (1996). Influence of child diagnosis on family and parental functioning: Down syndrome versus other disabilities. *American Journal on Mental Retardation, 101,* 149–160.

Carmichael, B., Pembrey, M., Turner, G., & Barnicoat, A. (1999). Diagnosis of fragile-X syndrome: The experiences of parents. *Journal of Intellectual Disability Research, 43,* 47–53.

Carr, J. (1988). Six weeks to twenty-one years old: A longitudinal study of children with Down's syndrome and their families. *Journal of Child Psychology and Psychiatry, 29,* 407–431.

Collins, V., Halliday, J., Kahler, S., & Williamson, R. (2001). Parents' experiences with genetic counseling after the birth of a baby with a genetic disorder: An exploratory study. *Journal of Genetic Counseling, 10,* 53–72.

Cummings, S.T. (1976). Impact of the child's deficiency on the father: A study of fathers of mentally retarded chronically ill children. *American Journal of Orthopsychiatry, 46,* 246–255.

Cummings, S.T., Bayley, H.C., & Rie, H.E. (1966). Effects of the child's deficiency on the mother: A study of mothers of mentally retarded, chronically ill, and neurotic children. *American Journal of Orthopsychiatry, 36,* 595–608.

Cunningham, C.C. (1996). Families of children with Down syndrome. *Down Syndrome Research and Practice, 4,* 87–95.

Cuskelly, M., & Dodds, M. (1992). Behavior problems in children with Down's syndrome and their siblings. *Journal of Child Psychology and Psychiatry, 33,* 749–761.

Cuskelly, M., & Gunn, P. (1993). Maternal reports of behaviour of siblings with children with Down syndrome. *American Journal on Mental Retardation, 97,* 521–529.

Dumas, J.E., Wolf, L.C., Fisman, S.N., & Culligan, A. (1991). Parenting stress, child behavior problems, and dysphoria in parents of children with autism, Down syndrome, behavior problems, and normal development. *Exceptionality, 2,* 97–110.

Dunn, M.E., Burbine, T., Bowers, C.A., & Tantleff-Dunn, S. (2001). Moderators of stress in parents of children with autism. *Community Mental Health Journal, 37,* 39–52.

Dykens, E.M. (1995). Measuring behavioral phenotypes: Provocations from the "new genetics." *American Journal on Mental Retardation, 99,* 522–532.

Dykens, E.M., Hodapp, R.M., & Finucane, B.M. (2000). *Genetics and mental retardation syndromes: A new look at behavior and interventions.* Baltimore: Paul H. Brookes Publishing Co.

Dyson, L.L. (1991). Families of young children with handicaps: Parental stress and family functioning. *American Journal on Mental Retardation, 95,* 623–629.

Dyson, L.L. (1993). Response to the presence of a child with disabilities: Parental stress and family functioning over time. *American Journal on Mental Retardation, 98,* 207–218.

Erickson, M., & Upsur, C.C. (1989). Caretaking burden and social support: Comparison of mothers of infants with and without disabilities. *American Journal on Mental Retardation, 94,* 250–258.

Fidler, D.J., Hodapp, R.M., & Dykens, E.M. (2000). Stress in families of young children with Down syndrome, Williams syndrome, and Smith-Magenis syndrome. *Early Education and Development, 11*, 395–406.

Fisman, S., Wolf, N., & Noh, S. (1989). Marital intimacy in parents of exceptional children. *Canadian Journal of Psychiatry, 34*, 519–525.

Forrester, M.B., & Merz, R.D. (1999). Prenatal diagnosis and elective termination of Down syndrome in a racially mixed population in Hawaii, 1987-1996. *Prenatal Diagnosis, 19*, 136–141.

Franke, P., Leboyer, M., Gansicke, M., Weiffenbach, O., Biancalana, V., Cornillet-Lefebre, P., et al. (1998). Genotype-phenotype relationship in female carriers of the permutation and full mutation of FMR-1. *Psychiatry Research, 80*, 113–127.

Franke, P., Leboyer, M., Hardt, J., Sohne, E., Weiffenbach, O., Biancalana, V., et al. (1999). Neuropsychological profiles of FMR-1 premutation and full-mutation carrier females. *Psychiatry Research, 87*, 223–231.

Franke, P., Maier, W., Hautzinger, M., Weiffenbach, O., Gänsicke, M., Iwers, B., et al. (1996). Fragile-X carrier females: Evidence for a distinct psychopathological phenotype? *American Journal of Medical Genetics, 64*, 334–339.

Friedrich, W.N., & Friedrich, N. (1981). Psychosocial assets of parents of handicapped and nonhandicapped children. *American Journal of Mental Deficiency, 90*, 130–139.

Gamble, W.C., & McHale, S.M. (1989). Coping with stress in sibling relationships: A comparison of children with disabled and nondisabled siblings. *Journal of Applied Developmental Psychology, 10*, 353–373.

Gath, A. (1977). The impact of an abnormal child upon the parents. *British Journal of Psychiatry, 130*, 405–410.

Gath, A. (1990). Down syndrome children and their families. *American Journal of Medical Genetics Supplement, 7*, 314–316.

Gath, A., & Gumley, D. (1984). Down's syndrome and the family: Follow-up of children first seen in infancy. *Developmental Medicine and Child Neurology, 26*, 500–508.

Gath, A., & Gumley, D. (1986). Family background of children with Down's syndrome and of children with a similar degree of mental retardation. *British Journal of Psychiatry, 149*, 161–171.

Gath, A., & Gumley, D. (1987). Retarded children and their siblings. *Journal of Child Psychology and Psychiatry, 28*, 715–730.

Gibbs, M.V., & Thorpe, J.G. (1983). Personality stereotype of noninstitutionalized Down syndrome children. *American Journal of Mental Deficiency, 87*, 601–605.

Glover, N.M., & Glover, S.J. (1996). Ethical and legal issues regarding selective abortion of fetuses with Down syndrome. *Mental Retardation, 34*, 207–214.

Gowen, J.W., Johnson-Martin, N., Goldman, B.D., & Appelbaum, M. (1989). Feelings of depression and parenting competence of mothers of handicapped and nonhandicapped infants: A longitudinal study. *American Journal on Mental Retardation, 94*, 259–271.

Graber, J.A., & Brooks-Gunn, J. (1996). Transitions and turning points: Navigating the passage from childhood through adolescence. *Developmental Psychology, 32*, 768–776.

Greenberg, J.S., Seltzer, M.M., Krauss, M.W., Chou, R.J., & Hong, J. (2004). The effect of quality of the relationship between mothers and adult children with schizophrenia, autism or Down syndrome on maternal well-being: The mediating role of optimism. *American Journal of Orthopsychiatry, 74*, 14–25.

Greenspan, S., & Delaney, K. (1983). Personal competence of institutionalized adult males with or without Down syndrome. *American Journal of Mental Deficiency, 88*, 218–220.

Hagerman, R.J. (1999). *Neurodevelopmental disorders*. Oxford: Oxford University Press.

Hagerman, R.J., & Lampe, M.E. (1999). Fragile X syndrome. In S. Goldstein & C.R. Reynolds (Eds.), *Handbook of neurodevelopmental and genetic disorders in children* (pp. 298–316). New York: The Guilford Press.

Hamburg, D.A., & Takanishi, R. (1989). Preparing for life: The critical transition of adolescence. *American Psychologist, 44*, 825–827.

Hanson, M., & Hanline, M.F. (1990). Parenting a child with a disability: A longitudinal study of parental stress and adaptation. *Journal of Early Intervention, 14*, 234–248.

Harris, V.S., & McHale, S.M. (1989). Family life problems, daily caregiving activities, and the psychological well-being of mothers of mentally retarded children. *American Journal on Mental Retardation, 94*, 231–239.

Harrison, P.L. (1987). Research with adaptive behavior scales. *Journal of Special Education, 21,* 37–68.

Hauser-Cram, P., Warfield, M.E., Shonkoff, J.P., & Krauss, M.W. (2001). Children with disabilities: A longitudinal study of child development and parent well-being. *Monographs of the Society for Research in Child Development, 66,* Serial No. 266.

Helm, D.T., Miranda, S., & Chedd, N.A. (1998). Prenatal diagnosis of Down syndrome: Mothers' reflections on supports needed from diagnosis to birth. *Mental Retardation, 36,* 55–61.

Hodapp, R.M. (1997). Direct and indirect behavioral effects of different genetic disorders of mental retardation. *American Journal on Mental Retardation, 102,* 67–79.

Hodapp, R.M., & Dykens, E.M. (1994). Mental retardation's two cultures of behavioral research. *American Journal on Mental Retardation, 98,* 675–687.

Hodapp, R.M., Ly, T.M., Fidler, D.J., & Ricci, L.A. (2001). Less stress, more rewarding: Parenting children with Down syndrome. *Parenting: Science & Practice, 1,* 317–337.

Holroyd, J., & McArthur, D. (1976). Mental retardation and stress on the parents: A contrast between Down's syndrome and childhood autism. *American Journal of Mental Deficiency, 80,* 431–436.

Hornby, G. (1995). Fathers' views of the effects on their families of children with Down syndrome. *Journal of Child and Family Studies, 4,* 103–117.

Houser, R., & Seligman, M. (1991). A comparison of stress and coping by fathers of adolescents with mental retardation and fathers of adolescents without mental retardation. *Research in Developmental Disabilities, 12,* 251–260.

Huang, L., Sadler, L., O'Riordan, M.A., & Robin, N.H. (2002). Delay in diagnosis of Williams syndrome. *Clinical Pediatrics, 41,* 257–261.

Jacquemont, S., Hagerman, R.J., Leehey, M.A., Hall, D.A., Levine, R.A., Brunberg, J.A., et al. (2004). Penetrance of the fragile-X associated tremor/ataxia syndrome in a premutation carrier population. *Journal of the American Medical Association, 291,* 460–469.

Johnston, C., Eliez, S., Dyer-Friedman, J., Hessl, D., Glaser, B., Blasey, C., et al. (2001). Neurobehavioral phenotype in carriers of the fragile X permutation. *American Journal of Medical Genetics, 103,* 314–319.

Johnston, C., Hessl, D., Blasey, C., Eliez, S., Erba, H., Dyer-Friedman, J., et al. (2003). Factors associated with parenting stress in mothers of children with fragile X syndrome. *Journal of Developmental and Behavioral Pediatrics, 24,* 267–275.

Kasari, C., & Bauminger, N. (1998). Social and emotional development in children with mental retardation. In J.A. Burack, R.M. Hodapp, & E. Zigler (Eds.), *Handbook of mental retardation and development* (pp. 411–433). New York: Cambridge University Press.

Kasari, C., & Sigman, M. (1997). Linking parental perceptions to interactions in young children with autism. *Journal of Autism and Developmental Disorders, 27,* 39–57.

Kay, E., & Kingston, H. (2002). Feelings associated with being a carrier and characteristics of reproductive decision making in women known to be carriers of X-linked conditions. *Journal of Health Psychology, 7,* 169–181.

Keysor, C.S., & Mazzocco, M.M.M. (2002). A developmental approach to understanding fragile X syndrome in females. *Microscopy Research and Technique, 57,* 179–186.

Koegel, R.L., Schreibman, L., O'Neill, L., & Burke, J.C. (1983). The personality and family interaction characteristics of parents of autistic children. *Journal of Consulting and Clinical Psychology, 51,* 683–692.

Krauss, M.W., & Seltzer, M.M. (1995). Long-term caring: Family experiences over the life course. In L. Nadel & D. Rosenthal (Eds.), *Down syndrome: Living and learning in the community* (pp. 91–98). New York: Wiley-Liss.

Krauss, M.W., & Seltzer, M.M. (1999). An unanticipated life: The impact of lifelong caregiving. In H. Bersani (Ed.), *Responding to the challenge: International trends and current issues in developmental disabilities* (pp. 173–188). Brookline, MA: Brookline Books.

Loveland, K.A., & Kelley, M.L. (1988). Development of adaptive behavior in adolescents and young adults with autism and Down syndrome. *American Journal on Mental Retardation, 93,* 84–92.

Ly, T.M., & Hodapp, R.M. (2002). Maternal attribution of child noncompliance in children with mental retardation: Down syndrome versus other causes. *Journal of Developmental and Behavioral Pediatrics, 23,* 322–329.

Marcovitch, S., Goldberg, S., MacGregor, D., & Lojkasek, M. (1986). Patterns of temperament in three groups of developmentally delayed preschool children: Mother and father ratings. *Developmental and Behavioral Pediatrics, 7,* 247–252.

McConkie-Rosell, A., Finucane, B., Cronister, A., Abrams, L., Bennett, R.L., & Pettersen, B.J. (2005). Genetic counseling for fragile X syndrome: Updated recommendations of the National Society of Genetic Counselors. *Journal of Genetic Counseling, 14,* 249–270.

McConkie-Rosell, A., Spiridigliozzi, G.A., Dawson, D.V., Sullivan, J.A., & Lachiewicz, A.M. (2001). Longitudinal study of the carrier testing process of fragile X syndrome: Perceptions and coping. *American Journal of Medical Genetics, 98,* 37–45.

McConkie-Rosell, A., Spiridigliozzi, G.A., Iafolla, T., Tarleton, J., & Lachiewicz, A.M. (1997). Carrier testing in the fragile X syndrome: Attitudes and opinions of obligate carriers. *American Journal of Medical Genetics, 68,* 62–69.

McKinney, B., & Peterson, R.A. (1987). Predictors of stress in parents of developmentally disabled children. *Journal of Pediatric Psychology, 12,* 133–150.

Mink, I.T., Nihira, E., & Meyers, C. E. (1983). Taxonomy of family life styles: In homes with TMR children. *American Journal of Mental Deficiency, 87,* 484–497.

Perry, A., Harris, K., & Minnes, P. (2004). Family environments and family harmony: An exploration across severity, age, and type of DD. *Journal on Developmental Disabilities, 11,* 17–29.

Piven, J., Chase, G., Landa, R., Wzorek, M., Gayle, J., Cloud, D., et al. (1991). Psychiatric disorders in parents of autistic individuals. *Journal of the American Academy of Child and Adolescent Psychiatry, 30,* 471–478.

Poehlmann, J., Clements, M., Abbeduto, L., & Farsad, V. (2005). Family experiences associated with a child's diagnosis of fragile X or Down syndrome: Evidence for disruption and resilience. *Mental Retardation, 43,* 255–267.

Pueschel, S.M. (1987). Health concerns in persons with Down syndrome. In S.M. Pueschel, C. Tingey, J.E. Rynders, A.C. Crocker, & D.M. Crutcher (Eds.), *New perspectives on Down syndrome* (pp. 113–133). Baltimore: Paul H. Brookes Publishing Co.

Pueschel, S.M. (1996). Young people with Down syndrome: Transition from childhood to adulthood. *Mental Retardation and Developmental Disabilities Research Reviews, 2,* 90–95.

Roach, M.A., Orsmond, G.I., & Barratt, M.S. (1999). Mothers and fathers of children with Down syndrome: Parental stress and involvement in childcare. *American Journal on Mental Retardation, 104,* 422–436.

Rodrigue, J.R., Morgan, S.B., & Geffken, G.R. (1990). Families of autistic children: Psychological functioning of mothers. *Journal of Clinical Child Psychology, 19,* 371–379.

Rodrigue, J.R., Morgan, S.B., & Geffken, G.R. (1992). Psychological adaptation of fathers of children with autism, Down syndrome and normal development. *Developmental Disorders, 22,* 249–263.

Romans-Clarkson, S.E., Clarkson, J.E., Dittmer, I.D., Flett, R., Linsell, C., Mullen, P.E., et al. (1986). Impact of a handicapped child on mental health of parents. *British Medical Journal, 293,* 1395–1397.

Roy, J.C., Johnsen, J., Breese, K., & Hagerman, R. (1995). Fragile X syndrome: What is the impact of diagnosis on families? *Developmental Brain Dysfunction, 8,* 327–335.

Ryde-Brandt, B. (1991). Now it is time for your child to go to school, how do you feel? *International Journal of Disability, Development and Education, 38,* 45–58.

Sanders, J.L., & Morgan, S.B. (1997). Family stress and adjustment as perceived by children with autism or Down syndrome: Implications for intervention. *Child and Family Behavior Therapy, 19,* 15–32.

Sarimski, K. (1997). Behavioural phenotypes and family stress in three mental retardation syndromes. *European Child and Adolescent Psychiatry, 6,* 26–31.

Schupf, N., Kapell, D., Lee, J.H., Ottman, R., & Mayeux, R. (1994). Increased risk of Alzheimer's disease in mothers of adults with Down's syndrome. *Lancet, 344,* 353–356.

Seltzer, M.M., Abbeduto, L., Krauss, M.W., Greenberg, J., & Swe, A. (2004). Comparison groups in autism research: Down syndrome, fragile X syndrome, and schizophrenia. *Journal of Autism and Developmental Disorders, 34,* 41–48.

Seltzer, M.M., Greenberg, J.S., Floyd, F.J., Pettee, Y., & Hong, J. (2001). Life course impacts of parenting a child with a disability. *American Journal on Mental Retardation, 106,* 265–286.

Seltzer, M.M., & Krauss, M.W. (1998). Families of adults with Down syndrome. In J.F. Miller, L.A. Leavitt, & M. Leddy (Eds.), *Communication development in young children with Down syndrome* (pp. 217–240). Baltimore: Paul H. Brookes Publishing Co.

Seltzer, M.M., Krauss, M.W., Orsmond, G.I., & Vestal, C. (2001). Families of adolescents and adults with autism: Uncharted territory. In L.M. Glidden (Ed.), *International review of research in mental retardation* (Vol. 23, pp. 267–294). San Diego: Academic Press.

Seltzer, M.M., Krauss, M.W., & Tsunematsu, N. (1993). Adults with Down syndrome and their aging mothers: Diagnostic group differences. *American Journal on Mental Retardation, 97,* 464–508.

Seltzer, M.M., Shattuck, P., Abbeduto, L., & Greenberg, J. (2004). The trajectory of development in adolescents and adults with autism. *Mental Retardation and Developmental Disabilities Research Reviews, 10,* 234–247.

Shonkoff, J.P., Hauser-Cram, P., Krauss, M.W., & Upshur, C. (1992). Development of infants with disabilities and their families: Implications for theory and service delivery. *Monographs of the Society for Research in Child Development, 57, Serial No. 6.*

Singhi, P.D., Goyal, L., Pershad, D., Singhi, S., & Walia, B.N.S. (1990). Psychological problems in families of disabled children. *British Journal of Medical Psychology, 63,* 173–182.

Skotko, B.G. (2005a). Mothers of children with Down syndrome reflect on their postnatal support. *Pediatrics, 115,* 64–77.

Skotko, B.G. (2005b). Prenatally diagnosed Down syndrome: Mothers who continued their pregnancies evaluate their health care providers. *American Journal of Obstetrics and Gynecology, 192,* 670–677.

Skotko, B.G., & Bedia, R.C. (2005). Postnatal support for mothers of children with Down syndrome. *Mental Retardation, 43,* 196–212.

Smith, T.B., Innocenti, M.S., Boyce, G.C., & Smith, C. (1993). Depressive symptomatology and interaction behaviors of mothers having a child with disabilities. *Psychological Reports, 73,* 1184–1186.

Steyaert, J., Legius, E., Borghgraef, M., & Fryns, J.-P. (2003). A distinct neurocognitive phenotype in female fragile-X premutation carriers assessed with visual attention tasks. *American Journal of Medical Genetics, 116A,* 44–51.

Stoneman, Z. (1997). Mental retardation and family adaptation. In W.E. MacLean (Ed.), *Ellis' handbook of mental deficiency, psychological theory and research* (pp. 405–437). Mahwah, NJ: Lawrence Erlbaum Associates.

Thayer, B., Ciarleglio, L., & Rucquoi, J. (1991). Prenatal diagnosis and pregnancy options: Termination support groups. *The Genetic Resource, 6,* 39–42.

Van Lieshout, C.F.M., de Meyer, R.E., Curfs, L.M.G., & Fryns, J.-P. (1998). Family contexts, parental behaviour, and personality profiles of children and adolescents with Prader-Willi, fragile-X, or Williams syndrome. *Journal of Child Psychology and Psychiatry, 39,* 699–710.

Van Riper, M. (1999). Living with Down syndrome: The family experience. *Down Syndrome Quarterly, 4,* 1–7.

Van Riper, M., Pridham, K., & Ryff, C. (1992). Symbolic interactionism: A perspective for understanding parent-nurse interactions following the birth of a child with Down syndrome. *Maternal Child Nursing Journal, 20,* 21–40.

Van Riper, M., Ryff, C., & Pridham, K. (1992). Parental and family well-being in families of children with Down syndrome: A comparative study. *Research in Nursing and Health, 15,* 227–235.

Van Riper, M., & Selder, F. (1989). Parental response to the birth of a child with Down syndrome. In J.D. Rainer, S.P. Rubin, M.K. Bartalos, J.E. Maidman, A.H. Kutscher, K. Anyane-Yeboa, et al. (Eds.), *Genetic disease: The unwanted inheritance* (pp. 59–76). New York: Haworth Press.

Williamson, P., Harris, R., Church, S., Fiddler, M., & Rhind, J. (1996). Prenatal genetic services for Down's syndrome: Access and provision in 1990-1991. *British Journal of Obstetrics and Gynecology, 103,* 676–683.

Wilton, K., & Renaut, J. (1986). Stress levels in families with intellectually handicapped preschool children and families with nonhandicapped preschool children. *Journal of Mental Deficiency Research, 30,* 163–169.

Zigman, W.B., Schupf, N., Lubin, R.A., & Silverman, W.P. (1987). Premature regression of adults with Down syndrome. *American Journal on Mental Deficiency, 92,* 161–168.

Professional Organizations

DOWN SYNDROME

Canadian Down Syndrome Society
Toll free (in Canada): 1-800-883-5608; telephone: 403-270-8500
E-mail: dsinfo@cdss.ca; http://www.cdss.ca/

Down Syndrome International
Telephone (outside United Kingdom): +44 845 230 0372
Telephone (within United Kingdom): 0845 230 0372
E-mail: enquiries@down-syndrome-int.org; http://www.down-syndrome-int.org/

Down Syndrome Research Foundation & Resource Centre
Toll free (in Canada): 888-464-DSRF (888-464-3773); telephone: 604-444-3773
http://www.dsrf.org

National Association for Down Syndrome
Telephone: 630-325-9112; e-mail: info@nads.org; http://www.nads.org/

National Down Syndrome Congress
Toll free: 800-232-NDSC (800-232-6372); telephone: 770-604-9500
E-mail: info@ndsccenter.org; http://www.ndsccenter.org/

National Down Syndrome Society
Toll free: 800-221-4602; e-mail: info@ndss.org; http://www.ndss.org/

The Down Syndrome Educational Trust
Telephone (outside United Kingdom): +44 23 9285 5330
Telephone (within United Kingdom): 023 9285 5330
E-mail: enquiries@downsed.org; http://www.downsed.org/

FRAGILE X SYNDROME

Conquer Fragile X Foundation
Telephone: 561-833-3457; e-mail: mail@cfxf.org; http://www.conquerfragilex.org/

FRAXA: The Fragile X Research Foundation
Telephone: 978-462-1866; e-mail: info@fraxa.org; http://www.fraxa.org/

The National Fragile X Foundation
Toll free: 800-688-8765; telephone: 925-938-9300
E-mail: NATLFX@FragileX.org; http://www.fragilex.org/

The Fragile X Society
Telephone (outside United Kingdom): +44 1371 875100
Telephone (within United Kingdom): 01371 875100
E-mail: info@fragilex.org.uk; http://www.fragilex.org.uk/

INTELLECTUAL DISABILITY

American Association on Intellectual and Developmental Disabilities
Toll free: 800-424-3688; http://www.aaidd.org

The Arc
Toll free: 800-433-5255; http://www.thearc.org

Index

Tables and figure are indicated by *t* and *f,* respectively.